The Addison-Wesley
PHOTO-ATLAS
OF
NURSING
PROCEDURES

Focus Group Advisors

Geraldine G. Allerman, R.N., Ed.D.
Assistant Professor
Lienhard School of Nursing
Pace University
New York, New York

**Diane M. Billings, R.N., B.S.N.,
M.S.Ed., Doctoral Candidate**
Associate Professor
School of Nursing
Indiana University
Indianapolis, Indiana

Patricia L. Cross, R.N., M.A.Ed.
Director of Educational Services
Medi-SHARE, Inc.
San Jose, California

Kathleen Deska Pagana, R.N., M.S.N.
Instructor, Department of Nursing
Lycoming College
Williamsport, Pennsylvania

Mary Hoyte Sizemore, R.N., Ed.D.
Assistant Professor
University of Texas at El Paso
College of Nursing and Allied Health
El Paso, Texas

The Addison-Wesley

PHOTO-ATLAS OF NURSING PROCEDURES

Pamela L. Swearingen, R.N.
Special Projects Editor

in association with

Indiana University School
of Nursing

Department of Nursing Services
Indiana University Hospitals

and the

Physical Therapy and Respiratory
Therapy Programs
Division of Allied Health Sciences
Indiana University School of Medicine
Indianapolis, Indiana

Addison-Wesley Publishing Company
Nursing Division • Menlo Park, California
Reading, Massachusetts • London
Amsterdam • Don Mills, Ontario • Sydney

Sponsoring Editor: Nancy Evans
Production Editor: Betty Duncan-Todd
Cover/Book Design and Page Layout: Janet Bollow
Photographer: Jeffry Collins
Artist: Jack P. Tandy
Copy Editor: Judith LaVigna
Proofreaders: Judith Hibbard, Fannie Toldi
Indexer: Lois Oster
Cover Photograph: Sepp Seitz/Woodfin Camp

Library of Congress Cataloging in Publication Data

Swearingen, Pamela.
   The Addison-Wesley photoatlas of nursing procedures.

   Includes index.
   1. Nursing—Pictorial works. I. Title. [DNLM:
1. Nursing—Atlases. WY 17 A227]
RT41.S96 1984   610.73′022′2   84–6305

ISBN 0–201–07868–6
ABCDEFGHIJ–KI–8987654

The author and publishers have exerted every effort to ensure that drug selection, dosage, and composition of formulas set forth in this text are in accord with current formulations, recommendations, and practice at the time of publication. However, in view of ongoing research, changes in government regulations, the reformulation of nutritional products, and the constant flow of information relating to drug therapy and drug reactions, the reader is urged to check product information or composition on the package insert for each drug for any change in indications of dosage and for added warnings and precautions. This is particularly important where the recommended agent is a new and/or infrequently employed drug.

Addison-Wesley Publishing Company
Nursing Division
2725 Sand Hill Road
Menlo Park, California 94025

For
Jessamin
and
Richard

Publisher's Foreword

At the core of the finest client care is a foundation of skills and procedures on which each nurse builds the unique network of experience, judgment, and sensitivity that defines nursing. As publishers, we believe these skills and procedures merit a professional presentation that reflects their essential importance in care; thus we offer *The Addison-Wesley Photo-Atlas of Nursing Procedures*. The first truly professional single-volume atlas for nurses, the *Photo-Atlas* will stand as a landmark in nursing publishing. We hope that all nurses who seek to achieve excellence in nursing practice will see this atlas as contributing to their effort.

The Addison-Wesley
Publishing Company
Nursing Division

Preface

Do you remember the anxiety that surrounded your first performance of a new procedure in the hospital—an injection, a catheterization, suctioning an airway? Most nurses never forget.

Mastering the procedures—the psychomotor skills that underlie day-to-day nursing care—is one of the most important and most difficult educational experiences in nursing. Performed correctly, as part of an overall plan of nursing care, these procedures help promote comfort and recovery for clients. Performed less than competently, some procedures can be life-threatening.

Procedures usually are learned by watching a skilled demonstration and then attempting a return demonstration. Because one on-site performance is seldom enough practice, methods and guidelines are needed to repeat the demonstrations until skills are mastered. *The Addison-Wesley Photo-Atlas of Nursing Procedures* offers you that extra assistance.

This single volume provides convenient access to realistic and detailed demonstrations of the procedures most frequently required of general duty staff nurses. It focuses on procedures directly involving a client; thus, such skills as bedmaking are not included. Critical care procedures are not included nor are those procedures that require a hands-on inservice demonstration to ensure safe client care. Because cardiopulmonary resuscitation is a basic technique taught to all hospital personnel, it is not included here.

Audience

Faculty, students, and practitioners alike will find this new two-color atlas a highly effective supplemental text for use in teaching, learning, or practice. New graduates, staff nurses, and nurses returning to practice will welcome its comprehensive reference value. This new atlas uses more than 1500 black-and-white photographs taken in a clinical setting to graphically present more than 300 guidelines and procedures. It assumes the reader's understanding of basic sciences and nursing fundamentals.

Organization and Approach

The *Photo-Atlas* is organized in two units: Unit One includes procedures basic to all nursing care; Unit Two includes procedures related to disorders of individual body systems. Since these are procedures that can be depicted by photography, psychosocial skills are not included.

Each body-system chapter begins with a review of anatomy and physiology, followed by a nursing assessment outline for that system. Where appropriate, variations of care throughout the life cycle are included in the narrative.

Every attempt has been made to include the necessary detail and rationale for each procedure while making each step easy to understand. The steps are within the nursing process framework, thus helping ensure optimal care of the client. The clear, profes-

sional tone of the presentation and the inclusion of rationale help establish an ideal climate for client teaching.

There are often several "correct" ways to perform a procedure based on agency practice and/or personal preference. This atlas depicts generic procedures that can be adapted to the materials and equipment available and to the method the reader has used successfully. Occasional use of identifiable commercial products in the photographs is not intended as product endorsement.

The photographs in this book represent the variety of nursing attire currently worn in hospitals and other health care settings around the nation. Thus, nurses are shown both with and without the traditional nursing cap and wearing many different styles of professional attire.

Reflects 1983 CDC Guidelines

All procedures depicted that relate to the prevention and control of infection conform to *1983 Guidelines for Infection Control in Hospitals* published by the Centers for Disease Control.

The Addison-Wesley Photo-Atlas of Nursing Procedures was created and developed to assist nurses at every level of practice as they learn, relearn, review and update their hands-on skills in client care. Ultimately this will enhance the quality of that care—a goal we all share.

Pamela L. Swearingen, R.N.
Special Projects Editor

Acknowledgments

The journey from idea to bound book is never solitary. On a project of this magnitude, the author requires assistance, encouragement, and support from many. I am fortunate to have found an abundance of all three requisites at every step.

The *Photo-Atlas* had its inception at one of the great teaching centers in nursing—Indiana University School of Nursing at Indianapolis. I am grateful to Dean Elizabeth Grossman and Associate Dean Magdelene Fuller from that school and to Sally Knox, Associate Director of Nursing for Indiana University Hospitals, for their support, for granting us the use of their excellent facilities, and for the opportunity to work with knowledgeable faculty and staff members. Deep appreciation is due also to Rebecca Porter of the Physical Therapy Program and Joanne Sprinkle of the Respiratory Therapy Program, both from the division of Allied Health Sciences at Indiana University Medical School. They and their staff helped tremendously.

Two people in particular have earned special thanks for their instrumental contribution to the photographic content of the book: Jeffry Collins, the talented photographer whose energy, perseverance, sense of humor, and wonderful "people skills" made completion of this monumental task not only possible but fun; and Jean Hutten, Learning Lab Coordinator at I.U. School of Nursing, whose unfailing support helped sustain me throughout the development of this book.

Our talented illustrator, Jack Tandy, merits particular recognition for his superb artwork showing interior structures. Jack's knowledge, skill, and caring make him one of publishing's most valued professionals.

Designer Janet Bollow has imbued this book from cover to cover with her customary excellence. Her ability to integrate text and photographs helped us achieve optimum usefulness and aesthetic appeal.

Among the many others who shared their time and expertise are: Mary Jane Shepherd, who offered expert assistance on the Z-track injection; the Indianapolis chapter of the United Ostomy Association, Inc.; Christine Scales of the Hollister Company; Richard Conwell of Abbott Laboratories; and Jerry McCord III of Johnson and Johnson, Orthopedic Division. In addition to our advisors, consultants, and reviewers, Dr. Evan Lehman, Jacqueline Jones, Carol Marshall, and Dr. Kenneth R. Woolling also proffered valuable advice.

I owe a special debt of gratitude to Cheryl Ashbaucher, Diane Billings, Ursula Easterday, Cheri Howard, and Kathy Pagana, whose efforts went far beyond the requirements of their jobs as advisors and consultants. Marguerite M. Jackson, Coordinator, Infection Control Team, University of California–San Diego Medical Center, has demonstrated far more interest in and commitment to this project than can reasonably be expected of any reviewer. Her expertise and thoroughness are reflected throughout this book.

Three other individuals deserve special recognition for their help in the planning and development of this book: Geraldine G. Allerman, Lienhard School of Nursing, Pace University; Mary Hoyte Sizemore, University of Texas at El Paso; and Patricia L. Cross, Medi-SHARE, Inc. I am grateful for their guidance and their insight.

Careful, thoughtful critiques from the following reviewers helped ensure the accuracy and clarity of the procedures depicted: Richard Barton, Presbyterian Hospital, San Francisco; Marilyn J. Bayne, University of Maryland; Margaret H. Birney, University of Delaware; Irene M. Bobak, San Francisco State University; Patricia Brown, Adelphi University, New York; Marge Cengiz and Sue Elster, University of Utah; Nancy Click, Riverside Methodist Hospital, Columbus, Ohio; Jeanne Flynt DeJoseph and Susan Eaton, Stanford University Hospital; Linda Duli, U.S. Army; Ezelia Goode and Mary Ann Fishburn, Kaiser Permanente, Los Angeles; Christine Farris, Tri-City Hospital, Oceanside, California; Loretta P. Higgins, Boston College; Nancy Hilt, University of Virginia; Daisy Hines, Long Beach City College; Barbara Huttmann, University of San Francisco; Alma Miles, Rush

University, Chicago; Judy Harr, Mary Lou Muswaswes, and Linda Winkler, University of California, San Francisco; Rosemary Murray, The Mt. Sinai School of Continuing Education in Nursing, New York; Sally B. Olds, Beth El School of Nursing, Colorado Springs, Colorado; Martha Orr, The New York Hospital; Patricia Parrott, Grady Memorial Hospital, Atlanta; Harriet Pilert, Church Hospital, Baltimore, Maryland; Dennis Ross, Castleton State College, Vermont; Martha Thompson, San Jose State University; and Betsy Todd, Drug Columnist, Geriatric Nursing, New York.

Finally I want to express my deepest thanks to the talented professionals with whom I have worked at Addison-Wesley: Nick Keefe, Margaret Moore, Betty Duncan-Todd, John Bratnober, Janice Kumano, and Nancy Evans—my friend, colleague, and editor, whose ability to find the right words, both spoken and written, has meant so much. Our shared experience has reaffirmed that the publishing process works best when author and publisher are partners from the idea onward rather than joining forces only at the completion of the manuscript. Together we have made this book better than it could have been had we each worked independently.

P.L.S.

Advisory Board

Contents in Brief

Contents

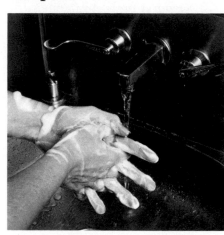
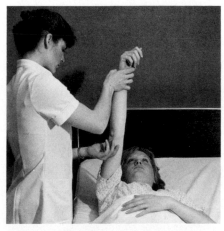

Chapter 3

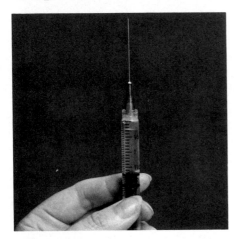

Administering Medications and Monitoring Fluids 91

UNIT II PERFORMING SPECIALIZED NURSING PROCEDURES 165

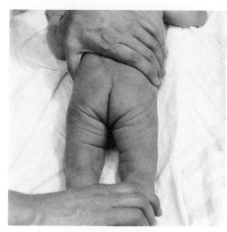
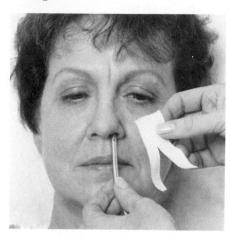

Chapter 6

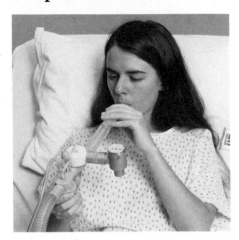

Managing Respiratory Procedures 303

Chapter 7

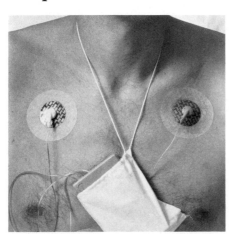

Managing Cardiovascular Procedures 379

Chapter 8

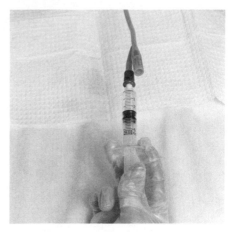

Managing Renal-Urinary Procedures 429

Chapter 9

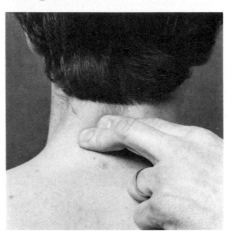

Managing Musculoskeletal Procedures 499

Chapter 10

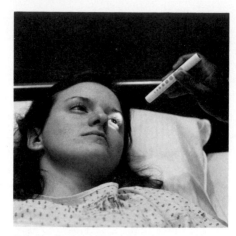

Managing Neurosensory Procedures 589

Unit I

Performing Basic Care Procedures

Chapter 1

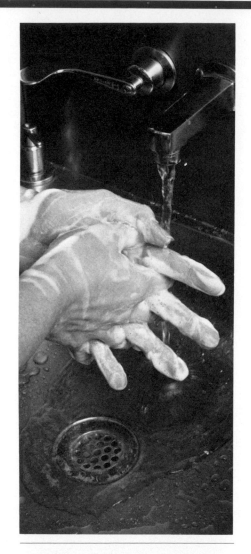

Employing
Techniques for
Infection
Prevention and
Control

CHAPTER OUTLINE

APPLYING BASIC
INFECTION CONTROL
MEASURES

Nursing Guidelines to
Protocols for Handwashing,
Cleansing Agents, and the Use
of Gloves

Reviewing Basic Handwashing

Using Isolation Precautions
   Applying isolation attire
   Removing isolation attire
   Double-bagging
     contaminated supplies

PREPARING FOR A STERILE
PROCEDURE

Applying Sterile Gloves

Establishing a Sterile Field
   Opening a sterile pack
   Dropping sterile supplies
     onto a sterile field
   Placing a sterile bowl onto
     the sterile field
   Pouring sterile solutions

Putting on Sterile Attire
(Including the Closed-Glove
Technique)

MANAGING SPECIAL
DRESSING CHANGE
TECHNIQUES

Packing a Wound (Using Wet
to Dry Dressings)

Changing the Dressing for a
Central Venous Catheter

Applying Basic Infection Control Measures

NURSING GUIDELINES TO PROTOCOLS FOR HANDWASHING, CLEANSING AGENTS, AND THE USE OF GLOVES

According to the Centers for Disease Control (CDC), in clinical situations in which *superficial* contact has been made with a client who is not suspected of being contaminated with virulent microorganisms, handwashing is generally not required. Superficial contact includes handshaking, measuring blood pressure, and handing medications or food to the client. However, handwashing is indicated when one has had prolonged and intense client contact. In addition, handwashing should be performed *before* invasive procedures; *before* caring for susceptible clients, such as newborns or clients in intensive care units; and *before* and *after* contact with wounds.

Hands should be washed *between* contact with different clients in intensive care units and newborn nurseries and *after* contact with sources that are suspected of being contaminated with virulent microorganisms or hospital pathogens. This includes contact with infected clients as well as contact with blood, secretions, or excretions from any client. The hands should be washed also between procedures for the same client (for example, if the urinary collection container is changed before feeding the client or changing a wound dressing), as well as upon leaving the room.

Generally, the decision for using soap and water versus an antimicrobial agent should be based on an assessment of the client, the client's susceptibility, and the potential for the spread of virulent organisms to oneself and to other clients. Antimicrobials are preferred when the resident skin flora of personnel is likely to cause disease after client contact, as with the newborn or clients in intensive care units who are severely compromised. An antimicrobial agent should be used when the hands might be contaminated with virulent organisms—for example, from a client in isolation precautions. For guidelines for the recommended cleansing agent and indications for the use of gloves, review Table 1-1.

Table 1-1   Recommended Agents for Preparing Hands and Cleaning Skin *Before** Nonsurgical and Surgical Procedures†

Procedure	Example	Handwashing	Gloves‡	Preparation of patient's skin	Comment
Nonsurgical					
Instruments used in procedure will come in contact with intact mucous membranes	Bronchoscopy, gastrointestinal endoscopy, and tracheal suction	Soap and water	Recommended	In general, none is required.	
	Cystoscopy, urinary tract catheterization	Soap and water	Sterile recommended	Antiseptics should be used to prepare urethral meatus.	

*Hands should be washed *after* all procedures when microbial contamination of the operator is likely to occur, especially those involving contact with mucous membranes, whether or not gloves are worn. Soap and water are adequate for such handwashing unless a virulent agent (e.g., *Shigella* or hepatitis B virus) is suspected of infecting the patient; then an antiseptic should be used.

†From Centers for Disease Control. 1981. Guideline for hospital environmental control: antiseptics, handwashing, and handwashing facilities. In *Guidelines for the prevention and control of nosocomial infections.* Atlanta, Ga.: U.S. Department of Health and Human Services.

‡Gloves protect the patient and the operator from potentially infectious microorganisms.

(Continued)

Table 1-1, *Continued*

Procedure	Example	Handwashing	Gloves‡	Preparation of patient's skin	Comment
Insertion of peripheral intravenous or arterial cannula	Intravenous therapy, arterial pressure monitoring	Soap and water or antiseptic	Not necessary but may be helpful in certain instances	Antiseptics should be used; a fast-acting one is desirable. Tincture of iodine is preferred, but alcohol is adequate if it is applied liberally and allowed to act for 30 seconds.	Most epidemics of infection associated with arterial pressure-monitoring devices appear to be caused by hospital-associated contamination of components external to the skin, such as transducer heads or domes.
Percutaneous insertion of a central catheter or wire	Hyperalimentation, central venous and capillary wedge pressure monitoring, angiography, cardiac pacemaker insertion	Antiseptic	Sterile recommended	Antiseptics should be used; a fast-acting one is desirable. Tincture of iodine is preferred. "Defatting" agents, such as acetone, are not recommended.	"Defatting" agents do not appear to decrease infections but can cause skin irritation.
Insertion (and prompt removal) of a sterile needle in deep tissues or body fluids, usually to obtain specimens or instill therapeutic agent	Spinal tap, thoracentesis, abdominal paracentesis	Soap and water or antiseptic	Sterile recommended	Antiseptics should be used; a fast-acting one is desirable. Tincture of iodine is preferred.	
Surgical					
Insertion of a sterile tube or device through tissue into normally sterile tissue or fluid	Chest tube insertion, culdoscopy, laparoscopy, peritoneal catheter insertion	Antiseptic	Sterile recommended	Antiseptics should be used. Hair should be clipped with scissors if hair removal is considered necessary.	
Minor skin surgery	Skin biopsy, suturing of small cuts, lancing boils, mole removal	Soap and water	Sterile recommended	Antiseptics should be used.	Gloves are usually worn for a short time and thus antiseptic handwashing is not usually necessary to suppress resident flora for these superficial procedures.
Other procedures (major and minor surgery) that enter tissue below skin	Hysterectomy, cholecystectomy, herniorrhaphy	Antiseptic	Sterile recommended	Antiseptics should be used after the site has been scrubbed with a detergent. The patient can be shaved immediately before the procedure although clipping hair or using a depilatory is preferred.	Handwashing before surgical procedures that enter deep tissue is usually prolonged to ensure that all areas that harbor bacteria are adequately cleaned.

REVIEWING BASIC HANDWASHING

According to CDC, frequent handwashing is the single most important procedure for reducing the transmission of potentially infectious agents.

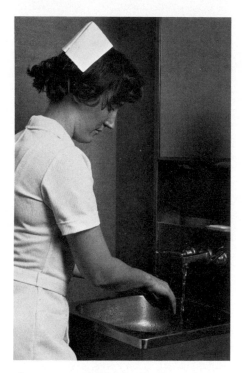

1 Before washing your hands, remove the rings from your fingers to facilitate thorough cleansing and drying. If your watch has an expansion band, slide it above your wrist. Adjust the water to a warm temperature, and rinse your hands.

2 Lather your hands thoroughly. Remember that it is the friction from rubbing your hands together that removes potentially infectious organisms from the skin. A 10-second vigorous handwashing will adequately remove most transient flora.

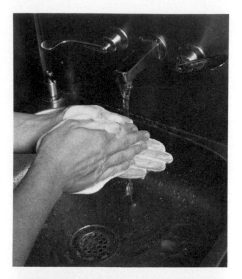

3 Wash each wrist by vigorously sliding the opposite hand around its surface area.

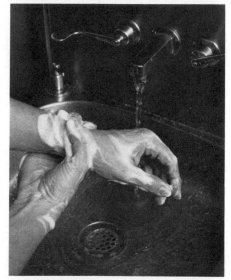

4 Interlace your fingers and thumbs, and slide them back and forth. Clean under your nails and around the nail beds with the fingertips and nails of the opposite hand.

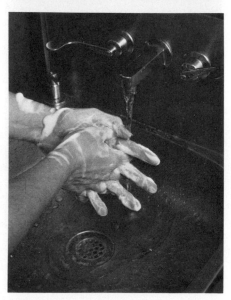

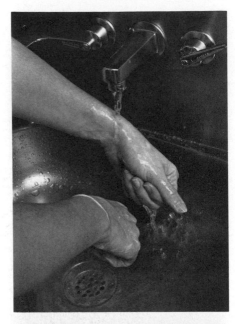

5 Thoroughly rinse each hand from the wrist down. If your hands were grossly soiled, repeat steps 2–5 above.

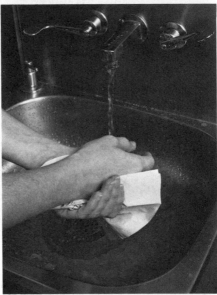

6 Dry your hands with disposable towels.

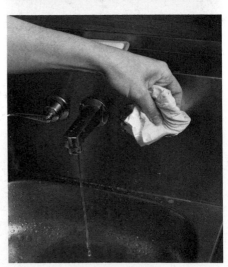

7 To protect your hands from the contaminated surface of the faucet handle, turn off the faucet by placing a dry section of your used towel over the handle.

USING ISOLATION PRECAUTIONS

There are many types of isolation precautions used in the hospital setting. The method used to interrupt the transmission of potentially infectious agents is determined by the agent's mode of transmission. It is essential, therefore, that nurses and other agency personnel assess the risk of infection to client, to self, and to other clients, and then implement a plan of care based on sound judgment. The following are general, but not exhaustive, CDC recommendations for the use of specific isolation attire.

Applying Isolation Attire
Applying a Gown

Gowns are worn to prevent soiling of clothing when caring for clients. They are indicated when caring for clients on isolation precautions if clothing is likely to be soiled with infective secretions or excretions, for example when changing the bed of an incontinent client. They are also indicated for all persons entering the rooms of clients who have infections that if spread could cause serious illness, even though gross soiling of clothing is not anticipated. These infectious conditions include diseases such as varicella (chickenpox) and disseminated zoster.

Applying a Mask

Masks are worn to prevent the transmission of infectious organisms through the air. In addition, masks help to prevent the transmission of infections that are spread through direct contact with mucous membranes by discouraging the wearer from contacting his or her own mouth, nose, or eyes until the hands have been washed and the mask removed. Disease conditions in which masks are indicated include varicella (chickenpox), disseminated zoster, and pharyngeal diphtheria. In addition, they should be worn when the caregiver has close contact with clients who have diseases such as rubella (German measles), mumps, pertussis, staphylococcal pneumonia, and streptococcal pneumonia.

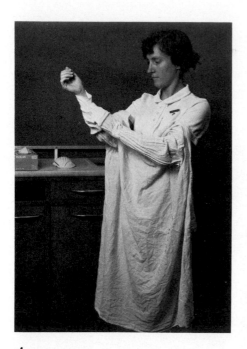

1 To put on a gown, slip your arms into the sleeves and then tie the strings at the back of the neck.

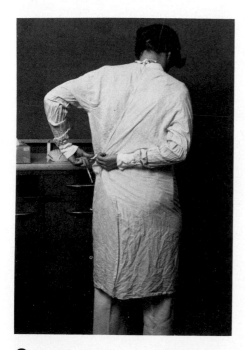

2 Overlap the gown in the back so that it covers the back of your clothing, and tie the strings at the waistline.

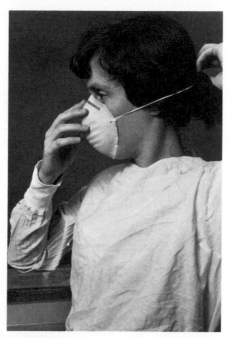

1 Generally, cup masks are worn in the isolation setting. To apply the mask, position the elastic strap securely around the back of your head. The mask should fit the face tightly enough to prevent venting at the sides.

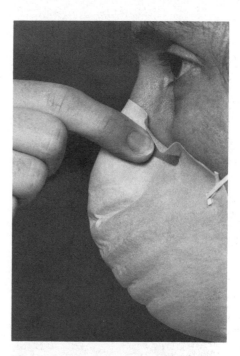

2 To minimize the gap between the mask and your nose, pinch the nose clip, as shown. Bring an extra mask into the room with you if you will be inside for longer than 20 minutes because a mask is ineffective when it becomes moist.

Applying Gloves

Gloves are worn for three reasons. First, they protect the wearer from becoming infected by microorganisms that are infecting the client. Second, they minimize the potential for the wearer to transmit his or her own resident microbial flora to the client; and third, they minimize the risk of cross-contamination from one client to another. Gloves are indicated when touching blood, secretions, excretions, or body fluids. Examples of disease states in which these situations can occur are: acquired immunodeficiency syndrome (AIDS), amebic or bacillary dysentery, varicella, conjunctivitis, coxsackievirus disease, gangrene, gastroenteritis, giardiasis, viral hepatitis, gonococcal ophthalmia neonatorum, disseminated zoster, rabies, and wound infections.

Removing Isolation Attire

When you have completed the care for your client under isolation precautions, remove your contaminated attire before leaving the room or after stepping into the anteroom if the isolation room has one. By following these steps, you will minimize the potential for contaminating your hands and garments.

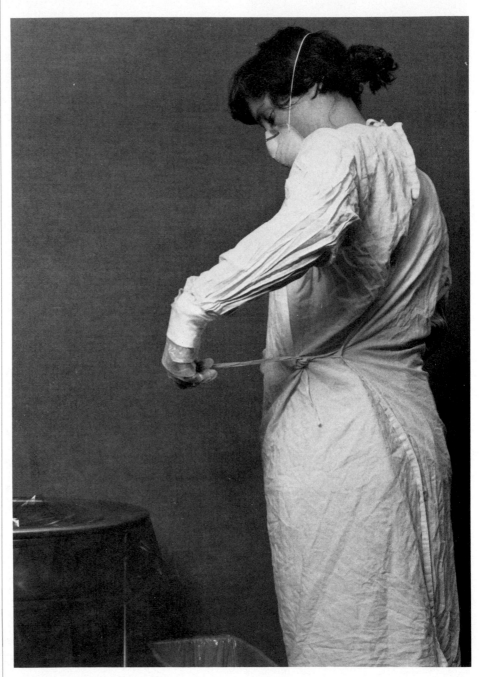

1 If you are wearing a gown, untie its waist strings.

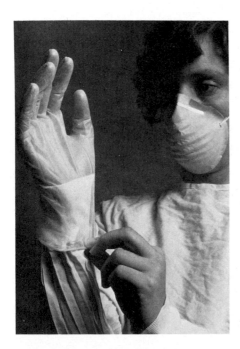

Put on the gloves, making sure they cover the cuffs of the isolation gown if the gown is also worn.

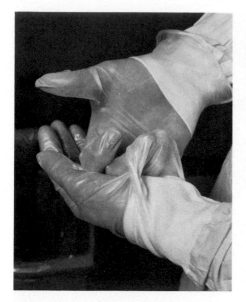

2 Remove your gloves: With your dominant hand, make a cuff by hooking gloved fingers into the lower outside edge of the other glove. Pull the glove inside out as you remove it, and then hold the glove in your gloved hand.

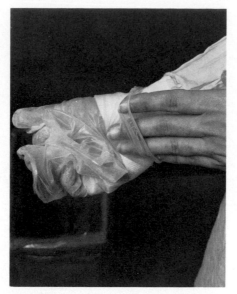

3 Tuck your ungloved fingers into the inside edge of the remaining glove. Remove that glove by pulling it inside out and encase the other glove as you do. Discard the gloves into the designated waste container. If you are wearing a gown, untie the neck strings next.

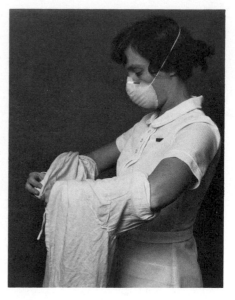

4 After untying the neck strings, remove the gown by turning it inside out during the process.

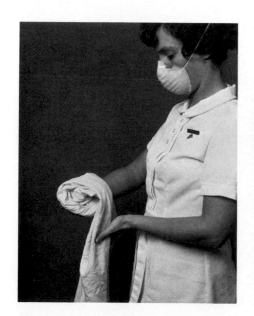

5 Hold the gown away from your body, and roll it up so that the contaminated side is innermost.

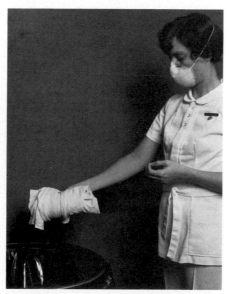

6 Place the gown in an impermeable bag that has been designated for contaminated laundry.

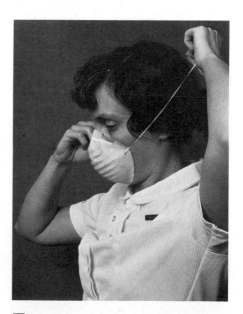

7 Finally, remove the mask by grasping it by the elastic strap and pulling it off. Dispose of it in the waste container, and wash your hands with antimicrobial soap before leaving the room.

Double-Bagging Contaminated Supplies

Articles may need to be enclosed in an impermeable bag before they are removed from the room of a client in isolation. This is done to protect personnel who may handle articles that are contaminated with infectious material. Most articles do not need to be bagged in this manner. Exceptions are articles from the room of a client in strict isolation or articles contaminated with infective material. A single bag is usually adequate if it is impermeable and sturdy and if the object can be placed in the bag without contaminating the outside of the bag. If the outside of the bag becomes contaminated, double-bagging should be done before the contents are placed outside the room for removal.

Put on the necessary isolation attire by following the steps on pp. 8–10. In many instances, gloves alone are adequate provided the contaminated inner bag can be handled without touching your clothing. Bring an impermeable isolation bag into the room with you and place it over a hamper or chairback. Remove the contaminated bag from its hamper and twist the open end into a tail, either knotting or securing it with a twist tie. Deposit the contaminated bag into the clean outer bag (as shown) by pointing the tied end downward to ensure that the dirtiest part of the bag is farthest from the top of the clean bag. Avoid touching the outside of the clean bag with the dirty bag. Remove your isolation attire, and wash your hands with an antimicrobial soap. Label the bag "isolation" if it is not already identified as such; discard it according to agency policy, or arrange for its removal.

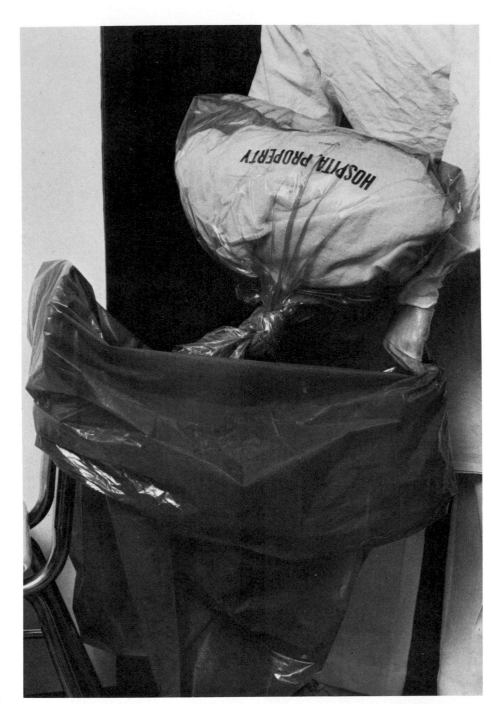

Preparing for a Sterile Procedure

APPLYING STERILE GLOVES

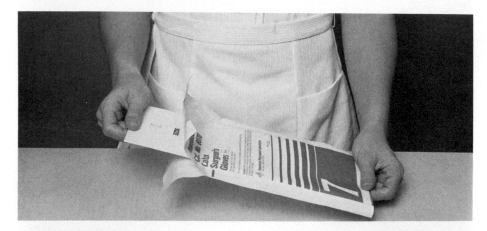

1 After washing your hands, open the outer wrap of the sterile glove pack and remove the inner wrap. Place the inner wrap on a clean, dry surface.

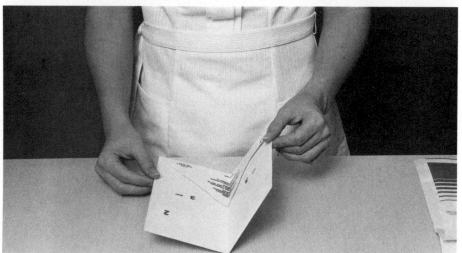

2 Carefully unfold the inner wrap, touching only the outside edges.

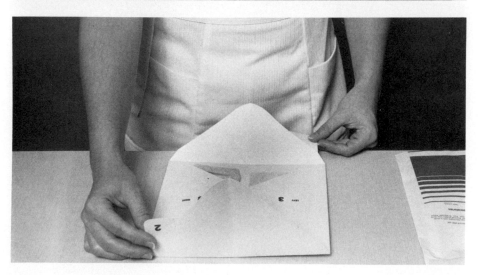

3 If the inner wrap has numbered flaps (as shown), open them numerically. Be sure to touch only the folded tabs. If the wrap is unnumbered, open the gloves by following the steps for opening a sterile pack on p. 16.

(Continued on p. 14)

4 With your dominant hand, grasp the opposite glove at the inner edge of the folded cuff.

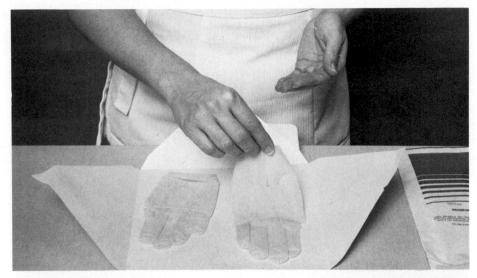

5 Carefully slip your hand into the glove.

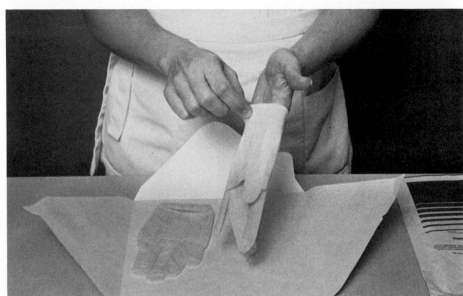

6 While still grasping the inner edge of the folded cuff, pull the glove over your hand.

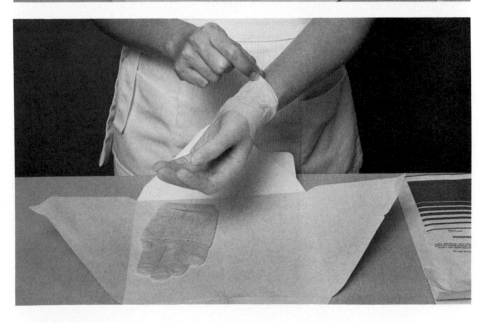

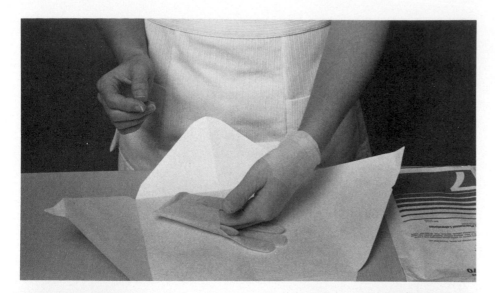

7 With your sterile gloved hand, slip your fingers into the folded cuff of the remaining glove.

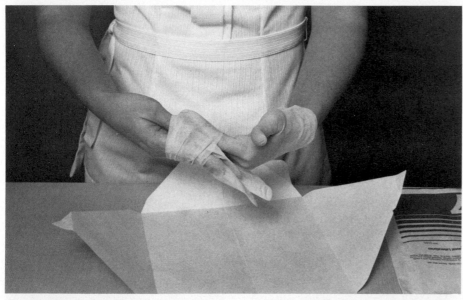

8 Carefully slip the glove over your fingers.

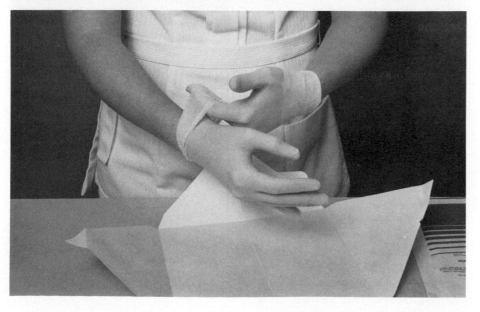

9 Pull the glove over your hand.

(Continued on p. 16)

10 Adjust each glove to ensure a snug fit over your hands and fingers. Carefully slide your fingers under each cuff and pull them up.

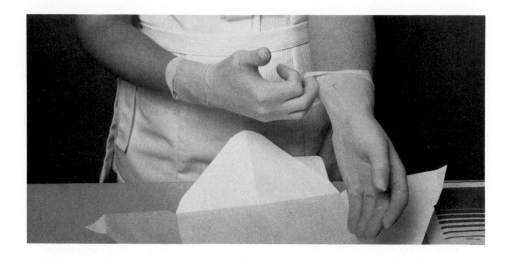

ESTABLISHING A STERILE FIELD

Opening a Sterile Pack

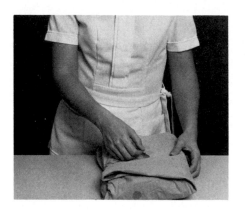
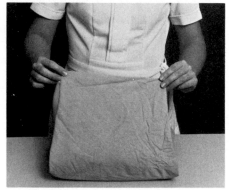
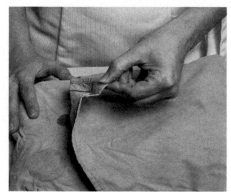
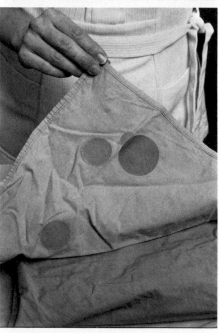

1 Wash your hands with an antimicrobial soap before opening the sterile pack. A sterile pack must be opened on a clean, dry surface. The outer wrap of commercially wrapped sterile packs should be inspected both for tears and for the sterility expiration date. Follow agency policy for returning outdated supplies. If the pack is agency-wrapped (as shown), ensure its sterility by inspecting the chemical indicator tape both for the integrity of its seal with the pack and for a change of colors, indicating it has been properly sterilized. Also check the sterility expiration date, which is written on the tape. Remove the indicator tape by pulling it from the center toward the outer edge of the pack.

2 Position the pack so that its outermost flap faces away from you. With your thumbs and index fingers, grasp the flap by small sections of its folded crease and lift it up and away from you. Hold your arms at the sides of the pack to avoid reaching over the sterile area.

3 Open the side flaps (top right). Grasp the folded corner of the uppermost flap by touching a small section with your thumb and index finger; lay the flap to the side. Do the same with the opposite flap. Lift the remaining flap toward you (bottom), stepping back 12.5–25 cm (5–10 in.) as you do, so that you do not contaminate the wrap with your clothing. If the pack has an inner wrap, repeat the above procedure to open it.

Dropping Sterile Supplies onto a Sterile Field

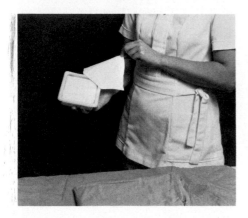

1 If your commercially wrapped sterile package is a peelback container (as shown), grasp the flap by its unsealed corner and pull the flap toward you. Position the pack so that its open end will face the sterile field.

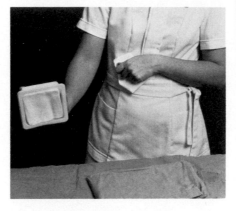

2 To prevent the container from contaminating the field, hold the opened pack 15 cm (6 in.) above the sterile field, and allow the contents to drop well within the sterile area. Remember that the 2.5 cm (1 in.) border along the edge of the field is considered contaminated.

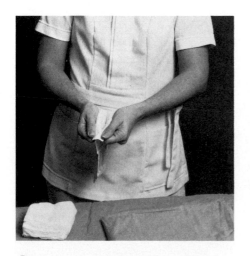

3 To open other types of commercially wrapped peelback containers such as glove packs or syringes (as shown), grasp both sides of the pack's unsealed edge and gently pull them apart.

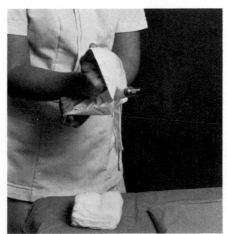

4 Hold the package so that its opened end is positioned away from your body and facing the sterile field. Carefully fold the sides back so that the outside wrap covers your hands and protects the contents. With the contents protected in this manner, allow it to drop onto the sterile field making sure it drops well within the sterile area.

Placing a Sterile Bowl onto the Sterile Field

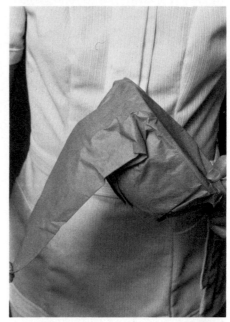

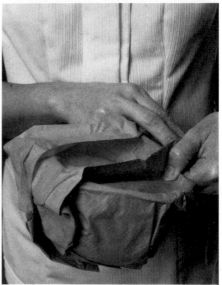

1 Hold a wrapped bowl at the rim with your thumb and index finger. Detach one of the corners (top) and bring it up and over the rim (bottom). Then hold the detached corner in place with your thumb and index finger.

(Continued on p. 18)

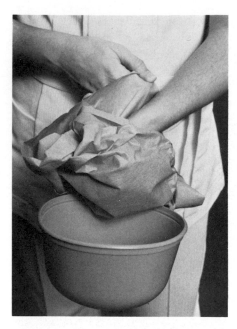

2 In the same manner, bring all the ends up to the rim; hold them in place with your thumb and index finger, confining the ends to a small area at the rim.

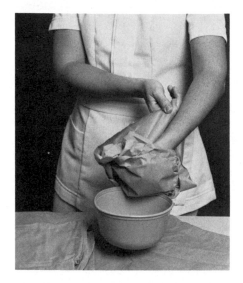

3 Place the bowl onto the sterile field. If it will be used to contain sterile solutions, place it near the edge of the field. This will enable you to pour the solution without reaching over a large section of the sterile area.

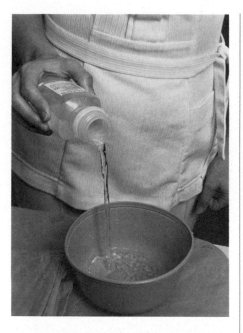

Pouring Sterile Solutions
Because the sterility of a solution cannot be ensured once its container has been opened, try to obtain a container with an amount of solution appropriate to the procedure. As you pour the solution, hold the container to the side of, and at an angle to, the sterile field so that your hand and arm do not reach over the sterile area. To minimize the risk of contamination, hold the container 10–15 cm (4–6 in.) above the bowl; pour slowly to avoid splashing the sterile drape and contaminating the sterile field.

PUTTING ON STERILE ATTIRE (INCLUDING THE CLOSED-GLOVE TECHNIQUE)

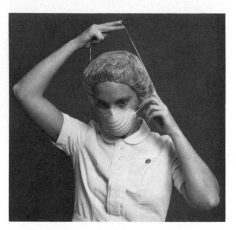

1 When you are required to wear sterile attire for procedures in which surgical asepsis is necessary, you must first wash your hands, put on a hair cover and face mask, and then open the sterile pack containing the sterile gown. (See steps on p. 16.)

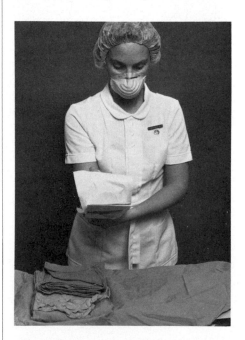

2 Remove the sterile gloves from their outer wrap and drop the inner wrap onto the sterile pack (as shown). Wash your hands with an antimicrobial soap and dry them thoroughly with the towel provided in the gown pack.

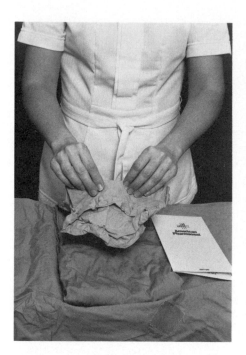

3 Grasp the sterile gown by its uppermost folded crease near the neckline.

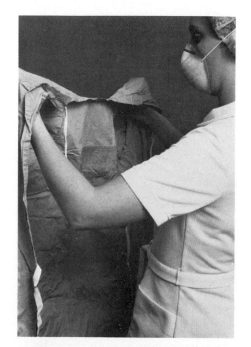

4 Step into an area in which you will have space to open the gown without contaminating it, and hold it away from you to allow the gown to unfold. Place your hands inside the gown and work your arms through the shoulders, being certain to touch the inside of the gown only.

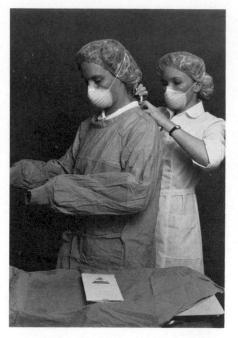

5 If you perform the closed-glove technique, advance your hands only as far as the proximal edge of the cuff (as shown). However, if you apply sterile gloves using the usual aseptic (open-glove) technique, extend your hands through the cuff, but do not touch the outside of the gown. Regardless of the gloving technique you use, a co-worker will be needed for assistance. The co-worker should first put on a mask and hair cover and then grasp the ties at the neckline area at the back of your gown and pull the gown up to cover the neckline of the front of your uniform. She will then tie the ties without touching the exterior of your gown.

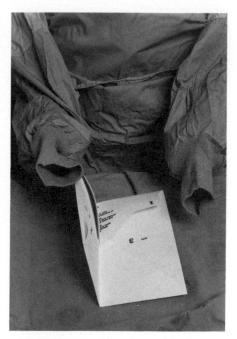

6 Unfold the inner wrap of the sterile gloves. If you are using the closed-glove technique, do this with your covered hands (as shown). Otherwise, follow the guidelines for applying sterile gloves using the technique described on pp. 13–16 and proceed to step 14.

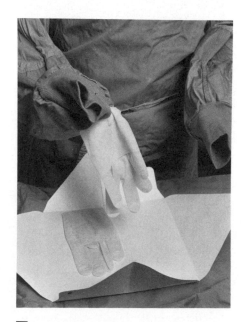

7 Grasp the first glove by manipulating your thumb and index finger through the fabric of the sleeve or cuff.

(Continued on p. 20)

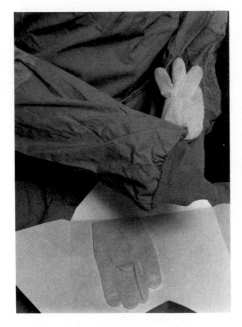

8 Place the glove palm down onto the cuff of your sterile gown. The fingers of the glove should point toward your elbow.

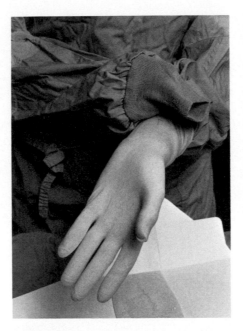

10 When the glove has been successfully pulled over the cuff, extend your fingers into the glove.

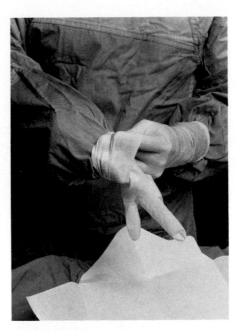

12 Position the glove over the closed cuff.

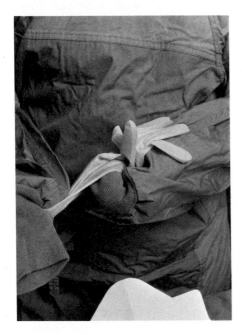

9 Manipulate your fingers within the cuff to firmly anchor the glove. With your other covered hand, stretch the glove over the entire cuff.

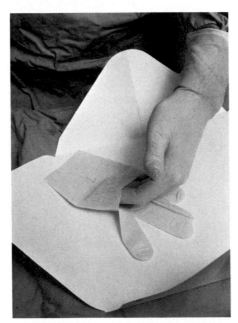

11 Place your gloved fingers within the folded cuff of the remaining glove.

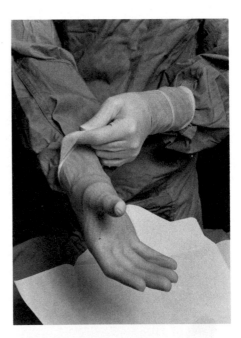

13 Pull the glove up over the gown's cuff as you extend your fingers through the glove. Adjust the glove to fit your fingers. Make sure both gloves cover the cuffs of the gown.

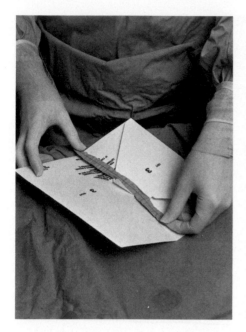

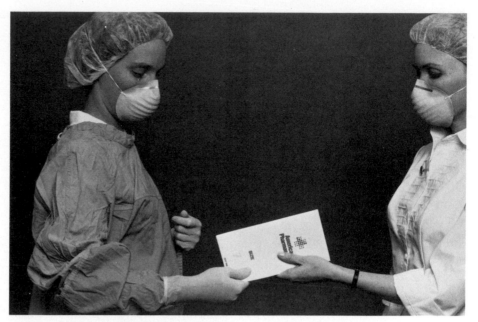

14 Place the back tie of the gown's waistband into the crease of the empty inner glove wrapper.

15 Close the wrapper and hand it to your co-worker. Instruct her to touch the outer wrap only.

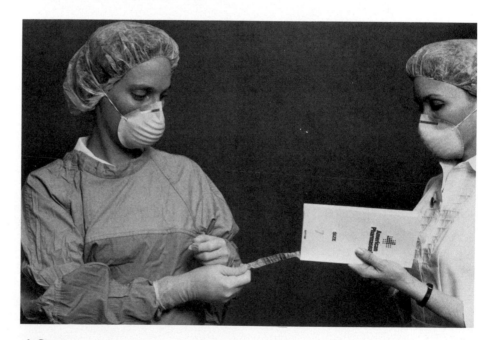

16 Make a three-quarter turn; then pull the tie from the wrapper and tie the gown at the front. *Note: If you prefer, your co-worker may instead put on a sterile glove and grasp the tie with her gloved hand while you make a three-quarter turn.*

Managing Special Dressing Change Techniques

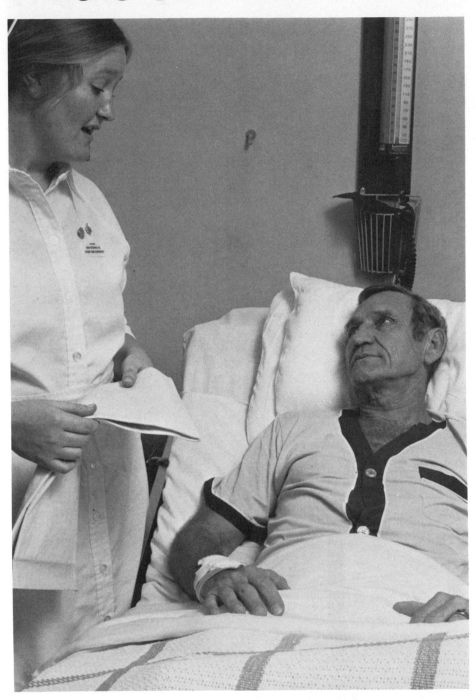

PACKING A WOUND (USING WET TO DRY DRESSINGS)

Assessing and Planning

1 Wash your hands and then explain the dressing change procedure to your client. Assess his level of comfort; if a pain medication has been prescribed, ask him whether he will need one for the procedure. If you do administer the medication, delay the procedure for 20 minutes until the medication takes effect. Position the bed at an optimal working height, provide privacy for the client, and place a bed-saver pad under the area of the wound to protect the bed linen. Inspect the dressing site and determine the approximate number of gauze pads you will need for the packing and outer dressing, as well as the need for either tape or fresh Montgomery straps. If the wound is a large one that requires deep packing, you will need sterile gloves or forceps to remove the packing. Packing from smaller wounds can be removed with clean gloves if it can be easily grasped by the outer dressing and pulled from the wound without direct contact with the clean glove. You may need to check the client's chart or care plan for additional information.

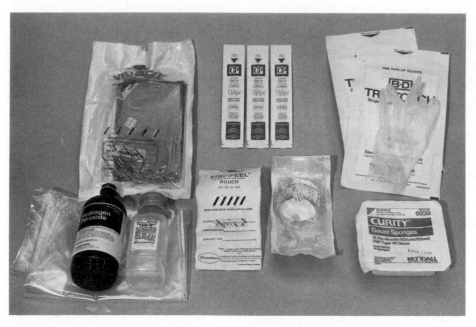

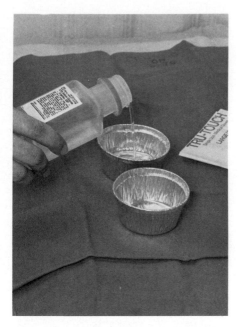

2 Assemble the following materials: sterile bowl(s)—the number will be determined by the number of different solutions to be used; sterile towels, drape, or a Mayo stand cover to make a sterile field; sterile normal saline and sterile hydrogen peroxide (or the prescribed cleansing and wetting solutions); sterile cotton swabs, three to four packs; clean gloves; sterile gloves, two to three pairs (depending on whether the packing can be grasped indirectly through the outer dressing or will require direct removal); sterile gauze pads; and an impermeable plastic bag for the disposal of contaminated waste. In addition, you will need tape if Montgomery straps are not used or a gauze roll if the wound is on an extremity.

(It is important that the gauze pads be unfilled and made of a fine mesh. A filled gauze pad has cotton fiber filling that can get left behind in the wound, and fine mesh is necessary for optimal wound debridement because larger mesh gauze may remove the healing granulation tissue.)

3 Place the impermeable plastic bag in a convenient place that is away from the dressing change site. Adjust the client's gown or remove it, and provide warmth and privacy. If the client is on contact isolation for a major wound infection, wash your hands with an antimicrobial soap and put on a mask and gown. If the client is on drainage/secretion precautions for a minor or limited wound infection, masks and gowns are not necessary. Prepare the sterile field at this time, following the steps on pp. 16–18. Carefully pour the prescribed solutions into the sterile bowls. For this procedure, the nurse will use one bowl for the cleansing and debriding solution (equal parts of normal saline and hydrogen peroxide) and the other bowl for the wetting solution (normal saline).

4 Put on the clean gloves and either untie the Montgomery straps to expose the dressing or loosen the tape.

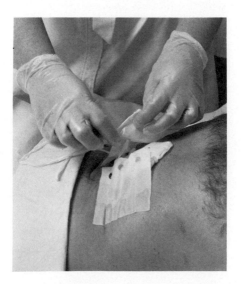

(Continued on p. 24)

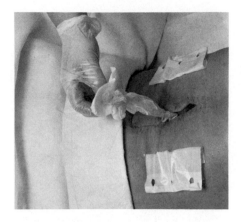

5 Grasp the gauze packing by securing it with the outer dressing that covers it. Pull gently to remove all the packing.
Caution: Use a sterile glove when removing the packing from a deeper wound. Packing from deep wounds usually can not be grasped easily through an outer dressing. To protect the client, use a sterile glove and grasp the packing directly with the gloved hand.

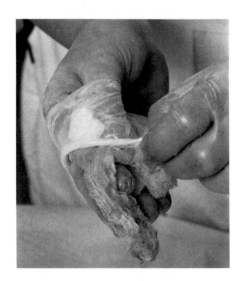

6 Inspect the contaminated dressing to assess the amount and color of debris and drainage; note if it has an odor, which may be indicative of an infection. Encase the dressing in your gloves as you remove them, and dispose of both in the impermeable plastic bag.

Implementing

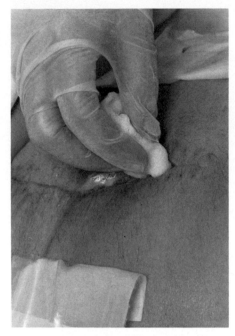

7 Put on a pair of sterile gloves and soak a gauze pad in the cleansing solution. At this time, designate one hand contaminated for cleaning and rinsing and the other sterile for contact with the sterile field. Before cleaning the site, inspect the wound and assess for swelling, size, color, odor, and drainage. Estimate the amount of healing granulation tissue. Saturate the wound from top to bottom with the cleansing solution, and dispose of the contaminated pad.

9 Moisten a cotton swab in the cleansing solution and clean the crevices of the wound. You may also use a fresh cotton swab to assess the depth of the crevice. This information will be important later when you pack the wound. Then, rinse the wound and surrounding area with the normal saline by following steps 5–7 above.

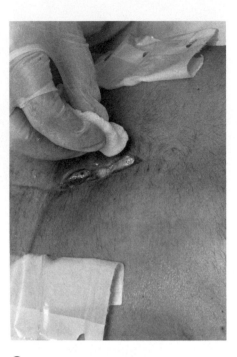

8 Soak another gauze pad in the cleansing solution and clean the area around the wound.

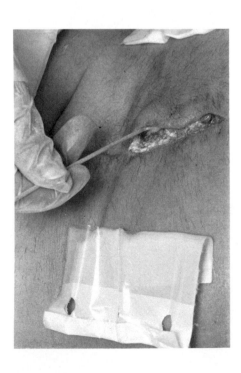

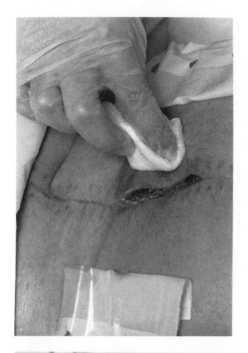

10 Use a dry gauze pad to blot the skin surrounding the wound. Remove your gloves and dispose of them along with the contaminated gauze and cotton swabs.

11 Apply a fresh pair of sterile gloves and prepare to pack the wound by moistening a gauze pad in the normal saline. Be certain to wring out the excess moisture because packing that is too wet will not debride the wound effectively. In addition, saturated packing could moisten the outer dressing and potentially draw infectious organisms into the wound.

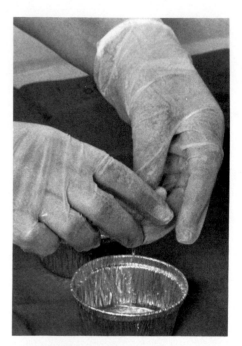

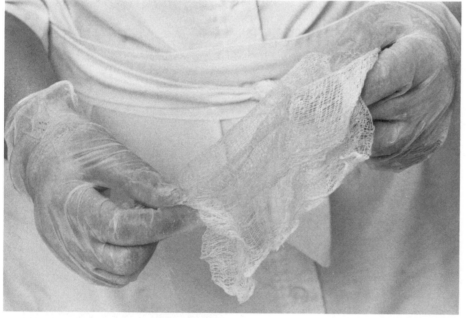

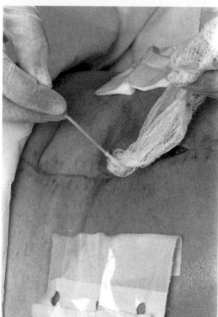

12 Unfold the moistened gauze pad to expand its surface area into a single layer.

13 Use a cotton swab to place the gauze into the crevices of the wound.

(Continued on p. 26)

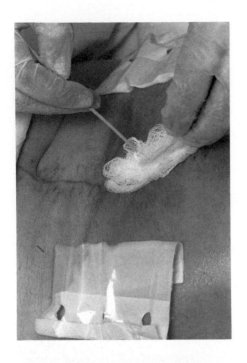

14 Completely fill the wound, adding more gauze as necessary.

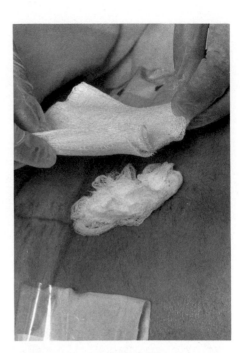

15 Cover the wet gauze with a dry dressing. Using the same number of dry pads for each wet pad that is used will allow enough air to circulate into the wound to dry the wet packing; it will also prevent the outer dressing from becoming saturated, thus reducing the potential for contamination.

16 Tape the dressing in place. If the wound is on an extremity, wrap the dressing with a strip of gauze roll to secure it. If Montgomery straps are used, change them if they are soiled, and then tie them securely (as shown).

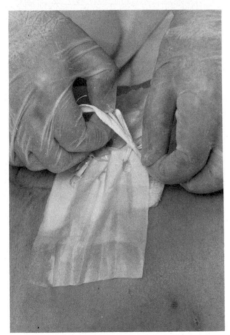

Evaluating

17 Return the client to a position of comfort and assist him with his gown if he is unable to do it himself. Securely tie off the impermeable plastic bag, remove it from the bedside, and dispose of it according to agency policy. Then, wash your hands. If your client is on isolation precautions, wash your hands with an antimicrobial soap. Finally, record the procedure in your nurse's notes. Document the appearance, size, and odor (if present) of the wound and describe the amount and quality of the drainage. Note the amount and appearance of the granulation tissue as well.

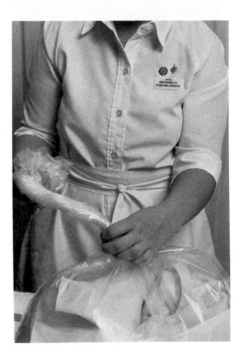

CHANGING THE DRESSING FOR A CENTRAL VENOUS CATHETER

Assessing and Planning

1 Wash your hands and explain the dressing change procedure to your client. Let her know that she will need to turn her head away from the insertion site during the dressing change so that she does not breathe on the area and possibly contaminate it. Assess the need for a mask if she is unable to keep her head turned to the side. Adjust the height of the bed to facilitate the dressing application. If your client's catheter will be disconnected for an IV tubing change, flattening the bed also helps to increase intrathoracic pressure thereby minimizing the risk of an air embolism.

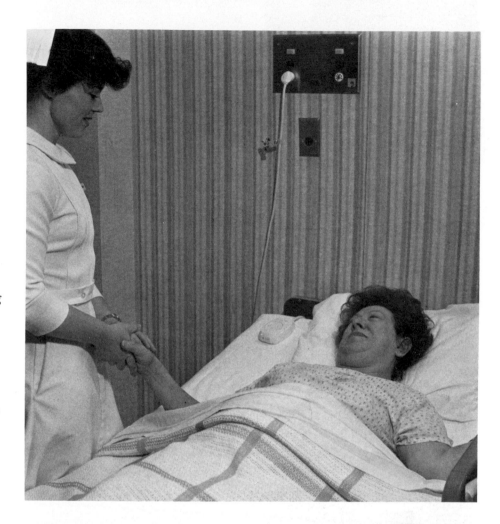

2 Assemble the following materials: three pairs of sterile gloves, sterile drapes to create a sterile field around the insertion site, clean gloves, and an impermeable plastic bag for the disposal of the contaminated supplies. If your agency considers changing the dressing on a central venous catheter to be a procedure requiring surgical asepsis, assemble a sterile gown, mask, and a hair cover. Some agencies believe a mask on both the nurse and the client reduces the risk of contamination of the catheter site and include this practice in their protocol for dressing changes. You will also need either a commercially prepared dressing change kit or a variation of the following materials: an overwrap for a sterile field, three iodophor swabsticks, povidone–iodine ointment, a nonadhering dressing pad, sterile gauze pads, a tincture of benzoin swabstick, elastic bandage, tape, scissors (sterile), and a dressing change label. Some agencies also use acetone to defat the skin. If this is the protocol you are following, obtain four acetone swabsticks also.

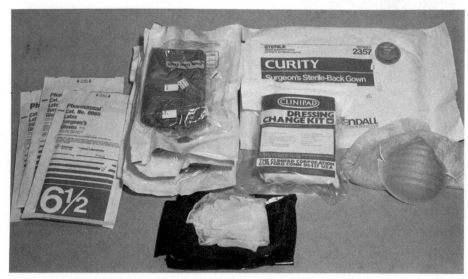

(Continued on p. 28)

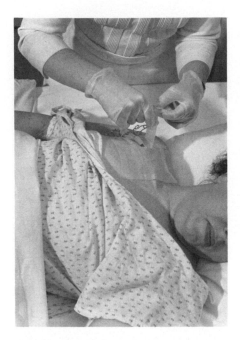 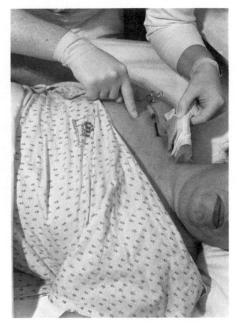 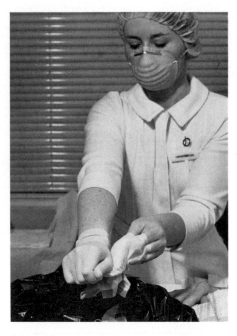

3 <u>Put on a head cover and a mask if it is required by agency policy.</u> Wash your hands and prepare your sterile field following the steps on pp. 16–18. Instruct the client to turn her head away from the insertion site. Then, lower the client's gown at the insertion site, put on clean gloves, and loosen the tape all around the dressing. Remove and deposit the used gloves in the impermeable bag.

4 Put on sterile gloves and gently remove the contaminated dressing. As you inspect the site, assess for redness, drainage, swelling, and odor—indicators that the client may have an infection. (Note that the central line in this photograph is not attached to an IV solution. It is used for hemodialysis, instead.)

5 Encase the dressing in your gloves and deposit them in the impermeable plastic bag. If your agency requires sterile gowning, put on a gown at this time. Then put on two pairs of sterile gloves, one pair on top of the other, so that you will not need to change gloves in the middle of the procedure. This can be done more easily if the outer gloves are a size larger than the inner gloves.

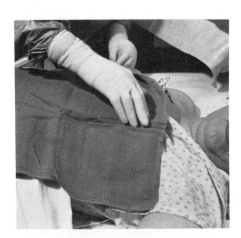

6 Drape the client to create a sterile field around the catheter insertion site. Position the first drape across the chest.
Note: In some agencies, draping might also be optional, depending on client compliance or the presence of exposed wounds such as tracheostomies. Follow agency policy.

7 Place a second drape over her turned head (as shown). Position a third drape superior to the insertion site (as shown in the next photo). The area enclosed by the sterile drapes should measure approximately 20 cm (8 in.) in diameter.

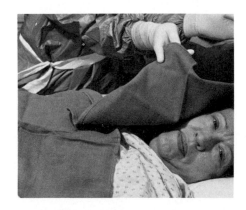

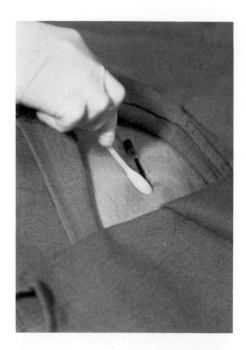

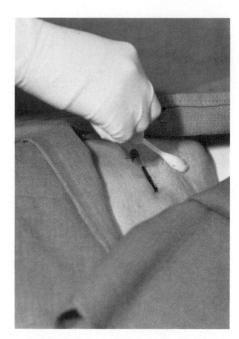

Implementing

8 Open all the swabstick packages (or prepare gauze pads with the solutions). Remove the acetone-soaked swab and apply it directly to the insertion site. Acetone will defat the skin, removing oil, blood, and perspiration that may harbor bacteria. It will also help remove the adhesive left from the previous dressing. The frequency and use of acetone, however, are determined by agency policy because its prolonged use can cause skin irritation.

9 From the insertion site, work outward in a circular fashion to cover a diameter approximately 15–20 cm (6–8 in.). Do not touch the same area more than once with the same swab.

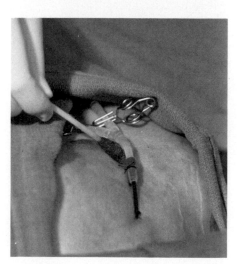

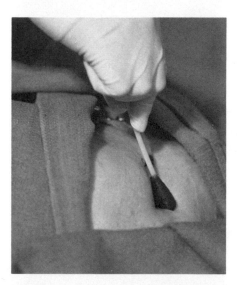

10 Use a fresh swab to cleanse the suture sites and the areas around and under the catheter.

11 Prepare the skin with the iodophor swabs in the same manner described in steps 8–10. Use moderate friction; allow the iodophor 2–3 minutes to dry, the time required for the antimicrobial agent to become effective.

12 When you swab around and under the catheter and suture sites, use care because these are especially sensitive areas for the client. Then carefully remove the outer pair of gloves and dispose of them in the impermeable plastic bag.

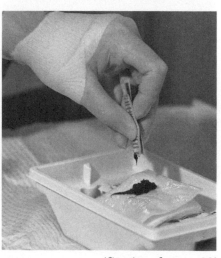

13 Squeeze the povidone–iodine ointment onto the nonadhering dressing pad.

(Continued on p. 30)

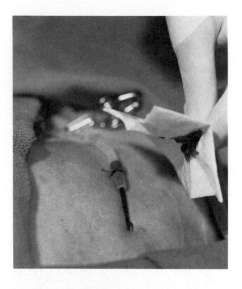

14 Place the ointment and pad directly over the insertion site. This will ensure added protection against bacterial and fungal growth.

15 Apply tincture of benzoin to the skin surrounding the nonadhering dressing. This will not only protect the skin from the tape, but it will also help ensure adherence of the dressing and minimize the potential for contamination. Allow the solution to dry.

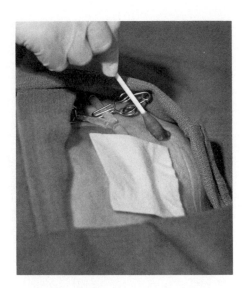

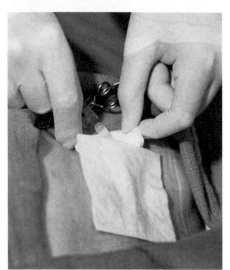

16 Some catheters will require support to prevent pressure on the skin and tissue surrounding the catheter hub. You can minimize the pressure, and hence the client's discomfort, by folding a sterile gauze pad and placing it under the hub to cushion it.

17 Trim the elastic bandage to fit the client's dressing, and make a slit to accommodate the catheter hub.

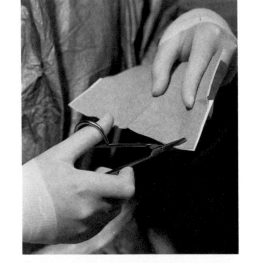

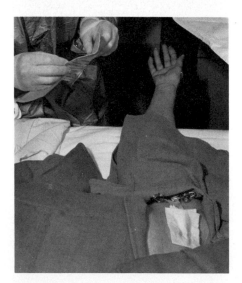

18 Before applying the bandage to the dressing, ask the client to abduct her arm. This will ensure full shoulder range of motion yet keep the tape's air-occlusive seal intact.

19 Remove the protective backing from one side of the elastic bandage and apply it to the dressing.

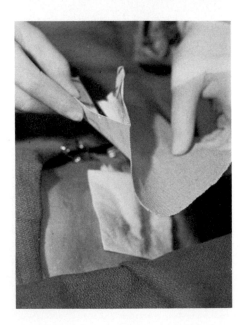

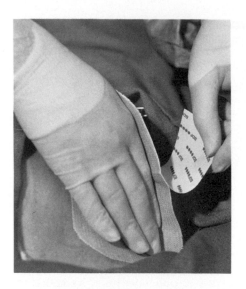

20 Remove the rest of the backing and adhere the bandage to the dressing and skin starting from the center and working outward.

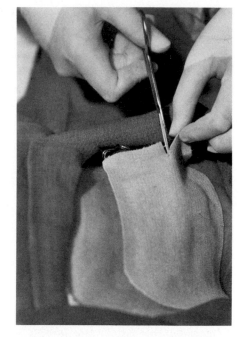

21 Trim the elastic bandage at the hub area more, if necessary, so that you can easily expose the hub. →

22 Adhere that section of the dressing to the skin.

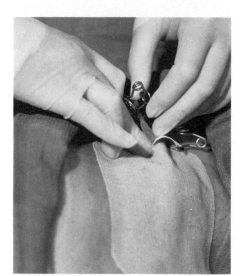

23 Remove your gloves, and tape around all four sides of the bandage with air-occlusive tape to make the dressing airtight. If your client is receiving an IV solution through the central catheter, change the tubing at this time, following the steps in Chapter 7. →

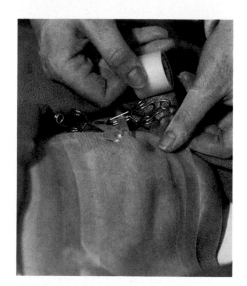

Evaluating

24 Initial and write the dates of both the catheter insertion and the dressing change on the label and adhere it to the dressing. Assist the client into a comfortable position. Remove the contaminated waste from the bedside and dispose of it according to agency policy; then wash your hands. Document the procedure in your nurse's notes, and record your assessment of the insertion site and the manner in which the client tolerated the procedure.

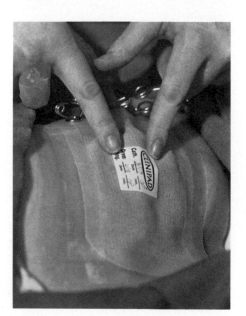

References

American Hospital Association. 1979. *Infection control in the hospital,* 4th ed. Chicago: The Association.

Association of Operating Room Nurses. 1978. *Standards of practice.* Denver, Colo.: The Association.

Bauman, B. Feb. 1982. Update your technique for changing dressings: wet to dry. *Nursing '82* 12:68–71.

Centers for Disease Control. 1981–1984. Guideline for hospital environmental control: antiseptics, handwashing, and handwashing facilities. In *Guidelines for the prevention and control of nosocomial infections.* Atlanta, Ga.: U.S. Department of Health and Human Services.

Centers for Disease Control. 1983. Guideline for isolation precautions in hospitals. In *Guidelines for prevention and control of nosocomial infections.* Atlanta, Ga.: U.S. Department of Health and Human Services.

Davis, J. et al. Dec. 1982. Sure-fire asepsis for your TPN patients. *RN* 45:39–41, 91.

Gruendemann, B. J., and Meeker, M. H. 1983. *Alexander's care of the patient in surgery,* 7th ed. St. Louis: C. V. Mosby.

Jackson, M. M., and Lynch, P. Feb. 1984. Infection control: too much or too little? *Am J Nurs* 84:208–210.

Kozier, B., and Erb, G. 1983. *Fundamentals of nursing,* 2nd ed. Menlo Park, Calif.: Addison-Wesley Publishing.

Nursing Photobook. 1981. *Controlling infection.* Horsham, Pa.: Intermed Communications.

Smith, S. F., and Duell, D. 1982. *Nursing skills and evaluation.* Los Altos, Calif.: National Nursing Review.

Sorensen, K. C., and Luckmann, J. 1979. *Basic nursing: a psychophysiologic approach.* Philadelphia: W. B. Saunders.

Soule, B. M. (editor). 1983. *The APIC curriculum for infection control practice.* Dubuque, Iowa: Kendall/Hunt Publishing.

Chapter 2

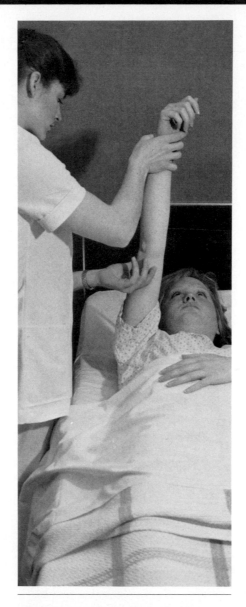

Using Proper Positioning, Mobilization, and Transferring Techniques

CHAPTER OUTLINE

ASSISTING THE CLIENT WITH POSITIONING AND MOBILIZATION

Performing Passive Range of Motion Exercises
  Performing traditional ROM exercises
  Performing proprioceptive neuromuscular facilitation exercises

Nursing Guidelines for Using Pressure-Relief Mattresses and Pads
  Sheepskin
  Eggcrate mattress
  Flotation pad
  Air mattress
  Lapidus airfloat system

Nursing Guidelines for Proper Client Positioning
  Supine
  Side-lying
  Prone
  Positioning aids

Assisting the Client with Crutches, Canes, and Walkers
  Checking for correct crutch height
  Guarding the client
  Assisting the client with crutches to sit in a chair

TRANSFERRING MOBILE AND IMMOBILE CLIENTS

Nursing Guidelines for Lifting and Transferring Clients

Moving the Client Up in Bed
  Assisting the mobile client
  Lifting the immobile client

Dangling the Client's Extremities on the Side of the Bed
  Assisting the mobile client
  Moving the immobile client

Moving the Client from the Stretcher to the Bed
  Teaching the segmental transfer technique
  Transferring the immobile client

Logrolling the Immobile Client

Assisting the Client from the Wheelchair (or Chair) to the Bed

Using a Mechanical Lifting Device

Assisting the Client with Positioning and Mobilization

PERFORMING PASSIVE RANGE OF MOTION EXERCISES

To prevent contractures (the shortening of soft tissues/muscles, ligaments, joint capsules, or fasciae) and ankylosis (the abnormal consolidation of a joint), nurses must ensure that range of motion (ROM) exercises are performed every day for all immobilized clients with *normal* joints. Modification may be necessary if the client has decreased tone (flaccidity), which is seen initially following spinal cord injury or cerebrovascular accident; if ROM is done incorrectly, the potential for subluxation increases. In addition, if the client has increased tone (spasticity), which may develop as the recovery sequence progresses in either of the above disorders, the use of routine exercise positions may actually enhance spasticity. If you lack experience with these disorders, consult with the physician, physical therapist, or occupational therapist to assist you in modifying the exercise plan for these clients. ROM is contraindicated during the inflammatory phase of rheumatologic diseases and for joints that are dislocated or fractured. However, after assessment of the client, the need for initiation of ROM is an independent nursing judgment, and it should be incorporated into the daily care plan of the immobilized client. Many of the movement patterns can be performed concurrent with position changes and bed baths. In addition, the principles of ROM can be applied when getting a client on and off the bed pan or while changing the hospital gown.

Before initiating ROM, familiarize yourself with the following terms:

- *Passive Range of Motion:* These exercises are performed by the nurse, therapist, or significant other to help the client maintain full joint movement and to prevent contractures. Because the client's muscles are not utilized to perform the exercise, muscle strength is neither maintained nor augmented.
- *Active Range of Motion:* These exercises are performed by the client, helping to maintain full joint movement. They also assist in the maintenance of muscle strength.
- *Assisted Range of Motion:* The client moves the part through some portion of the range of motion, with the nurse, therapist, or significant other assisting in completing the movement. The degree of the client's participation in the exercise will determine the degree to which the muscle strength will be maintained.
- *Abduction:* Moving a limb away from the body's midline
- *Adduction:* Moving a limb toward the body's midline
- *Extension:* Straightening of a bent part (increasing the angle between two bones at a joint)
- *Flexion:* Bending (decreasing the angle of two bones at a joint)
- *Hyperextension:* Moving a body part beyond the plane of the body
- *Opposition:* Combination of abduction, rotation, and flexion of the thumb so that the tip of the thumb can touch the fingers
- *Radial Deviation:* Moving the hand toward the radial (thumb) side of the wrist while the hand and forearm stay in the same plane
- *Ulnar Deviation:* Moving the hand toward the ulnar (fifth-finger) side of the wrist while the hand and forearm stay in the same plane
- *Rotation:* Turning of a body part on its vertical axis

Performing Traditional ROM Exercises

The exercises in the following procedures are passive and employed when the client is unable to move the specified body part. Adapt these exercises for situations in which the client has partial body movement and requires assisted ROM. When active ROM is desired, you can teach these exercises to the client. You may also teach these exercises to clients who are capable of exercising their paralyzed sides with the assistance of their stronger sides. Remember to include family members and significant others so that they, too, can help exercise the client.

Before starting the exercises, explain them to the client, and obtain a sheet or bath blanket for warmth and privacy. Remove the pillow to allow full movement of the client's head and shoulders.

Unless it is contraindicated, assist the client into a supine position. Perform the exercises from head to toe, completing them on one side of the body before moving to the other side of the body. Then assist the client into a prone position and perform the exercises that are indicated for that position. Never push a movement beyond the point at which the client complains of discomfort or at which you feel resistance to the movement. If possible, consult with a physical therapist or occupational therapist to assist you with modifying the exercise on a joint in which you have elicited pain, tremors, or spasms. To avoid straining your back, elevate the bed to an optimal working level; move the client to the right side of the bed before exercising the right side of the body (and vice versa). Be sure to allow room at the head of the bed for the neck and arm movements. To assist you with proper hand positioning, we have shown the neutral (start) position for the exercises. For convenience, all the exercises have been demonstrated on the right side of the client's body. Be certain that you practice correct body mechanics when performing all exercises. Repeat each exercise at least three to five times.

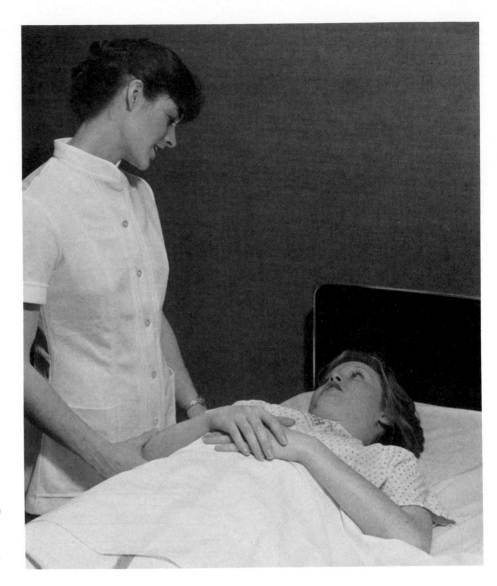

Exercising the Neck

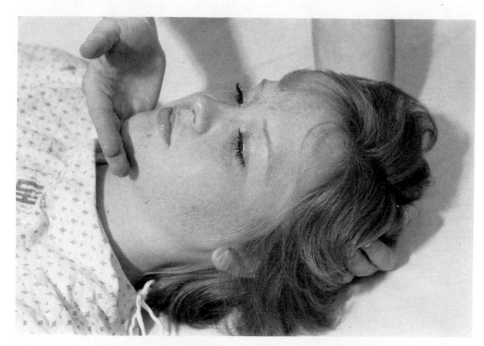

1 To begin the neck exercises, cup the client's chin with your right hand and support the back of the head with your left hand. Be sure to position your right hand high enough on the chin to avoid putting pressure on the trachea during the flexion exercises. *Caution: Do not force any of the neck movements.*

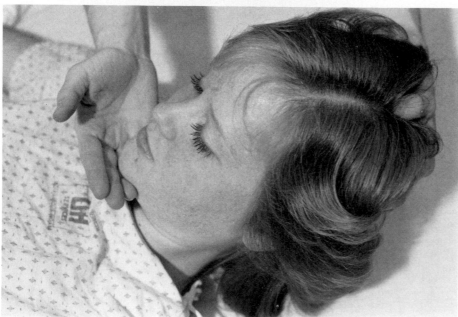

2 To flex the neck, gently tilt the back of the head forward and move the chin toward the chest, touching it if possible.

(Continued on p. 38)

3 Extend the neck by gently tilting the chin upward and moving the head back as far as it will comfortably go without forcing the movement. Return to the neutral position.

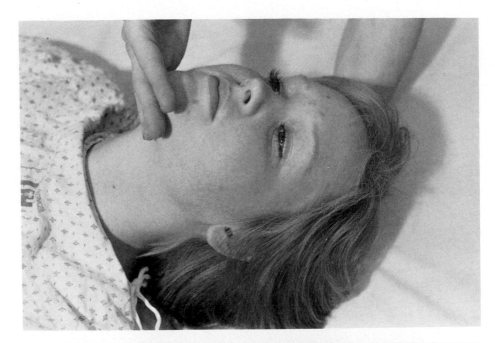

4 To rotate the neck, slowly and gently turn the head to the left (as shown), and touch the left ear to the mattress, if possible. Then rotate the neck to the right in the same manner.

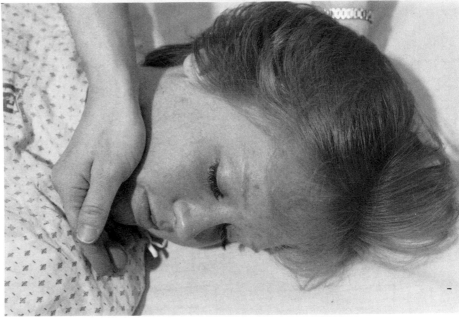

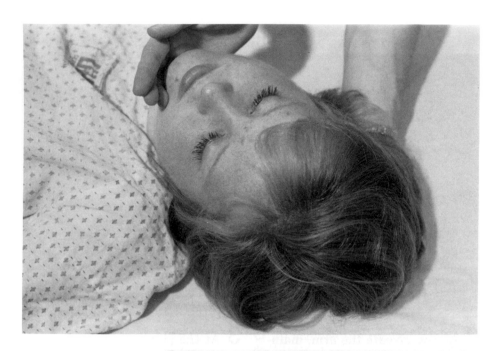

5 To laterally flex the neck, gently guide the ear toward the left shoulder keeping the client's nose pointing toward the ceiling (as shown); then guide the ear toward the right shoulder.

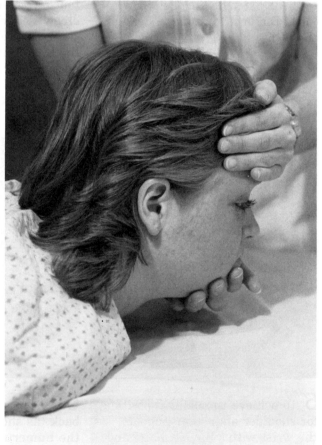

6 When the client is prone, you may extend the neck by supporting the chin with your right hand and gently pushing back on the forehead with your left hand. Move the back of the head toward the spine as far as it will *comfortably go without forcing the movement.*

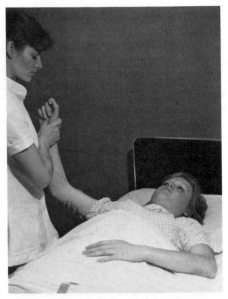

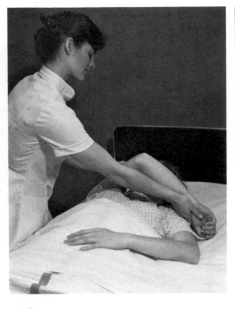

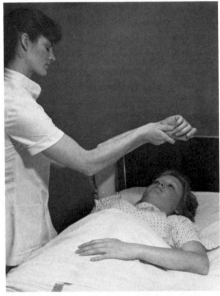

Exercising the Elbows

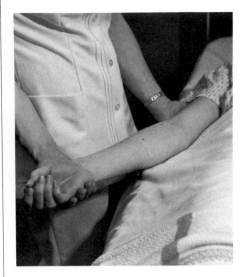

12 To complete the horizontal adduction, move the arm as far across the body as possible. Allow the elbow to extend slightly so that the contact of the hand with the bed does not block the motion of the humerus.

11 To achieve the neutral position for horizontal shoulder adduction, support the upper arm with your left hand and the hand and wrist with your right hand (top). Hold the arm with the elbow flexed at a 45°–90° angle to the body. Slowly guide the arm across the body toward the left side of the bed (bottom).

1 To achieve the neutral position for flexing the elbow with the forearm in supination, support the wrist with your right hand and the upper arm with your left hand. The arm should be slightly abducted from the body with the elbow extended and the palm turned up.

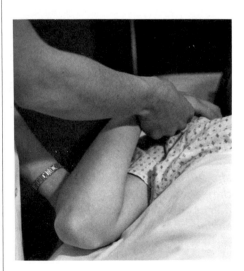

2 Guide the palm toward the shoulder. The degree of elbow flexion will be determined by the amount of upper arm musculature. (The greater the musculature, the less the degree of flexion.) Return to the neutral position while maintaining support of the upper arm and wrist.

Exercising the Wrists and Fingers

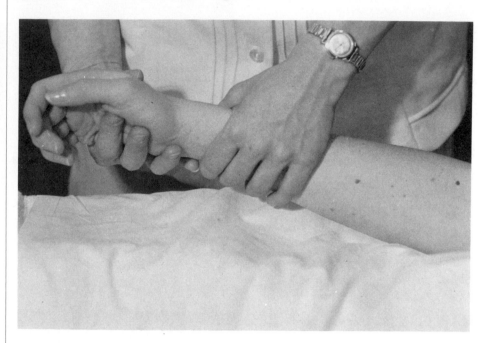

1 To achieve the neutral position for wrist flexion and extension, support the forearm proximal to the wrist with your left hand. Support the hand distal to the wrist with your right hand.

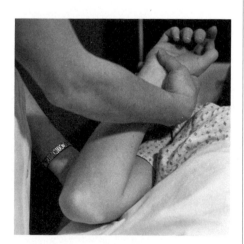

3 To achieve the neutral position for flexing the elbow with the forearm in pronation, support the wrist with your right hand and the upper arm with your left hand. The arm should be slightly abducted from the body with the elbow extended and the palm turned down.

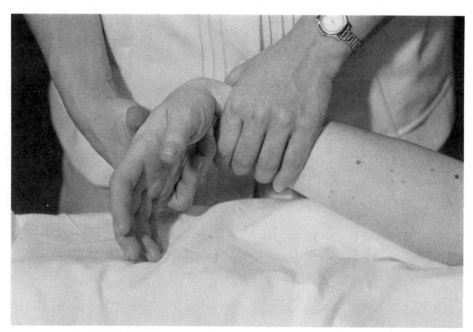

2 To flex the wrist (palmarflexion), gently push down on the dorsum of the hand.

4 Flex the elbow and guide the dorsum of the hand toward the shoulder. Again, the degree of elbow flexion will be determined by the amount of upper arm musculature. Return to the neutral position. Alternating flexion with supination and flexion with pronation allows you to perform the elbow and forearm movements simultaneously.

(Continued on p. 44)

3 Extend the wrist (dorsiflexion) by gently pushing up on the palmar surface of the hand.

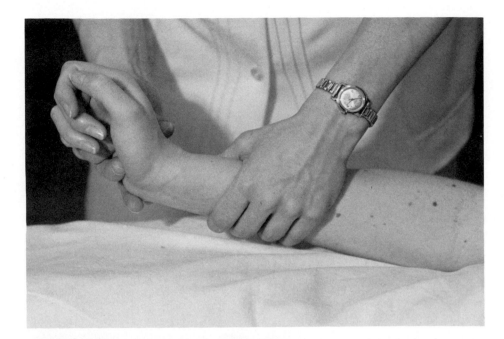

4 To achieve the neutral position for radial and ulnar deviation, support the hand with your right hand and the wrist with your left hand. The hand and wrist should be in the same plane.

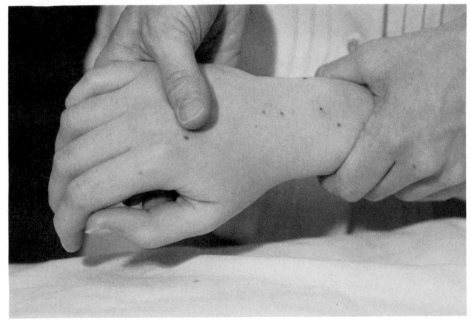

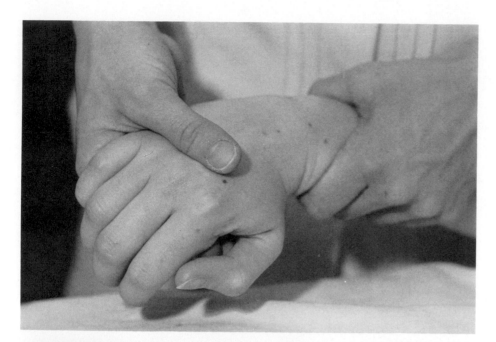

5 For radial deviation, gently guide the thumb side of the hand toward the wrist.

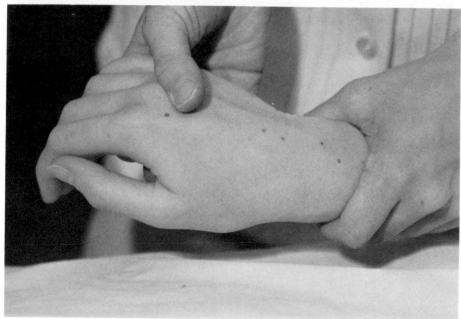

6 Gently guide the fifth-finger side of the hand toward the wrist for ulnar deviation.

(Continued on p. 46)

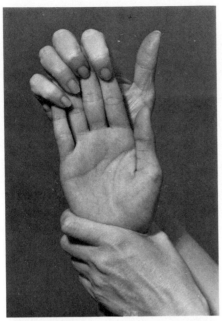

7 Extend the fingers by gently straightening them with your right hand while you support the wrist with your left hand. Do not pull the fingers beyond the plane of the hand.

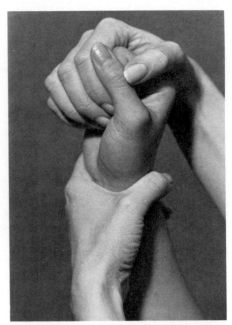

8 Flex the fingers by gently curling them with your fingers.   →

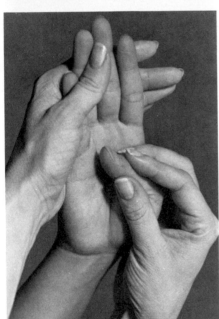

9 With the fingers extended, oppose the thumb to the base of the fifth finger.

10 Extend the thumb.   →

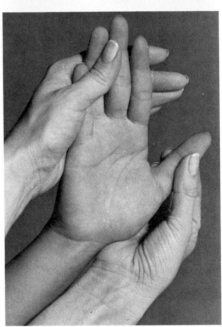

Exercising the Hips and Knees

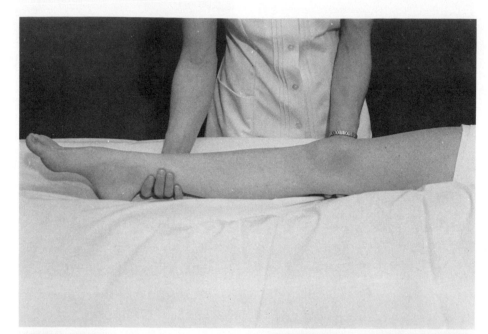

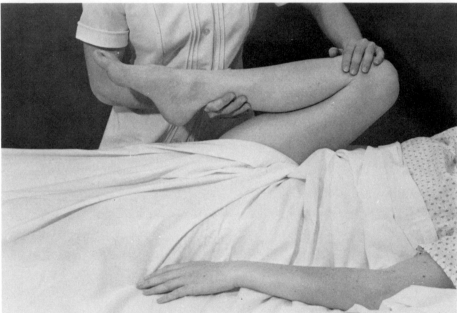

1 To achieve the neutral position for hip and knee flexion and extension, place your left hand under the knee and your right hand under the ankle (as shown). Lift the leg so that it bends at the hip and knee, and move the thigh as close to the trunk as possible (bottom). To avoid blocking the flexion at the knee, place your left hand on top of the knee as you complete the above movement.

(Continued on p. 48)

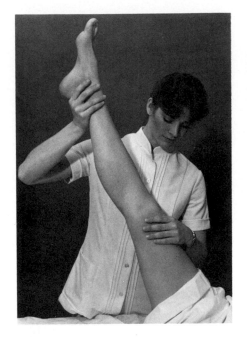

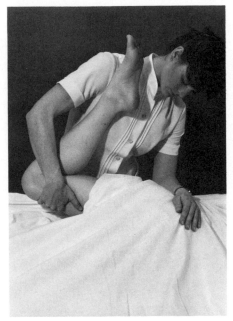

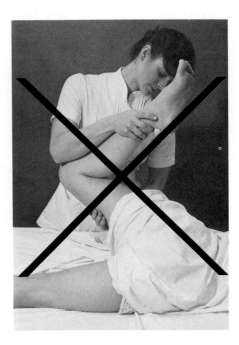

2 To flex the hip with the knee extended, return to the neutral position. Then gently lift up on the ankle with your right hand while keeping the knee straight with your left hand. You have reached the client's full range when you feel the knee begin to bend or when the client complains of a pulling sensation in the back of the knee.

3 When the client is prone, you may extend the hip while flexing the knee. To do this, stabilize the pelvis with your left hand and support the anterior thigh with your right hand. Lift gently on the anterior thigh, no more than 7.5–12.5 cm (3–5 in.), depending on the client's range.

Note: This photo depicts incorrect hip extension. The movement is occurring in the lumbar joints because the nurse is lifting the thigh too high.

4 To achieve the neutral position for internal and external rotation of the hip with the hip and knee extended, support the ankle with your right hand and place your left hand proximal to the knee. The knee should point toward the ceiling.

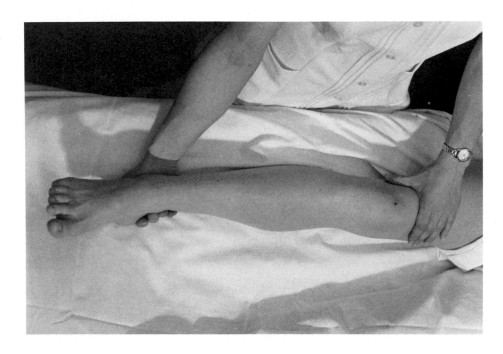

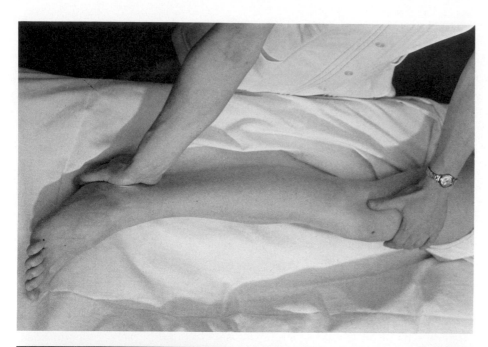

5 To internally rotate the hip, gently turn the leg toward the midline of the client's body.

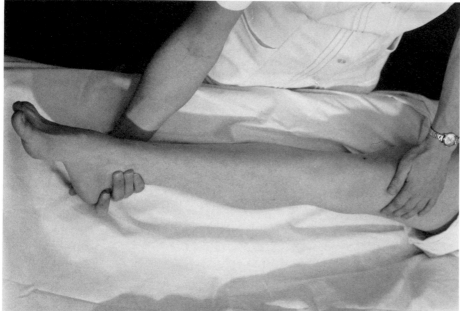

6 Turn the leg toward yourself (laterally) for external rotation.

(Continued on p. 50)

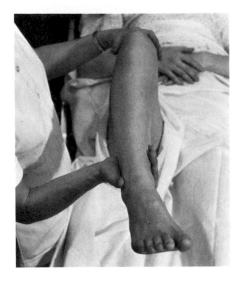

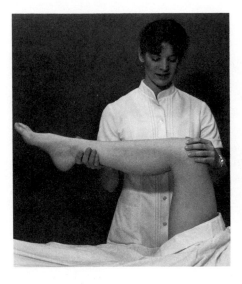

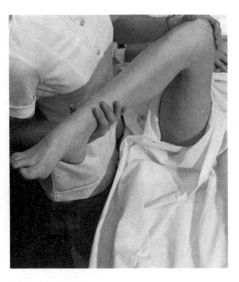

7 This photo depicts the neutral position for internal and external rotation of the hip with the hip and knee flexed. Position the femur at a 90° angle to the body

(see above), and flex the knee at a 90° angle to the femur. Place your left hand on the knee, and support the ankle with your right hand.

8 To externally rotate the hip, gently guide the client's foot toward yourself. Remember to keep the knee and dorsum of the foot pointing toward the ceiling to ensure that you do not change the vertical position of the femur.

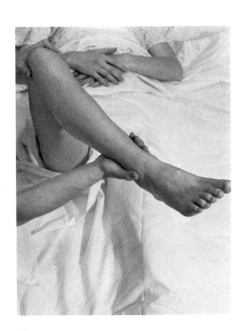

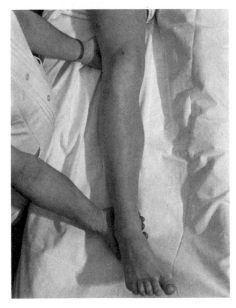

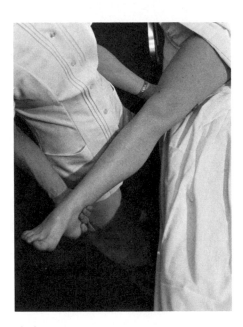

9 To internally rotate the hip, guide the foot toward the client's midline.

10 This photo depicts the neutral position for hip abduction and adduction. Position your left hand under the knee and your right hand under the ankle.

11 To abduct the hip, simultaneously move the leg off the bed as you step back with your right foot and pivot onto your left foot. Keep the client's toes and knee pointing toward the ceiling as you move the leg. Then, adduct the hip by returning the leg to the midline.

Exercising the Ankles and Toes

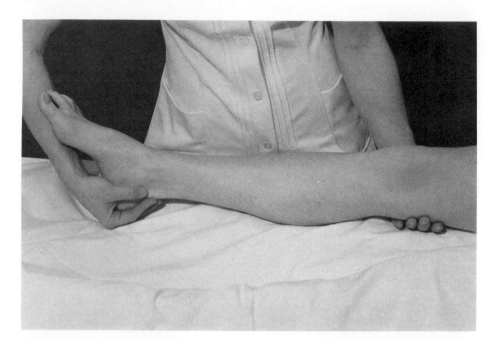

1 To achieve the neutral position for ankle dorsiflexion, place your left hand under the knee and cradle the foot with your right hand and forearm.

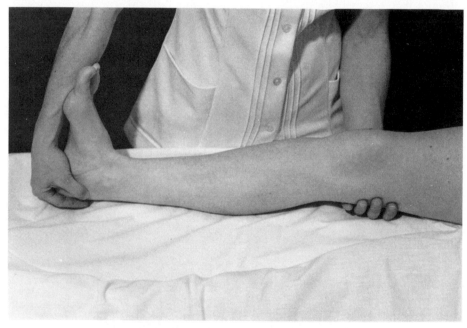

2 To dorsiflex the ankle, shift your weight onto your left leg and push against the ball of the client's foot with your right forearm. As you do this, pull the heel in the opposite direction with your right hand.

(Continued on p. 52)

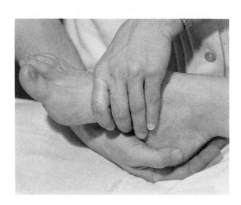

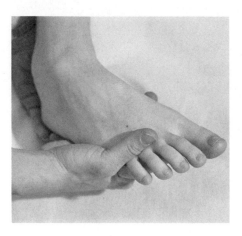

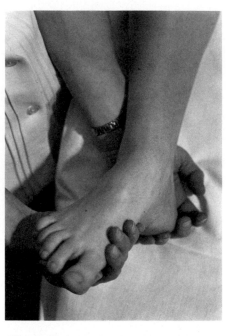

3 It is seldom necessary to plantarflex the ankles because in bed, feet posture naturally in this position. However, if the client can pull the toes up but can not push them down, you must also plantarflex the ankles. To do this, cradle the heel with your right hand and press gently on the dorsum of the foot with your right hand.

4 To invert the ankle, turn the client's foot toward the midline without changing the position of the heel.

5 Evert the ankle by turning the foot laterally toward yourself. Normally, your client will have more range with inversion than with eversion.

6 To extend the toes, support the forefoot with your left hand and gently guide the toes toward the dorsum of the foot with your right hand.

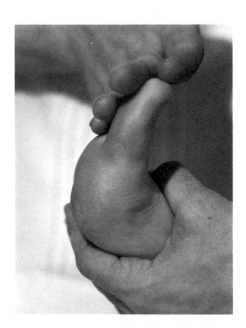

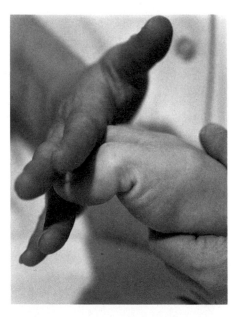

7 Flex the toes by bending them toward the sole of the foot with your opened fingers.

Performing Proprioceptive Neuromuscular Facilitation Exercises

The movement patterns described below provide an alternative to the traditional passive ROM exercises. Their advantage over the latter is that they combine movements at several joints simultaneously thereby reducing the amount of time necessary to complete the series. To achieve this end, each exercise is performed on the diagonal. For example, one movement pattern (diagonal) for the upper extremities combines components of flexion, abduction, and external rotation of the shoulder. To help you understand both the movement components occurring at each joint and the correct hand positioning for the involved joints, review the steps for the traditional ROM exercises. Consult with your agency's occupational or physical therapist for added information if these exercises are new to you.

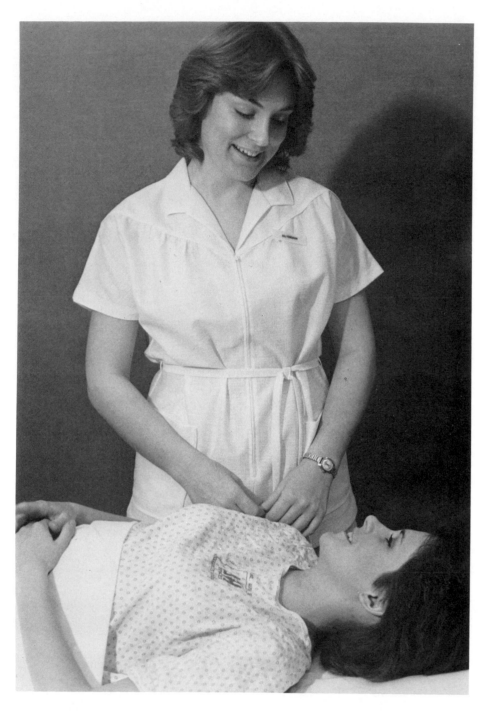

Explain the exercises to your client, and provide a drape for warmth and privacy. Elevate the bed to an optimal working level, and then remove the pillow and position the client so that she is flat on her back. If you will exercise her right side first, move her to the right side of the bed. Never push the movement beyond the client's range; and modify the exercise on a joint in which you elicit pain, spasms, or tremors. Remember to use proper body mechanics. Repeat each movement three to five times.

Exercising the Neck

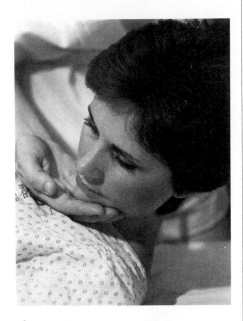

1 For the first diagonal movement, position the client's head so that her neck is flexed and rotated to the left, as if she were looking down at her left elbow.

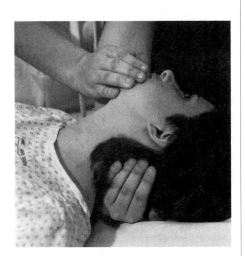

2 Extend the neck while you rotate it to the right, so that she is looking up and over her right shoulder. The second diagonal is the direct opposite of the first. Position the client so that the neck is flexed and rotated to the right, as if she were looking at her right elbow. Extend her neck while rotating it to the left, so that she is looking up and over her left shoulder.

Exercising the Upper Extremities

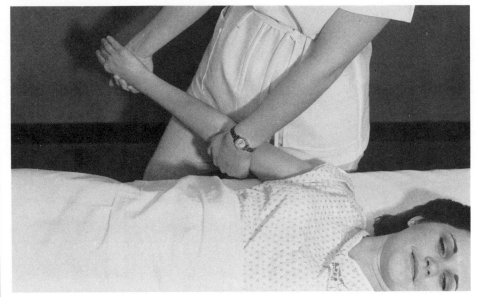

1 To perform the Diagonal-One (D-1) movements, start with the arm extended, abducted, and internally rotated at the shoulder so that the client's thumb points toward the floor. If you are exercising the right upper extremity, your right hand will guide the movement of the client's hand while your left hand will support and guide the movement of the humerus.

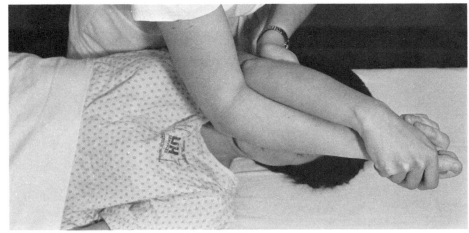

2 Move the arm diagonally up and across her nose as if she were reaching for the opposite corner of the bed. This movement results in shoulder flexion, adduction, and external rotation with the elbow extended.

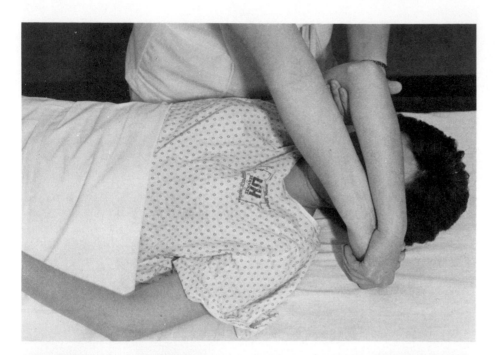

3 Return to the start position for D-1, and perform the same shoulder movements, but allow the elbow to flex as the shoulder flexes.

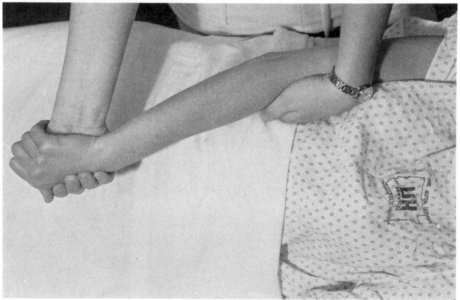

4 For Diagonal-Two (D-2) movements, start with the arm extended, adducted, and internally rotated at the shoulder. The client's thumb should be resting against her left anterior iliac crest.

(Continued on p. 56)

5 Lift the arm up and across the client's body so that her hand points toward the opposite corner of the room and the thumb points downward. This completed diagonal flexes, abducts, and externally rotates the shoulder with the elbow extended.

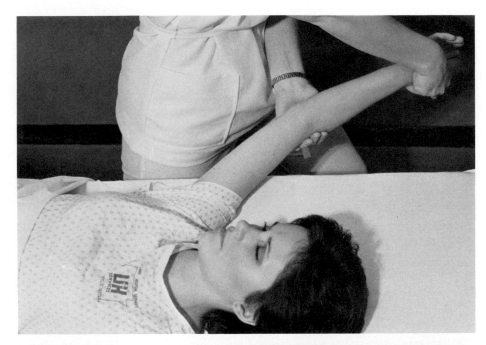

6 Return to the start position for D-2 and perform the same shoulder movements, but this time allow the elbow to flex as you flex the shoulder.

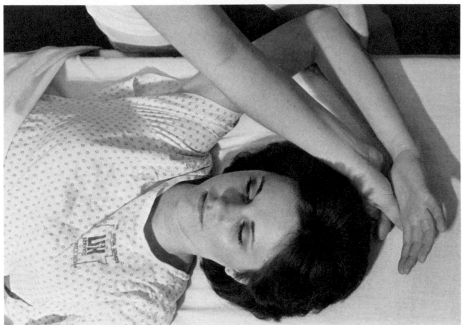

Exercising the Lower Extremities

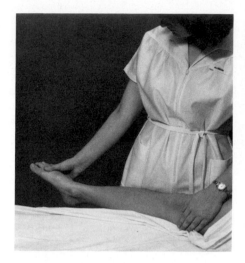

1 To perform D-1 movements, start with the hip extended, abducted, and internally rotated. The knee should be extended and the ankle plantarflexed (as shown). Your right hand will support and guide the movement of the lower leg while your left hand will guide the movement of the thigh.

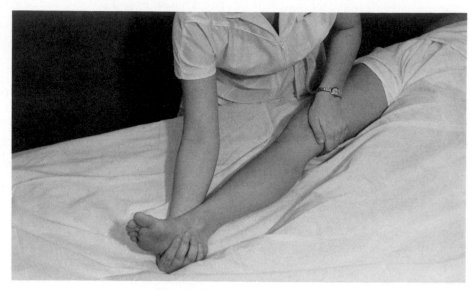

3 For D-2 movements, start with the client's hip extended, adducted, and externally rotated with the knee extended and the foot plantarflexed.

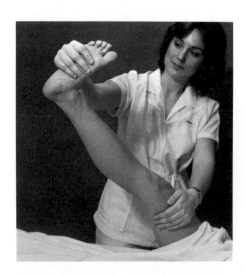

2 Lift up on the leg and move it along the diagonal into a position of hip flexion, adduction, and external rotation with the ankle moving into dorsiflexion and inversion. The completed diagonal is similar to a soccer kick in which the ball is kicked with the inner aspect of the foot. Return to the start position.

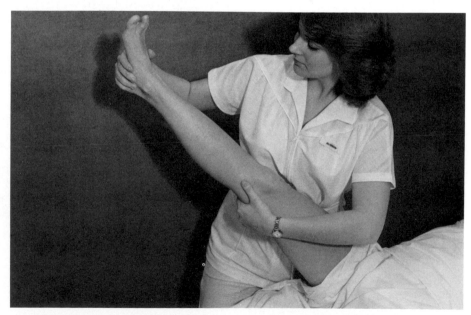

4 Move into a position in which the client's hip is flexed, abducted, and internally rotated with the knee extended and the foot moving into dorsiflexion. This diagonal can be compared to kicking a ball with the outer aspect of the foot. Return to the start position. Now assist the client to the left side of the bed and perform the exercises on her left side. *Note: Knee flexion also can be performed along with the hip flexion patterns, or it can be done separately.*

Nursing Guidelines for Using Pressure-Relief Mattresses and Pads

Sheepskin

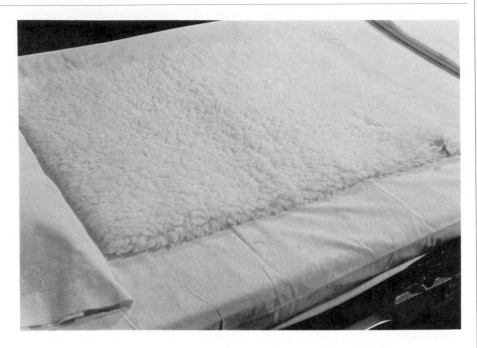

Use

The cushionlike fibers pad the body to distribute the pressure around the bony prominences and minimize the potential for skin breakdown. The sheepskin also improves air circulation and enhances the drying of perspiration to prevent skin maceration, potentially caused by continued exposure to moisture.

Nursing Considerations

- Change the pad whenever it becomes wet or soiled. Larger pads are impractical for the incontinent client. For incontinent clients, consider the use of smaller pads placed under heels or shoulders.
- Because the client buys the sheepskin, make sure it is properly labeled prior to each laundering.
- Pads made from synthetic fabrics launder better than natural sheepskin.
- Place the pad on top of the bottom sheet so that it has immediate contact with the client's skin.

Eggcrate Mattress

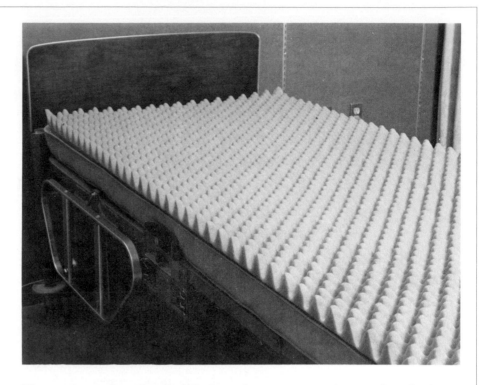

Use

The corrugated surface minimizes the pressure points under the bony prominences. In addition, it promotes better air circulation to help prevent skin breakdown.

Nursing Considerations

- To keep the bottom sheet taut and wrinkle-free, knot each corner (see below).
- If the client is diaphoretic, consider using a thin bath blanket rather than a bottom sheet.
- If the mattress becomes soiled, wash the soiled area with soap and water. Let it dry thoroughly before replacing it on the client's bed.

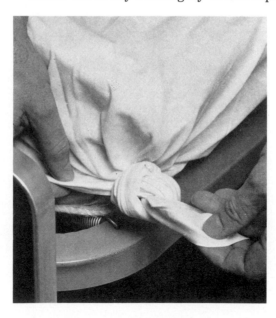

(Continued on p. 60)

Flotation Pad

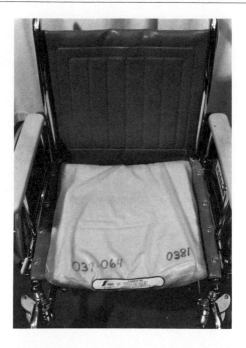

Use

The gel-like inner substance molds to the client's body to help minimize pressure over the bony prominences. The smaller pad (as shown) fits in a chair or wheelchair.

Nursing Considerations

- Keep pins, needles, and other sharp objects away from the pad.
- Cover the pad with nothing thicker than a sheet or pillow case so that you do not diminish its effectiveness.
- The pad's plastic outer surface may promote increased perspiration that could lead to skin maceration. Inspect the client's skin frequently.

Air Mattress

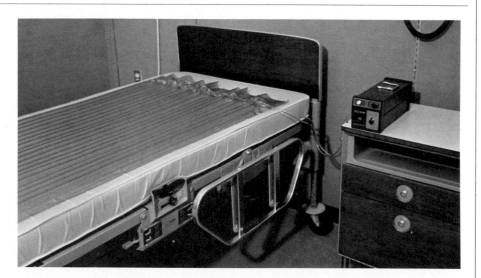

Use

The air in the mattress displaces the client's weight and minimizes the pressure over the bony prominences.

Nursing Considerations

- To ensure adequate mattress inflation, indent the plastic surface with your fingertip. Adjust the pressure if you can indent more or less than 1.25 cm (½ in.). Remember that underinflation can promote hip flexion contractures and protraction of the shoulder girdle, and overinflation may cause pressure to the bony prominences.
- To prevent damage to the mattress, keep needles, pins, and other sharp objects away from its surface.
- The noise of the machine may become a sensory problem, especially for neurologic clients.
- Unless the manufacturer provides a sponge pad for covering the mattress, keep only a bottom sheet or a thin bath blanket between the client and the mattress.
- Keep the electrical cord out of the path of the client and agency personnel.
- Some units provide alternating pressure, which also enhances peripheral circulation while relieving pressure.
- Even though immobilized clients on these mattresses may require fewer position changes, it is important that ROM exercises are continued to prevent contractures and ankylosis.
- Assess the client's skin for increased perspiration and potential maceration caused by the plastic surface of the mattress.

Lapidus Airfloat System

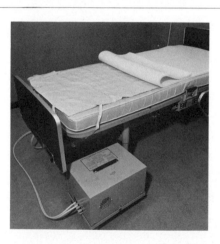

Use

This mattress changes its pressure points over the body every 15 seconds, aerates the skin through tiny air holes in the mattress, and rapidly circulates air in a wavelike fashion. These features prevent decubiti, absorb perspiration thereby preventing skin maceration, and stimulate peripheral circulation.

Nursing Considerations

- Always use the system with its 2.5 cm (1 in.) foam pad that absorbs moisture. The foam pad dries spontaneously by means of the circulating air flow underneath it.
- A 50 × 50 cm (20 × 20 in.) pad can connect to the same power supply for use on a wheelchair or chair.
- Keep the power box and electric cord out of the path of the client and agency personnel.

Nursing Guidelines for Proper Client Positioning

In addition to ROM exercises, meticulous skin care, and frequent turning, the immobilized client also requires carefully planned positioning to prevent the complications of prolonged bed rest. Proper positioning will minimize pressure to the bony prominences, maintain correct body alignment to reduce stress and strain to the joints, ensure maximal chest expansion for proper breathing, and prevent the formation of contractures.

For most clients a good rule of thumb for positioning in bed is to try to achieve the proper standing alignment. The head should therefore be neutral or slightly flexed on the neck, the hips should be extended, the knees extended or minimally flexed, and the feet should be at 90° angles to the legs. If pillows are unavailable for maintaining your client's position, consider substituting blankets, towels, or spreads. Review the following general procedures to assist you in positioning immobile clients.

Supine

Lower Body

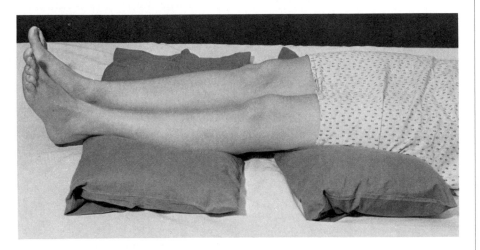

- To take pressure off the lower back, slightly flex the client's hips by placing a thin pillow under the thighs. The pillow should not extend into the popliteal area, nor should it be placed directly under the knees because it could occlude the popliteal arteries.
- To prevent hip flexion contractures, ensure that the client is side-lying or prone with the hips extended for the approximate amount of time she is supine.
- Placing a pillow under the thighs is contraindicated for clients with inflammatory joint diseases because they have a tendency to posture in flexion due to pain. It is important that you attempt to maintain their hips and knees in extension with every position change.
- Place a thin pillow under the client's ankles and lower legs to keep the heels off the bed's surface thereby preventing pressure. As an alternative, use sheepskin or heel protectors; or, if possible, use a pressure-relief mattress or pad.

Upper Body

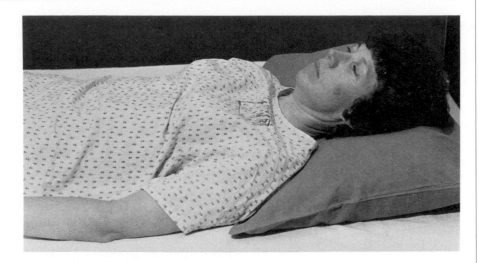

Unless a flat position is required (for example, for neck pain or neck injury), support the client's head and shoulders with a small pillow so that the head is neutral or slightly flexed on the neck.

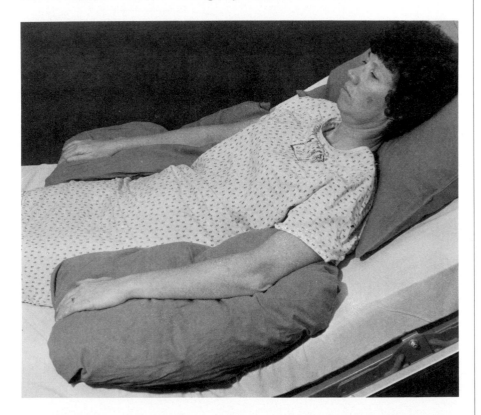

Semi-Fowler's position (30° head elevation) When the head must be elevated, extend the shoulders and support the arms on each side of the body with pillows. Allow the fingertips to extend over the edges of the pillows to maintain the normal arching of the hands. Because this position places the client in hip flexion, ensure that alternate positions, with the client's hips in extension, are also used.

(Continued on p. 64)

Side-Lying

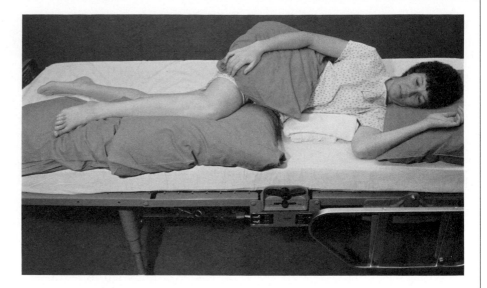

- Ensure that the client's spinal column is in straight alignment from the head to the coccyx.
- Place a pillow under the head to maintain its normal alignment with the body. The pillow should be just thick enough to accommodate the space between the bed and the head.
- For curvaceous clients, a pad positioned between the iliac crest and the axilla will help to maintain proper spine alignment. It should be thick enough to prevent the vertebral column from sagging into the bed and wide enough so that the pressure it may potentially produce in the soft tissues can be evenly distributed over the entire rib cage.
- Place a pillow under the upper arm to prevent shoulder adduction and internal rotation. To ensure optimal chest expansion for proper breathing, the weight of the upper arm and pillow should be centered over the pelvis rather than over the rib cage.
- The upper leg should be flexed at the hip and knee and supported by a thick pillow to prevent both internal rotation and adduction of the hip and pressure to the patella. Ensure that the thigh is well supported and that the pillow does not touch the lower leg.
- If necessary, place a second pillow under the upper foot to prevent its inversion and to maintain its alignment with the rest of the leg.
- This is an optimal time to position the lower leg in extension from the hip. You may slightly flex the knee for the client's comfort.
- It may be necessary to support the client's position by placing a pillow behind the back.

Prone

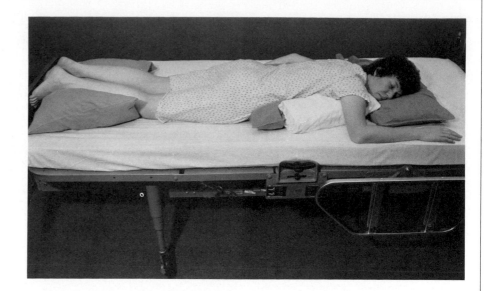

Caution: This position is contraindicated for clients with tracheostomies, cervical injuries, or breathing difficulties.

- Turn the client's head to the side and place a flat pillow under the head and shoulders to prevent hyperextension of the neck.
- Place thin pads under the angles of the axillae and the lateral aspects of the clavicles. This will prevent internal rotation of the shoulders, maintain the anatomic position of the shoulder girdle, and promote optimal chest expansion for breathing.
- Position one arm so that it is flexed at the shoulder and elbow and the other arm so that it is extended from the shoulder with the palm flat on the bed. Periodically reposition the arms to prevent joint stiffness.
- Place a flat pillow (the darker pillow in the photo) under the waist-line so that it cushions the anterior superior iliac spines and prevents pressure to the area. It will also minimize strain to the lower back, promote chest expansion, allow room for breast tissue, and prevent a lordotic posture (swayback).
- To minimally flex the knees, position a thin pillow under the lower legs. This will minimize pressure to the patellae and keep the toes off the mattress as well. Be certain that the toes clear the pillow.
- To prevent plantarflexion and hip rotation and to prevent injury to the toes and heels, move the client to the end of the bed to allow her feet to recline between the edge of the mattress and the footboard. Position the feet so that they are as close to a 90° angle from the legs as possible.

Positioning Aids

Trochanter Rolls

To prevent abduction and external rotation of the hip, position the client on a large towel or bath blanket that has been folded so that it extends from the client's waist to the midthigh (below left). The material should drape equally on either side of the body. Turn the fabric as the nurse is doing in the photo (below right) so that the roll is undermost.

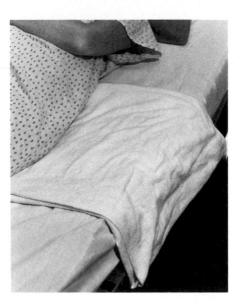
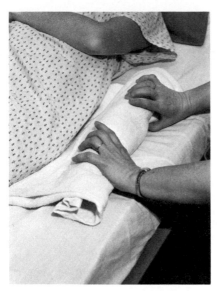

Tuck the roll tightly against the client's hips, and do the same on the opposite side. Ensure that the lower legs and feet internally rotate toward the client's midline.

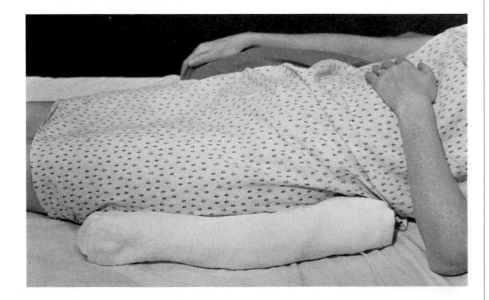

Sand Bags

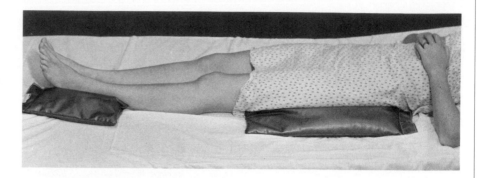

Sand bags are another positioning aid that prevent abduction and external rotation of the hips. Although smaller clients might be properly supported by placing only the larger sand bags at the hip area, bigger or more flaccid clients requiring added support will benefit from two sets of sand bags (as shown). Place the larger bags from the waist to the midthighs and the smaller bags along the lower legs. The bags are positioned correctly if the legs and feet are internally rotated toward the midline. For client comfort, wrap the sand bags with pillow cases or towels.

Foot Supports

Caution: Foot supports might be contraindicated for clients who are hypertonic (spastic), for example those with head injuries, multiple sclerosis, or in the spastic recovery phase of a cerebrovascular accident. Experts contend that the contact of the foot's surface on the board may actually trigger spasticity and hence reinforce plantarflexion (Farber 1982:172). Your spastic clients might benefit instead from foot cradles, which keep bed linen off their feet, or from more frequent ROM exercises. Another option is to cut off a pair of high-top tennis shoes so that each shoe ends just proximal to the head of the client's metatarsals. These shoes will maintain dorsiflexion, yet prevent contact of the balls of the feet with a hard surface. However, clients without spasticity usually are helped with foot supports such as the device in the photo. This foot support not only prevents plantarflexion, but prevents external rotation of the hips as well. Pad these devices with fleece, a blanket, or a towel to prevent the formation of decubiti on the soles of the feet.

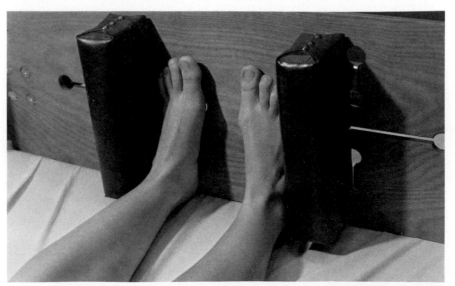

(Continued on p. 68)

Hand Rolls

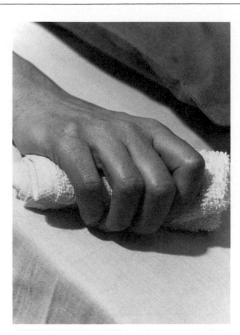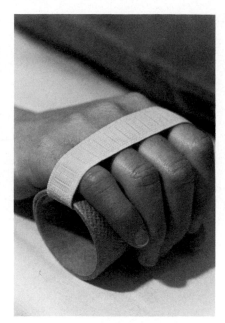

Hypotonic (flaccid) clients (for example, those with spinal cord injuries) may benefit from positioning devices such as a rolled washcloth (above left) placed within their grasp. This will place the hand, wrist, and fingers in a position that maintains a functional grasp. The thumb is positioned so that it opposes the tip of the index finger. Spastic clients, on the other hand, may require the firm surface of a splint or a cone (above right). The hard surface of these devices presses on the muscles to inhibit spasticity (Farber 1982:152). In addition, the elastic band that secures the cone to the hand stimulates the extensor muscles, thus encouraging finger extension.

ASSISTING THE CLIENT WITH CRUTCHES, CANES, AND WALKERS

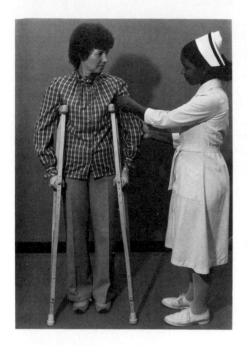

Checking for Correct Crutch Height

Before assisting your client with crutch walking, it is important to ensure that the crutches are the correct height. With the client's elbows flexed 20°–30°, the shoulders in a relaxed position, and the crutches placed approximately 15 cm (6 in.) anterolateral from the toes, you should be able to place two fingers comfortably between the axillae and the axillary bars (as shown). Adjust the crutches if you find either too much or too little space at the axillary area. Advise the client never to rest the axillae on the axillary bars because this could injure the brachial plexus (the nerves in the axillae that supply the arm and shoulder area). Terminate ambulation and recheck the crutch height if the client complains of numbness or tingling in the hands or arms.

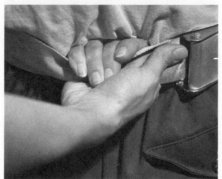

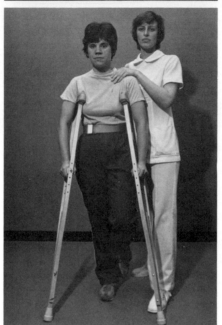

Canes: If your client is walking with a cane, stand at the affected side and guard her by grasping the security belt and positioning your free hand at the shoulder area. This is the same stance used in crutch walking. Remind the client to place the cane on the unaffected side so that the cane and the weaker leg can work together with each step. The top of the cane should reach the level of the greater trochanter of the client's femur.

Guarding the Client

Note: For your client's safety, always inspect the rubber tips of the assistive device to make sure they are not worn; also ensure that the client wears appropriate shoes with nonslip soles.

Crutches: When walking with clients who are using crutches, stand on the affected side and grasp the security belt in the midspine area at the small of the back (top center). Position your free hand at the shoulder area so that you can pull the client toward you in the event that there is a fall forward. Make sure, however, that you do not obstruct the movement of the humerus. Instruct the client to look up and outward toward the destination rather than at her feet.

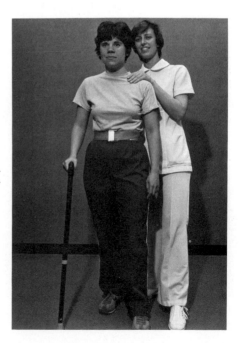

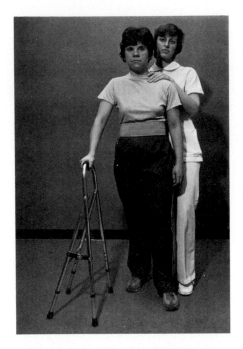

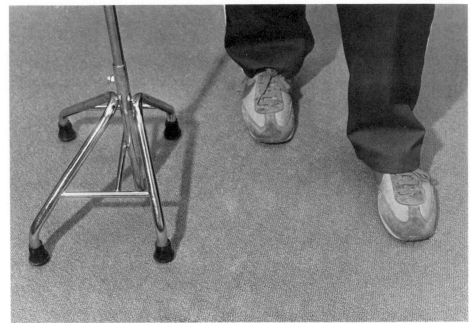

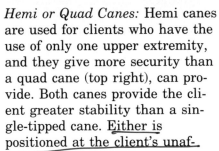

Hemi or Quad Canes: Hemi canes are used for clients who have the use of only one upper extremity, and they give more security than a quad cane (top right), can provide. Both canes provide the client greater stability than a single-tipped cane. Either is positioned at the client's unaf-fected side, with the straight, nonangled side adjacent to the body. The canes should be positioned approximately 15 cm (6 in.) from the client's side with the hand grips level with the greater trochanter of the femur. Guard the client as you would if she were using a single-tipped cane.

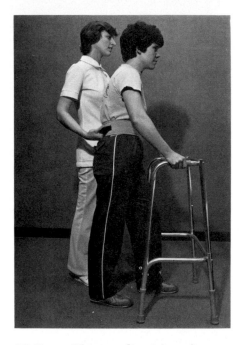

Walkers: If your client is using a walker, guard her as you would a client using a cane or crutches, and stand adjacent to her affected side. Instruct the client to put all four points of the walker flat on the floor before putting weight on the hand pieces. This will prevent stress cracks in the walker and ensure the client's safety. Instruct her to move the walker forward and walk into it and then repeat the movement.

Assisting the Client with Crutches to Sit in a Chair

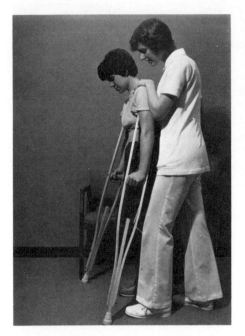

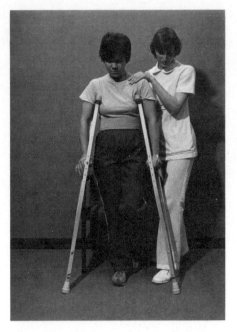

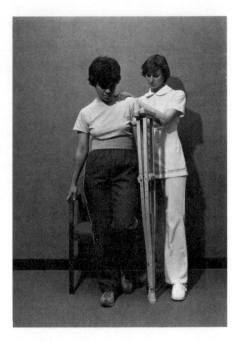

1 Before the client sits in a chair, you must first secure the chair by bracing it against a wall. Then instruct her to walk toward the chair and when she reaches it to begin her turn (as shown) so that ultimately the chair will be directly behind her.

2 She should place her unaffected leg against the front of the chair.

3 Instruct the client to move the crutches to her affected side and to grasp the chair's arm with the hand on the unaffected side.

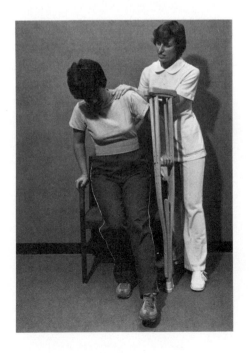

4 Tell her to flex the knee of her unaffected leg to lower herself into the chair. Advise the client to place her affected leg straight out in front of her to ensure that it remains nonweight bearing, if this is appropriate.

5 Once she has been seated, she should slide back into the chair so that she is in a good sitting posture. Place a support under the foot if the knee must remain extended while the client is sitting. Reverse these steps to assist her to stand from a sitting position.

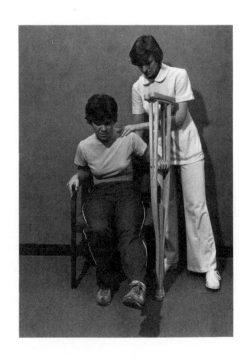

Transferring Mobile and Immobile Clients

Nursing Guidelines for Lifting and Transferring Clients

- To promote your clients' independence and to help maintain their muscular strength, always encourage them to move themselves, or to participate in the move as much as possible.
- Whenever possible, use mechanical lifting devices to transfer immobile clients, especially those who are obese.
- Always adjust the height of the bed to a level that enables you to maintain a vertical back while lifting and transferring.
- To avoid bending your back or stretching across the bed, position the client as close to you as possible.
- Instead of using the muscles in your upper body for lifting, flex your knees and utilize your larger leg and hip muscles; straighten your knees as you lift.
- Before initiating a lift or transfer, spread your feet apart to provide a wide base of support. One foot should be positioned slightly in front of the other.
- As you move the client from one position to another, shift your weight in the direction of the move.

MOVING THE CLIENT UP IN BED

Assisting the Mobile Client

If your client is strong enough to both lift up with her arms and push down on her feet, teach her how to move herself up in the bed. This is important because it will promote independence, help to maintain her physical strength, and minimize the strain on your own back as well.

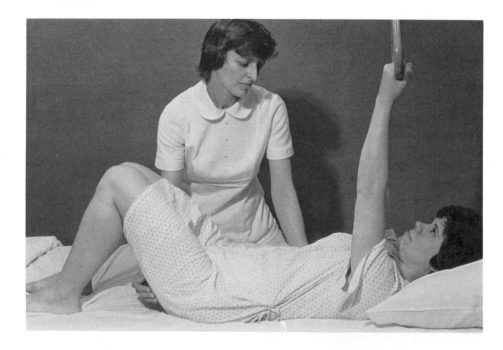

1 Flatten the bed, and adjust its height to an optimal working level. Instruct the client to bend her knees and to reach up and grasp the trapeze. (In most agencies, it is not necessary to obtain an order for a trapeze.) Place your right hand under her buttocks so that you can guide her during the move.

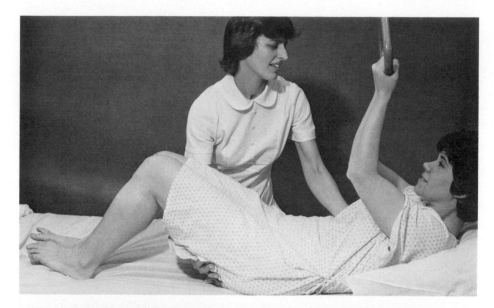

2 Instruct her to push down on her feet and to lift her upper body with her arms. As you guide her, face the direction of the move; shift your weight to the leg that is closer to the head of the bed.

Lifting the Immobile Client

1 If your client is immobile, ask one or more helpers to assist you with the lift. Position her on a draw sheet that extends from her head to her midthighs. Cross her arms across her chest to prevent them from dragging across the bed; then roll the draw sheet close to her body. With two movers each would stand on opposite sides of the bed and grasp the sheet at the head and buttocks area. With three movers (as shown) the nurses on the same side will cross their adjacent arms to more evenly distribute the client's weight between them.

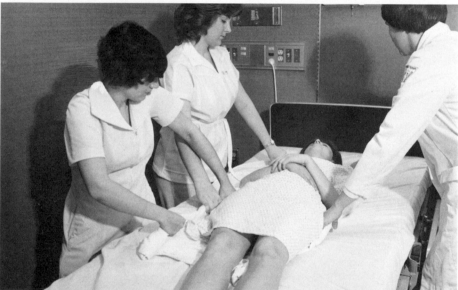

2 On a predetermined signal, shift your weight back and away from the client as if you were pulling the sheet apart. In this way, the taut sheet will elevate the client just enough to make the move to the head of the bed easier. To avoid injuring your back, it is important that you keep the natural curve in your back and avoid extending it as you pull back. As soon as the client has been elevated, shift your weight to the foot closer to the head of the bed and move the client forward.

Note: When the movers are of different heights, all will not be at an optimal working height with the bed.

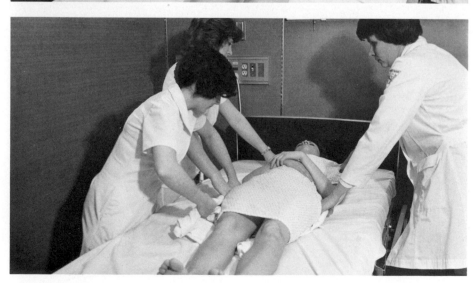

DANGLING THE CLIENT'S EXTREMITIES ON THE SIDE OF THE BED

Assisting the Mobile Client

1 On the day of surgery, most clients are required to sit on the side of the bed and dangle their legs before getting out of bed. If your client has mobility, encourage her to do most of the moving and lifting with your assistance. Explain the procedure to her and raise the height of the bed to a comfortable working level. The procedure described next will be performed in stages to protect the client's back, minimize the strain to an abdominal or perineal incision, and exercise the upper extremities as well. With the client flat on her back, place a hand on her far hip to guide her. Explain that she should roll toward you next (bottom).

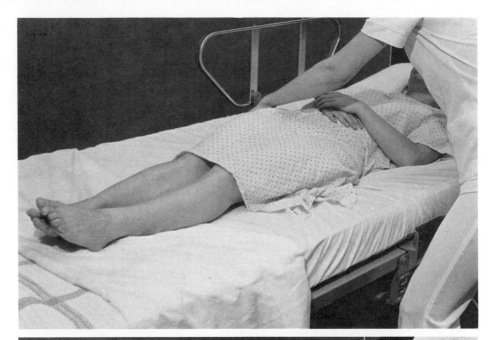

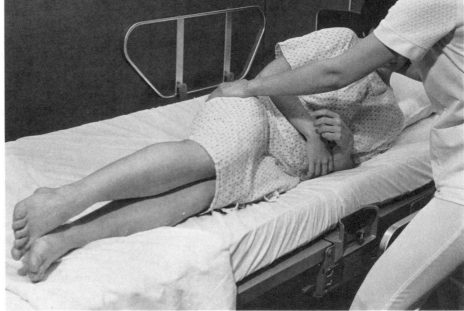

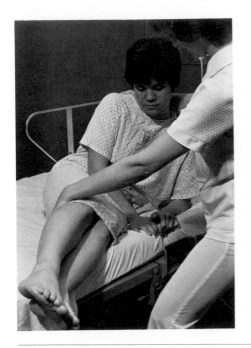

2 Once she is on her side, instruct her to flex her knees slightly and slide her legs off the side of the bed as she pushes up with her arms. You may assist her by guiding her legs and supporting her shoulders.

3 Support her at the edge of the bed until she feels comfortable and stable. Once she is secure, lower the bed so that her feet can dangle on the floor, or put a foot stool under her feet.

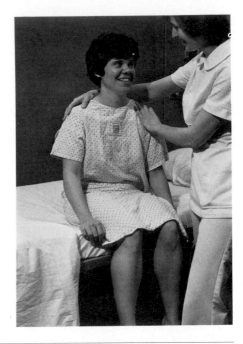

Moving the Immobile Client

1 To dangle the extremities of the immobile client, you will need to do most of the lifting and moving yourself. Explain the procedure to the client and ask her to assist you as much as possible. Raise the bed to a comfortable working level, and place your hand under her knees so that you can flex them and lift her feet off the bed (bottom).

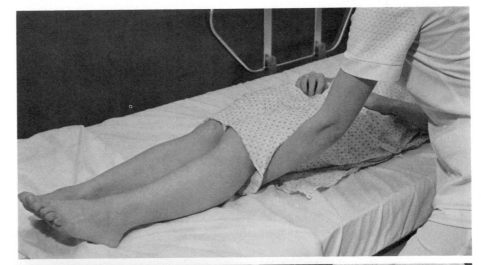

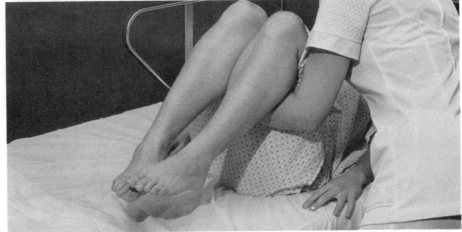

(Continued on p. 76)

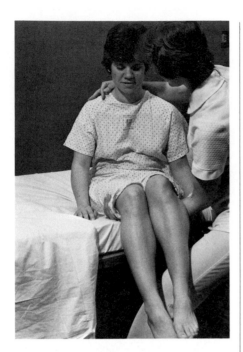

2 Place your right arm around her shoulders and pivot her upper body up and around as you lower her legs over the side of the bed. For your own stability and safety, place your feet apart and pivot your weight from your right foot to your left foot as you lower her legs over the side. *Note: As an alternative, you can raise the head of the bed 90° and pivot the client to the side of the bed, using the same hand positioning depicted in this photo.* Because she may experience dizziness for a while, continue to support her until she is stable enough for you to rest her feet on a foot stool or to lower the bed for her feet to rest on the floor.

MOVING THE CLIENT FROM THE STRETCHER TO THE BED

Teaching the Segmental Transfer Technique

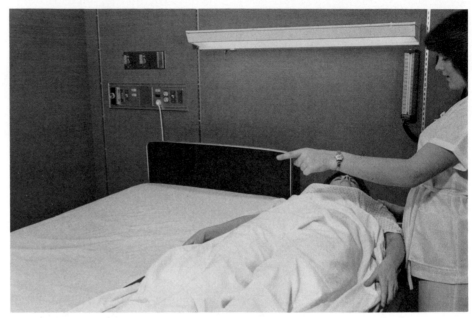

1 If your client can assist in the transfer, you can instruct her to move onto the bed from the stretcher by employing the segmental transfer technique. Before she begins the move, ensure that both the bed and the stretcher are locked in place to prevent them from separating during the move; adjust the bed to a height as close to that of the stretcher as possible. Explain to the client that she will move her head, trunk, and feet in stages.

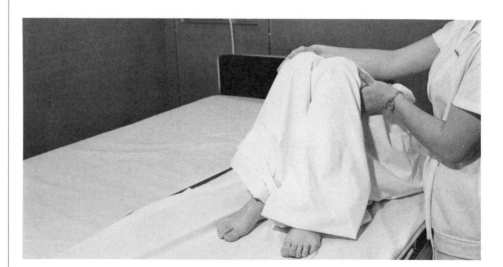

2 Ask her to flex her hips and knees so that her feet are flat on the stretcher.

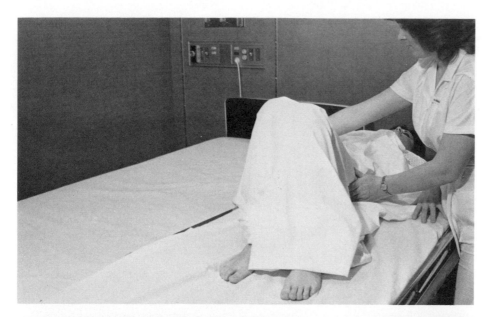

3 She should press down on her feet and slide her trunk, buttocks, and then her head over to the side of the stretcher.

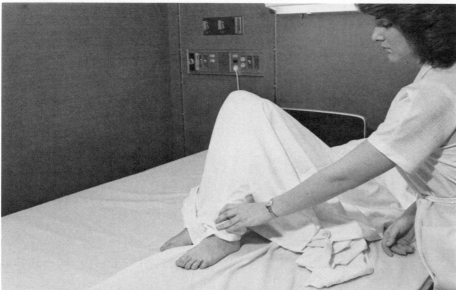

4 Instruct her to lift her feet and move them to the edge of the stretcher.

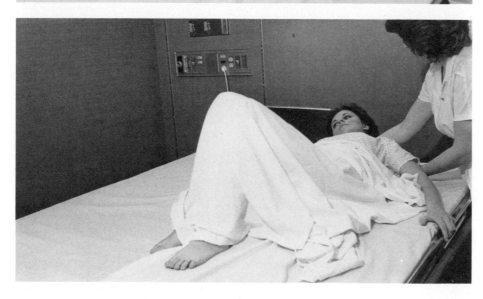

5 She should move her trunk and then her head as close to the edge of the stretcher as possible.

(Continued on p. 78)

6 Tell her to place her feet on the side of the bed.

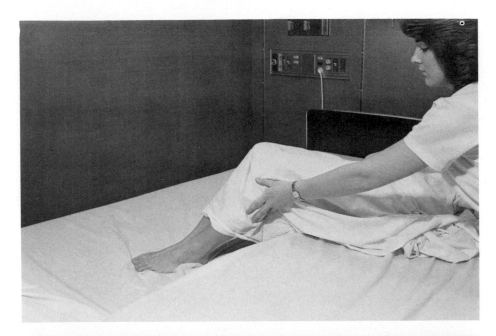

7 Instruct her to make a bridge with her trunk by lifting her pelvis off the stretcher.

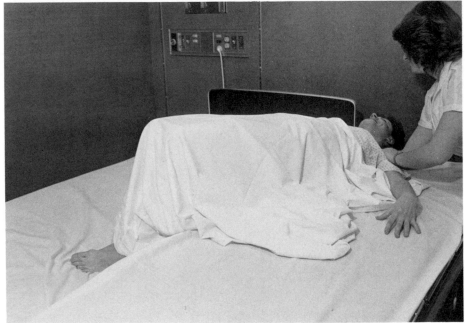

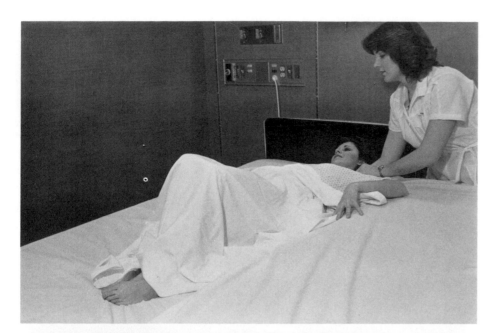

8 She will then move her pelvis and trunk onto the bed.

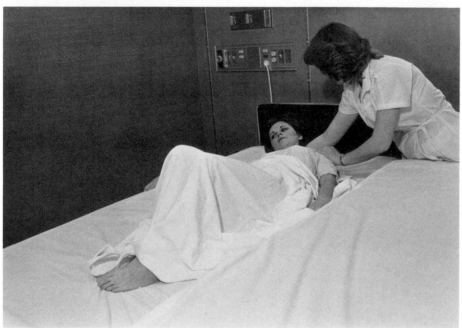

9 While her knees are still flexed, instruct her to press down on her feet to move her trunk and then her head to the center of the bed.

5 Remove the stretcher and move the client from the edge of the bed to the center of the bed following the same technique.

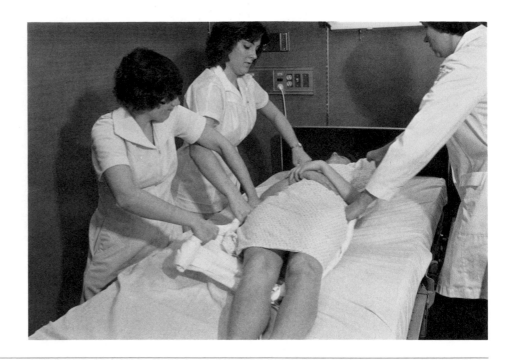

LOGROLLING THE IMMOBILE CLIENT

1 If your client has a neck injury or a spinal disorder, it will be necessary for you to logroll her when you change her position so that you maintain the alignment of her vertebral column during the turn. Logrolling is also indicated for clients with hip pinnings or hip prostheses to keep the hips in extension. Seek the assistance of a helper, and explain the procedure to your client. Raise the bed to an optimal working level, and using a drawsheet, move the client to the edge of the bed opposite the side toward which she will be turned. (Review the steps in the preceding procedure.)

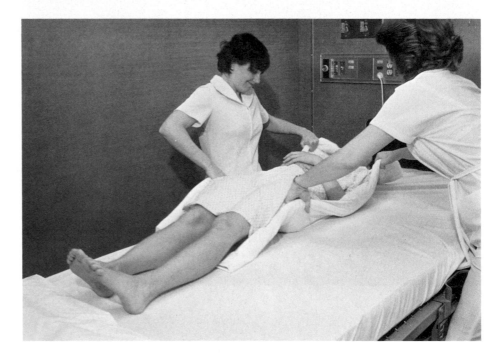

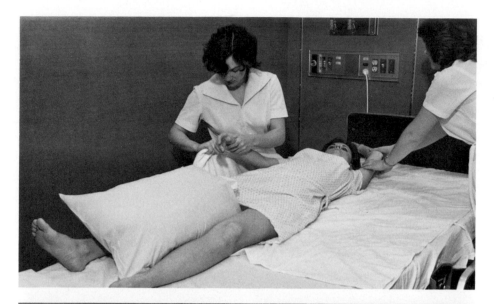

2 Straighten the draw sheet on the side to which the client will be turned, and place a pillow between her legs to maintain the position of the lower extremities. To roll the client toward the left side of the bed, you should first place her right arm beside her body; then flex her left arm over her head so that she will not roll over it during the turn. However, if your client has limited shoulder movement, keep the arm in extension next to the body. *Caution: If your client has a neck injury, you will need a second helper at this point to support the neck during the turn.*

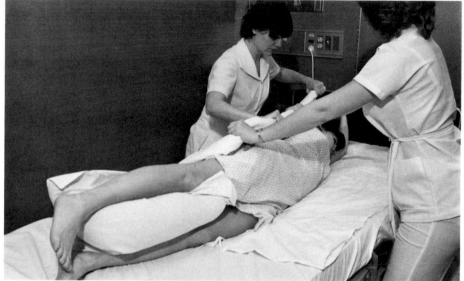

3 The nurse on the left side of the bed will flex her knees, maintain a wide base of support with her feet, and then grasp and lift up on the rolled draw sheet to guide the client toward herself. The nurse on the right side of the bed will maintain tension on the sheet to ensure the client's proper alignment. Note that the nurses' hands are alternated on the sheet to evenly distribute the client's weight. Either support the client in a side-lying position (see steps, p. 64) or continue to the prone position (as shown in step 4).

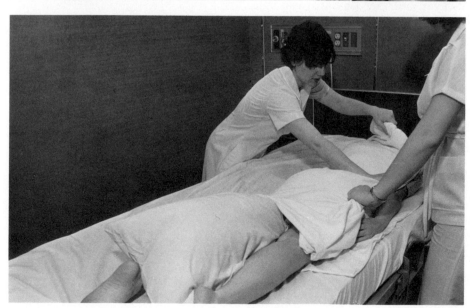

4 Continue the turn with the nurse on the right side of the bed guiding the client onto her abdomen. Place the client in a proper prone position (see steps, p. 65).

ASSISTING THE CLIENT FROM THE WHEELCHAIR (OR CHAIR) TO THE BED

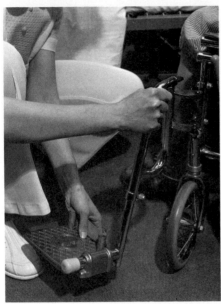 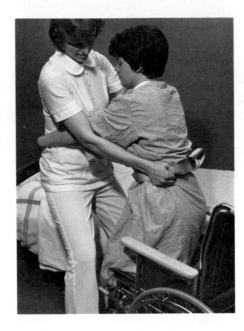 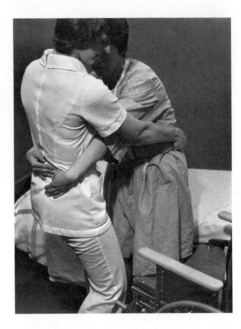

1 Clients who have enough mobility to help support themselves during the transfer may be assisted from the wheelchair or chair to the bed with the standing-pivot technique. Position the wheelchair at a 45° angle to the bed and lock both the wheelchair and bed to ensure their stability. If the client will be transferred from a chair, make sure it is stable and will not slide on the floor. It is important to either remove the wheelchair's leg rests or swing them out of the way so that they will not obstruct the move. Explain the procedure to the client and ensure that she understands each step and her role during the transfer. Encourage her to assume as much of the lifting and weightbearing as she can comfortably handle, using her stronger leg, if this is appropriate. Before starting, however, you must ensure that her transfer belt is securely fastened around her waist.

2 Flex your knees and position your feet into a wide base of support with one foot slightly in front of the other. Grasp the client's transfer belt, and instruct her to position her arms around your waist. On the cue to stand, the client will prepare to stand on her stronger leg as you assist her into the standing position by pulling her trunk forward and up. As you pull her forward, transfer your weight from your forward leg to your back leg.

3 To ensure the stability of your client's stronger leg, position the side of your knee against the side of her knee to maintain it in extension. Pivot the client and guide her until the backs of her legs are positioned against the bed. Keep your knees flexed and your back straight.

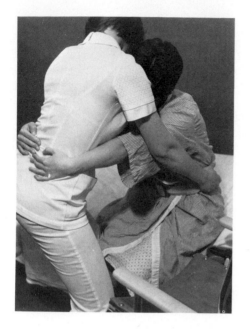

4 Assist the client in lowering herself to the sitting position by using a slow bending of your knees to control the rate of descent.

5 Support her until she is stable and comfortable. Then remove the transfer belt and robe and assist her into bed. Reverse the procedure to move her from the bed to the chair.

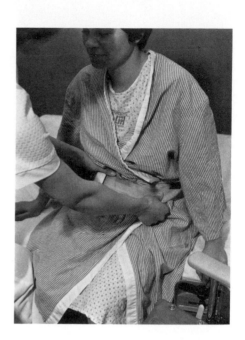

USING A MECHANICAL LIFTING DEVICE

Mechanical lifts, such as the Hoyer, are excellent devices for lifting and transferring the immobile client. They are, however, contraindicated for clients with certain types of spinal disorders that require the vertebral column to be maintained in static alignment.

1 Be sure to read the operating instructions for the mechanical lifting device your agency employs. Be certain that the client's weight does not exceed the device's weight limit. Although it is possible to use the lift alone, a helper will both facilitate the process and ensure the client's safety by guarding him during the lifting procedure. First, explain the procedure to the client and assure him that he will be safe and comfortable during the transfer. Then, adjust the bed to a comfortable working height and roll the client into a side-lying position. Place the canvas sling along the client's body, extending it from his head to no farther than the popliteal fossa of his knees. While your helper supports the client's position, fan-fold (accordian-pleat) the sling.

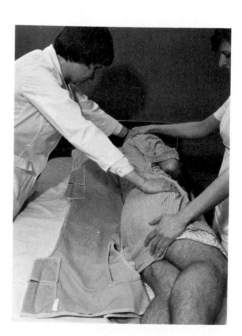

(Continued on p. 86)

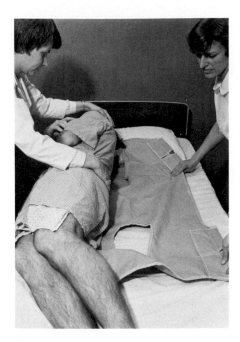

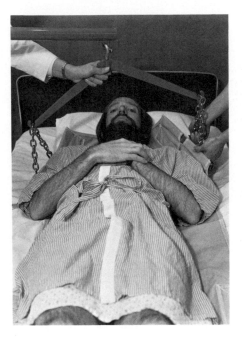

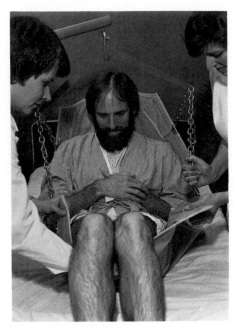

2 Roll the client to his opposite side and straighten the sling.

3 Return the client to his back and cross his arms across his chest. Move the lift to the side of the bed. Center the boom over the sling so that the chains can be attached to its upper section.

4 Elevate the boom slightly so that the chains can be attached to the lower section of the sling. While one nurse attaches the chains, the other should support and flex the client's knees. Ensure that the client's weight is evenly distributed in the sling.

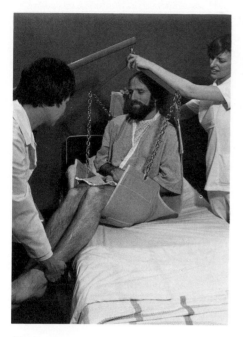

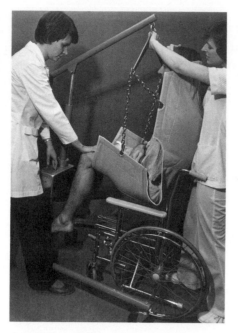

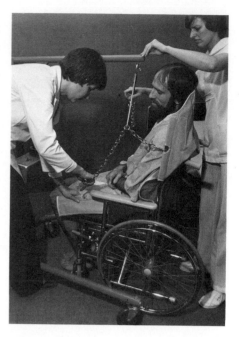

5 Either elevate the lift slightly, or lower the bed just enough so that you can clear the client of the bed and guide his legs over the side.

6 Move the client and the lift away from the bed and push a wheelchair or other transfer device under the client. Lock the wheelchair and then lower the lift so that the client is seated securely in the wheelchair. Protect his head as the boom is being lowered. Instruct the client to keep his arms folded during the transfer. This keeps the device balanced and prevents the client's arms from striking against the chair.

7 Unhook the chains, and either remove the sling if the client will be in the chair for an extended period of time or adjust it to remove the wrinkles. Place a security belt around the client's pelvis to ensure his stability in the chair.

(Continued on p. 88)

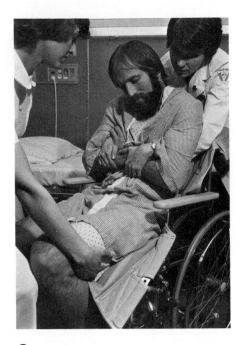

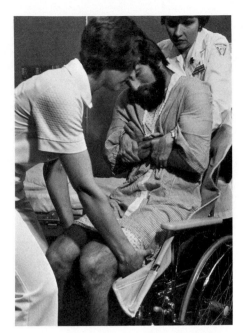

8 If your client slides down in his chair and is sitting on his sacrum, it will be necessary for you to lift him up so that he is positioned correctly. To do this, first cross his arms across his chest. Then, while one nurse stabilizes his legs and feet and prepares to push his pelvis back into the chair, the other stands behind the chair and positions her arms under the client's axillae and grasps his forearms. By grasping the crossed forearms rather than under the axillae, you will avoid the application of a force that could potentially separate the humerus from the glenoid fossa.

9 On a predetermined signal, the person behind the wheelchair will pull the client back and up in the chair while the nurse in front pushes his legs toward the back of the wheelchair to slide his pelvis into the correct position.

References

Basmajian, J.V. 1978. *Therapeutic exercise,* 3rd ed. Baltimore: Williams & Wilkins.

Farber, S.D. 1982. *Neurorehabilitation: a multisensory approach.* Philadelphia: W.B. Saunders.

Getz, P.A., and Blossom, B.M. Dec. 1982. Preventing contractures: the little "extras" that help so much. *RN* 45:45–48.

Hilt, N.E., and Cogburn, S.B. 1980. *Manual of orthopedics.* St. Louis: C.V. Mosby.

Kozier, B., and Erb, G. 1983. *Fundamentals of nursing,* 2nd ed. Menlo Park, Calif.: Addison-Wesley Publishing.

Nursing Photobook. 1981. *Providing early mobility.* Horsham, Pa.: Intermed Communications.

Rantz, M.F., and Courtial, D. 1981. *Lifting, moving, and transferring patients,* 2nd ed. St. Louis: C.V. Mosby.

Sorensen, K.C., and Luckmann, J. 1979. *Basic nursing: a psychophysiologic approach.* Philadelphia: W.B. Saunders.

Sullivan, P.E., et al. 1982. *An integrated approach to therapeutic exercise.* Reston, Va.: Reston Publishing.

Chapter 3

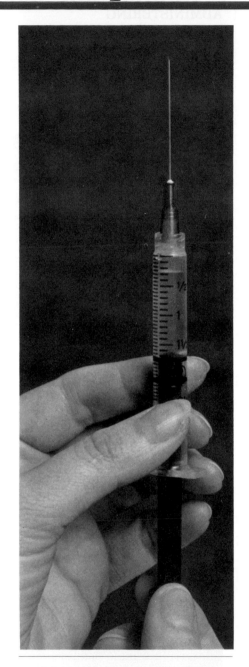

Administering Medications and Monitoring Fluids

Instilling Drops

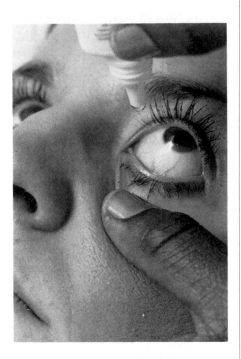

INSTILLING EAR DROPS

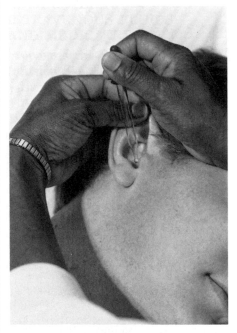

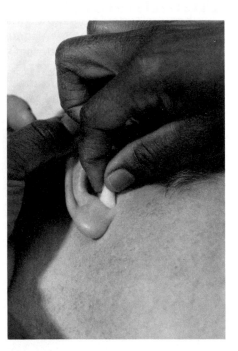

Review the preceding technique for instilling ointment. Follow the same guidelines, but dropper the medication into the center of the conjunctival sac (as shown). After administering the medication, instruct the client to close the eyelid and to move the eye around to distribute the medication. At the same time, apply gentle pressure to the inner canthus for 30 seconds to 1 minute to minimize the potential for systemic absorption through the tear ducts.

1 For your client's comfort, make sure the medication has been warmed to body temperature; then fill the dropper with the prescribed amount of medication. Ask your client to turn his head to the side so that the affected ear is uppermost. With your nondominant hand, pull up and back on the auricle to straighten the auditory canal. For an infant, pull down and back on the earlobe instead. Rest the wrist of your dominant hand on the client's head. This will allow your hand to move with the client rather than potentially injure the ear with the dropper, should he jerk during the instillation. Administer the medication, aiming it toward the walls of the canal rather than directly onto the eardrum. This will make the instillation less startling and hence more comfortable and safe for the client.

2 Unless the physician requests that the solution drain freely from the ear, you may insert a small piece of cotton loosely into the external auditory canal. Instruct the client to remain with the affected ear uppermost for 10–15 minutes to retain the solution.

INSTILLING NOSE DROPS

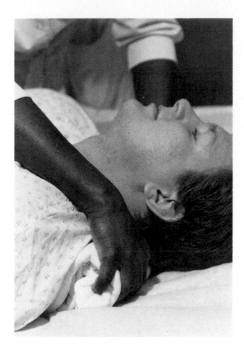 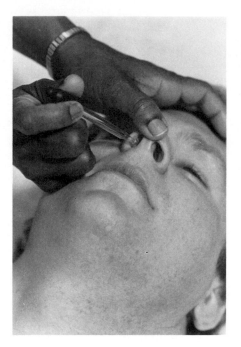 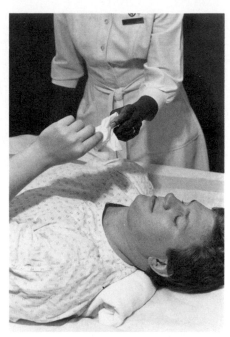

1 Instruct your client to gently blow his nose. Assist him into a supine position with his head tilted back. It may be helpful to place a small pillow or a rolled towel under the shoulders to help maintain this position.

2 With your nondominant hand, press back gently on the tip of the nose to open the nares. Rest your dominant hand lightly on the face so that your hand will move along with the client should he move suddenly. This will prevent the dropper from accidently injuring the nasal mucosa. Insert the dropper just inside the naris and instill the prescribed medication.

3 To ensure that the medication has time to drain through the nasal passages, encourage the client to maintain this position for a few minutes. Provide him with tissues in which to expectorate the solution that drains into the throat and mouth.

GIVING INHALANT MEDICATIONS VIA A NEBULIZER

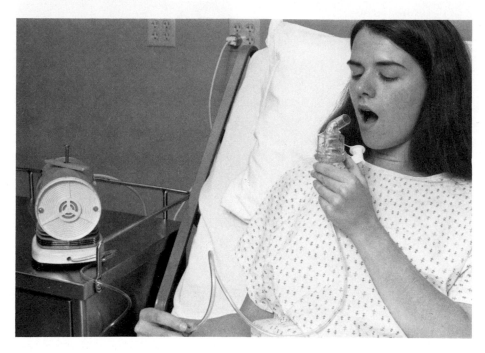

If your client has a pulmonary disorder, it may be necessary for you to use a nebulizer to administer an inhalant solution. The prescribed amount of solution is poured or droppered into the nebulizer (in the client's left hand as shown). The compressor (on the bedside table) is then plugged in. With the client sitting upright to enhance chest expansion, instruct her to hold the nebulizer 2.5– 5 cm (1–2 in.) from her mouth. She should first exhale and then inhale as she closes off the finger valve (adjacent to the client's right index finger) to deliver the fine mist into the alveoli or other areas of the lung. Explain that she should hold her breath for 3

seconds, and then repeat the process until all the medication has been delivered from the nebulizer. *Caution: Some bronchodilators, such as isoproterenol and isoetharine, significantly elevate the heart rate. Monitor the client's pulse rate frequently throughout the therapy and record the pretreatment and posttreatment measurements. Be sure to stay with the client throughout the treatment.* Ensure that the nebulizer and tubing are thoroughly cleaned and dried daily, according to your agency's guidelines. This practice reduces the likelihood that the nebulizer will become a reservoir for bacteria.

GIVING NITROGLYCERIN

Applying Nitroglycerin Ointment

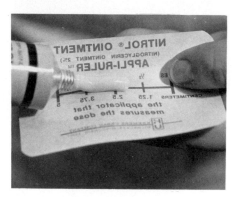

1 Nitroglycerin ointment is applied directly to the skin of clients with angina pectoris and cardiac ischemia to produce systemic vasodilation. This results in a decreased cardiac workload and improved myocardial tissue perfusion for a period of 4–6 hours. Before administering the medication, take your client's blood pressure and apical pulse to establish a baseline for subsequent comparison. Squeeze the prescribed dose directly onto the manufacturer's applicator paper. To ensure an accurate dosage, use an even pressure to produce a continuous column of medication. *Caution: Be sure to avoid direct contact with the nitroglycerin because it could give you a headache if it is absorbed through your skin. Wash your skin immediately with soap and water if this occurs.* Remove any residual ointment from previous applications prior to applying this dose.

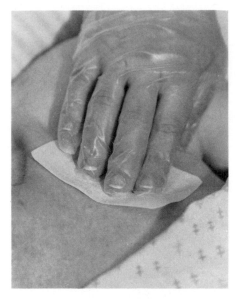 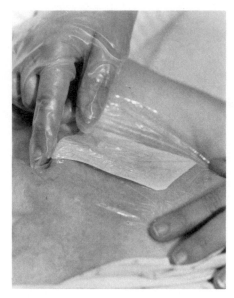 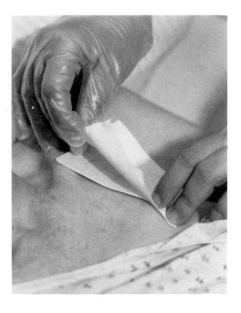

2 If desired, put on a clean glove to protect yourself from potential contact with the medication. Apply the ointment via the applicator paper directly to your client's skin. For optimal absorption, apply the ointment to skin that is hairless and dry. Application sites commonly used are shoulders, anterior and posterior chest, abdomen, and legs. Be sure to rotate application sites to prevent sensitization and dermal inflammation.

3 If the client is not receiving the desired effect from the medication, the physician may request that you cover the applicator paper with an occlusive plastic wrap (as shown) or with a wide strip of air-occlusive tape (right). Either will enhance absorption.

However, if your client is achieving the desired effect without an air-occlusive dressing, avoid applying one because the increased absorption from the dressing could result in headache and dizziness.

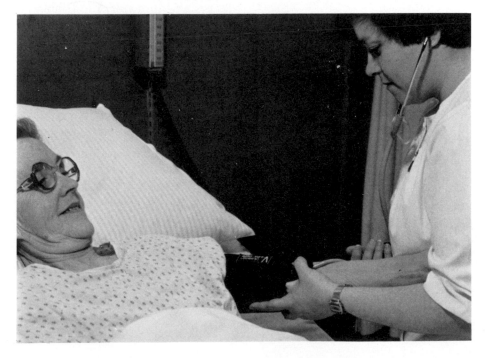

4 Check your client's blood pressure a few minutes after applying the ointment. There should be a moderate decline in the systolic pressure. Continue to monitor your client for headaches, faintness, or dizziness. If these symptoms occur, alert the physician, who will probably decrease the dosage until the client develops a tolerance to the side effects of the drug.

Applying a Nitroglycerin Disk

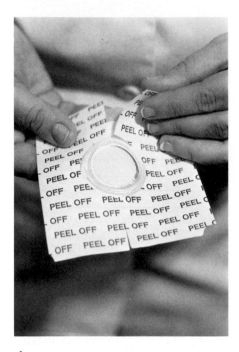

1 Review the previous steps for applying nitroglycerin ointment because the principles for application and usage are similar to the disk's. The advantages in using the disk are its neatness, dose accuracy, and its known duration of action. In addition, it poses less of a hazard for the person administering the drug. Disks produce a continuous release of medication over approximately a 24-hour period, starting approximately 30 minutes after application. To apply the disk, peel off the strip of protective paper backing from one side of the disk.

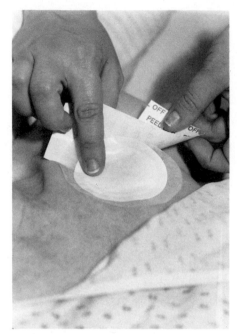

2 Adhere that side of the disk to a dry, hairless area of your client's skin. Then remove the remaining protective paper strip.

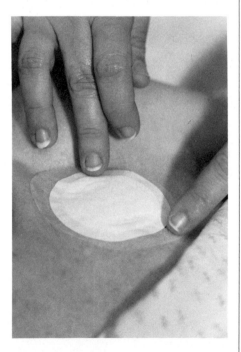

3 Securely adhere the disk's sticky surface to the client's skin.

ADMINISTERING MEDICATIONS THROUGH A NASOGASTRIC TUBE

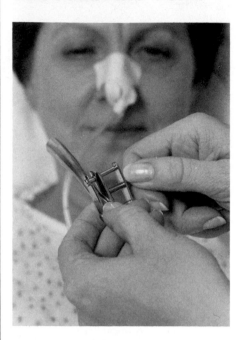

1 Have medications been prescribed that must be instilled into your client's stomach via a nasogastric tube? This can be done easily with the aid of a large (50 mL) piston or bulb syringe, an emesis basin, bed-saver pad, and 30 mL of tap water. First, however, you must confirm that the distal end of the tube is properly positioned in the stomach. After preparing the prescribed medication, position the client in high Fowler's, or in a slightly elevated right side-lying position if Fowler's is contraindicated. Either position will minimize the potential for aspiration and facilitate gravity flow into the stomach. Remove the tube plug, or detach the Hoffman clamp (as shown).

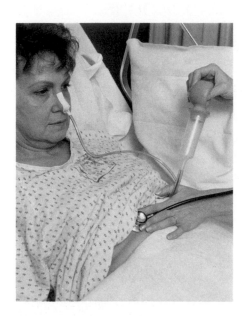

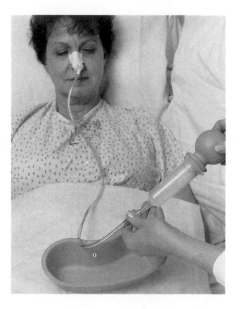

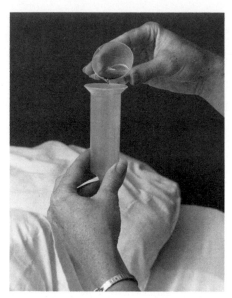

2 One method for confirming the correct position of the tube is to attach the large syringe to the proximal end of the tube. Then listen at the epigastric area as you instill 10–20 mL of air. A "whoosh" indicates that the tube is correctly positioned. If the client eructates (belches), the tube may be in the esophagus and will require repositioning into the stomach.

3 Another way to confirm correct placement of the tube is to aspirate for stomach contents. Place a bed-saver pad and emesis basin under the tube's proximal end. Then squeeze the bulb (as shown) or pull back on the piston to aspirate stomach contents. *Caution: Do not proceed with the instillation unless these tests confirm that the tube is in the stomach.*

4 To prevent loss of electrolytes and gastric juices, allow the stomach contents to flow back into the stomach. Remove the bulb or piston, hold the barrel 30–45 cm (12–18 in.) above the abdomen, and allow the aspirated contents to flow back through the tube via gravity flow. Then instill the medication into the barrel (as shown) and allow it to drain into the stomach. *Note: Use liquid dosage forms whenever you administer medications into a nasogastric tube. Crushing tablets or opening capsules changes the product form and may alter therapeutic effects.*

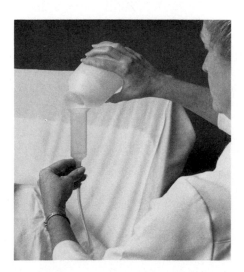

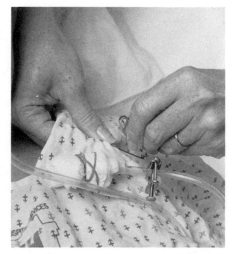

5 Instill approximately 30 mL of tap water into the barrel to ensure that residual medication does not adhere to the tubing.

←

6 Remove the syringe barrel and reinsert the tube plug or attach the Hoffman clamp to the end of the tube. Secure the tube to the client's gown (as shown). For optimal absorption, have your client remain in this position for 30 minutes. Wash and dry the syringe and return it to its container at the bedside. If intake and output records are being kept for your client, be sure to chart the nasogastric instillation.

PERFORMING A VAGINAL IRRIGATION (DOUCHE)

Vaginal irrigations are prescribed for preoperative cleansing—for example, with a povidone-iodine solution—for soothing inflamed vaginal mucosa and for applying heat or medications to the vaginal mucosa and cervix. They are contraindicated in late pregnancy and during postpartum and menstruation. Use clean technique and wear clean gloves for your own protection unless the client has an open wound. In that case, use sterile technique to protect the client from the potential spread of infection.

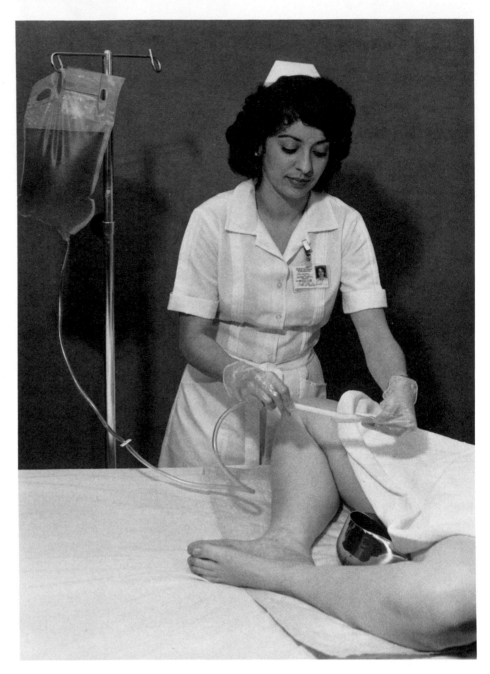

1 Prepare the prescribed solution, and check the solution's temperature with a thermometer to ensure that it is not too hot. Usually, 40.5 C (105 F) is the recommended temperature. Bring the solution and equipment to your client's room and hang the container on an IV pole 30–45 cm (12–18 in.) above the level of the client's vagina. This height will provide an adequate gravity flow yet prevent the solution from entering the vagina with too great a force. Explain the procedure to the client and ask her to void if she hasn't recently done so. An empty bladder will make the procedure more comfortable and allow greater expansion of the vaginal canal. Provide privacy, and drape her with a bath blanket or bed sheet. Assist her into a dorsal recumbent position, and place a bed-saver pad and bed pan under her buttocks. Her knees should be flexed and separated (as shown). Remove the protective cap from the nozzle, and inspect the nozzle for cracks or other irregularities that could potentially harm the vaginal mucosa.

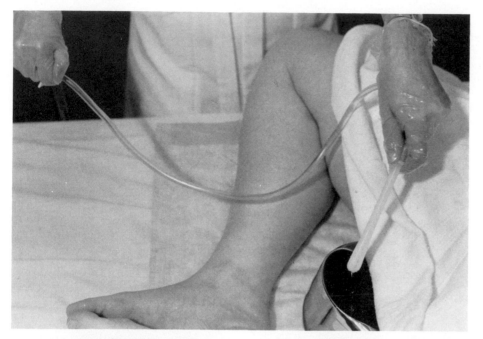

2 Direct the nozzle over the bed pan and then open the tubing clamp to run the solution to the end of the nozzle. This will flush the tubing of air and lubricate the nozzle to facilitate its insertion into the vagina.

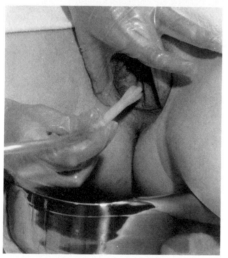

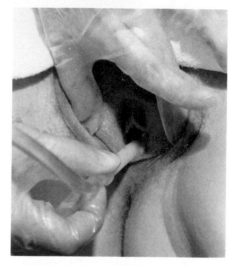

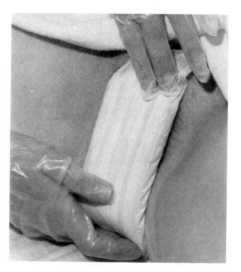

3 Separate the labia and allow the solution to flow over the external genitalia and vulva to prevent the introduction of contaminants into the vagina and uterus. Then close the clamp. *Note: If the client has copious discharge, cleanse the area with cotton balls soaked in a soapy solution. Use a fresh cotton ball for each single downward stroke. Gently insert the nozzle into the vagina.*

4 Direct the nozzle approximately 5–7.5 cm (2–3 in.) into the vagina angling it toward the sacrum to follow the anatomic structure of the vagina. Open the clamp again and allow the solution to flow. Unless the client has had cervical or vaginal surgery, gently rotate the nozzle to irrigate all the vaginal surfaces. When the solution has drained from the container, clamp the tubing and remove the nozzle. Then raise the head of the bed to permit the solution to drain out into the bed pan.

5 Dry the perineum with tissues, wiping from the front toward the anus. Then apply a sterile peripad to the perineum to absorb the residual solution and protect the clothing or bed linen from the irrigant. Remove the equipment from the bedside and either dispose of it or clean it according to agency procedure.

GIVING RECTAL MEDICATIONS

Inserting a Suppository

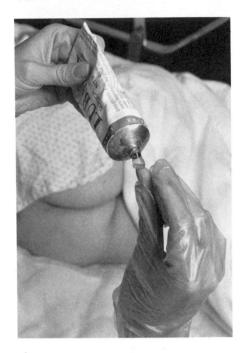

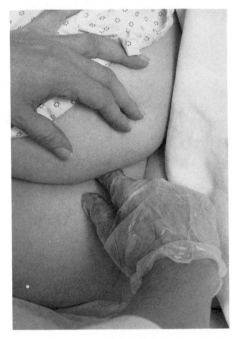

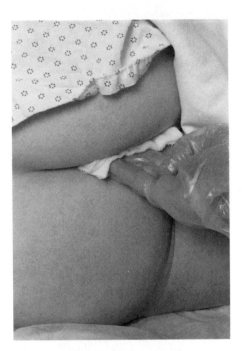

1 To insert a suppository, provide privacy, and assist the client into a position in which the rectum is easily accessible, for example, a side-lying position with the upper leg flexed (Sims) as shown. Put on a clean glove or a finger cot and generously lubricate the suppository with a water-soluble lubricant.

2 With your free hand, gently lift the uppermost buttock. With your gloved index finger, guide the suppository into the anus, directing it along the rectal wall and away from fecal masses. To prevent immediate expulsion, be sure to insert the suppository beyond the internal sphincter.

3 With a tissue or gauze pad, press gently on the anus for a few moments to help the client retain the medication; then clean the rectal area with the tissue or pad. Encourage the client to retain the suppository for at least 20 minutes before using the bed pan or going to the bathroom, if it is appropriate for the suppository to be expelled.

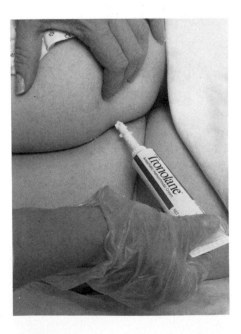

Instilling Ointment

Review the preceding technique for inserting a rectal suppository. To lubricate the applicator, remove its protective cover and squeeze the tube (as shown). This will push the ointment through the small openings on the applicator and facilitate its insertion into the rectum. Insert the applicator gently to avoid injury to the rectal canal or to hemorrhoids. Squeeze the prescribed amount of ointment. Clean the rectal area with tissues and assist your client to a position of comfort.

Administering Injectable Medications

GIVING INTRADERMAL INJECTIONS

Locating the Site

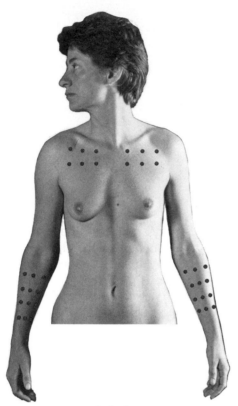

Anterior

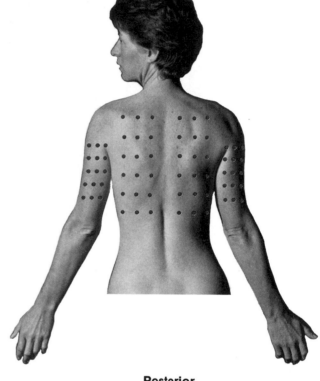

Posterior

Review these anatomic overlays to assist you in locating the proper sites for intradermal injections. The most common uses for intradermal injections are tuberculin skin testing (Mantoux test) and allergy testing.

The most frequently injected site is the ventral aspect of the forearm. To locate an appropriate injection site for this area, measure a hand's breadth from the antecubital space and a hand's breadth from the wrist. You can safely inject into the ventral area bordered by your two hands, provided the site is not scarred, covered with hair follicles, or inflamed, because these conditions would interfere with the reading.

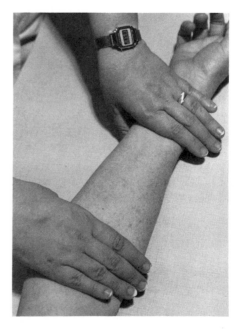

Injecting the Medication

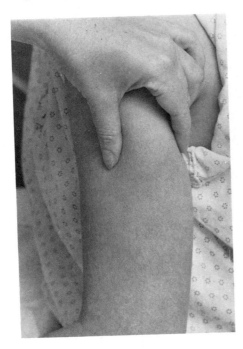 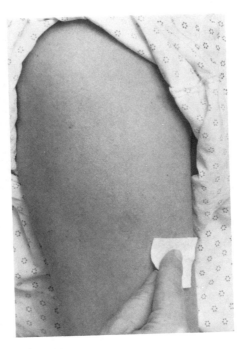 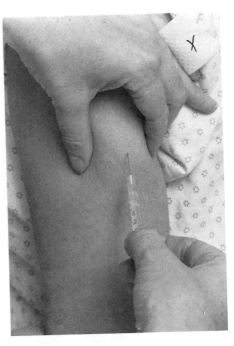

1 A subcutaneous injection is properly given into the layer of tissue that is above the muscle and below the skin and fat. To effectively reach this layer, you will need to assess each client to help you determine the correct angle of insertion and, occasionally, the need for a longer or shorter needle. With a ⅝-in. needle, you can usually vary the angle of insertion to correctly penetrate the subcutaneous layer. However, for very obese clients, a ⅝-in. needle may not be long enough to penetrate past the fatty layer. The same needle may be too long for children or very thin clients. Form a skin fold (as shown) to assess the amount of fat at the selected injection site and to determine the correct angle of insertion for reaching the subcutaneous tissue. If your client has an average build, a 45° angle is usually effective. An obese client may require a 90° angle, and a thin client may require an angle ranging from 15°–45°.

2 Draw up the prescribed medication into a 2–3 mL syringe with a 25-gauge, ⅝-in. (or the correct length) needle. The use of an air bubble should be determined by your agency's policy to ensure consistency in the amount of medication routinely delivered to each client. For example, if you use an air bubble and your co-worker does not, the amount of medication you deliver to your client will be slightly more than that delivered by your co-worker, because the air will clear the needle of medication. Consistency is especially crucial for diabetic clients receiving insulin. Prepare the site with an alcohol sponge. Start at the insertion site and work your way outward from the center in a circular fashion to cover an area 5 cm (2 in.) in diameter. Allow the alcohol to dry.

3 Bunch the skin between your thumb and index finger. This will minimize your client's discomfort as the needle is inserted. Insert the needle with the bevel up, at the angle appropriate for your client.

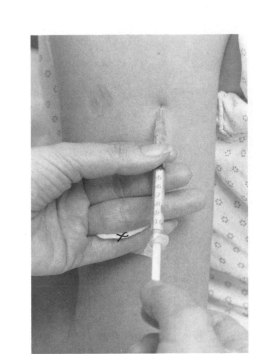

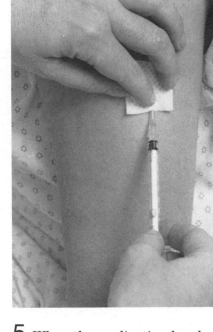

4 If t
and pa
marks.
rior ili
this la
as a di
can als
ridge a
(1–2 in
superio
buttock

4 <u>Release the skin and pull</u> back <u>on the plunger (as shown)</u> to <u>aspirate for blood</u>. If you do aspirate blood, withdraw the needle because injecting a medication into a vascular area could result in a systemic reaction to the medication. Obtain a new syringe and needle, as well as new medication, and try again. When you are certain you are in a nonvascular layer of subcutaneous tissue, slowly inject the medication. *Caution: Do not aspirate if you are injecting heparin because it could cause a hematoma to form at the injection site.*

5 When the medication has been injected, withdraw the needle at the same angle in which it was inserted to minimize trauma to the tissues. <u>Apply pressure with an alcohol sponge at the insertion site to avert bleeding</u>. If massage has not been contraindicated, as it would be with heparin, it can be employed to facilitate absorption of the medication.

GI

Ma
Do

1

of t
glut
cati
jecti
com
mus
scia
Noti
of th
agor
post
the g
femu
site f
have
devel
This
dicat
bile c
could

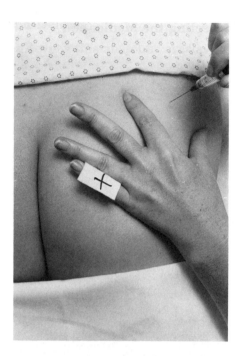

2 Spread the tissue between your thumb and index finger to make the skin taut, and then insert the needle in a quick dart-like motion. It is helpful to hold an alcohol swab between the last two fingers so that is readily available after the needle has been withdrawn.

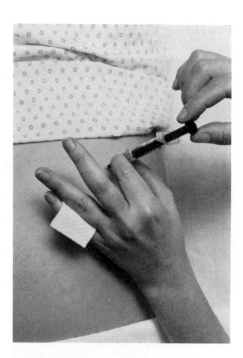

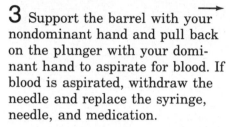

3 Support the barrel with your →
nondominant hand and pull back on the plunger with your dominant hand to aspirate for blood. If blood is aspirated, withdraw the needle and replace the syringe, needle, and medication.

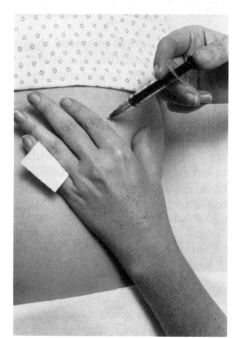

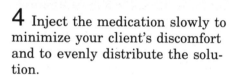

4 Inject the medication slowly to minimize your client's discomfort and to evenly distribute the solution.

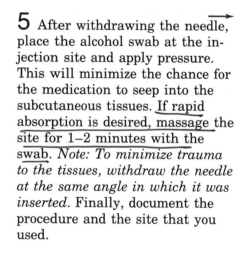

5 After withdrawing the needle, →
place the alcohol swab at the injection site and apply pressure. This will minimize the chance for the medication to seep into the subcutaneous tissues. If rapid absorption is desired, massage the site for 1–2 minutes with the swab. *Note: To minimize trauma to the tissues, withdraw the needle at the same angle in which it was inserted.* Finally, document the procedure and the site that you used.

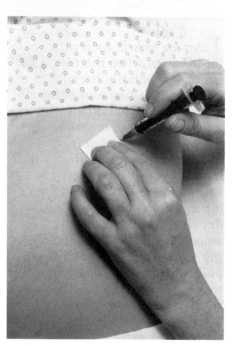

Performing the Z-Track Technique

Z-track injections are indicated when complete absorption of the medication is crucial or when medications such as iron preparations may potentially seep into the injection tract and stain the skin or surrounding tissues. Some agencies require the Z-track method for all injections into the gluteal muscle. The tissue is displaced downward and toward the median before, during, and after the injection so that when the tissue is released, the needle tract that would normally have formed becomes instead a broken, noncontinuous line. This method keeps the medication deep in the muscle by preventing its seepage up through the tissues.

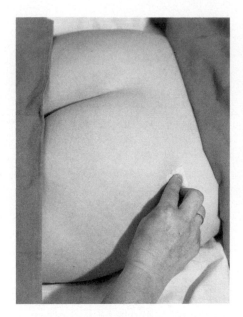

1 Draw up the medication, and then change the needle to one that is at least 5 cm (2 in.) long (for the average adult). Because you will need to inject deeply to reach the muscle, the size of the needle will depend on the size of the client. Draw up a 0.5-mL air bubble (or larger, depending on the length and gauge of the needle). This will enable you to clear all the medication from the needle as well as eject the residual medication from the needle's end to prevent tracking the solution as the needle is withdrawn. Now, you are ready to prepare the site with an alcohol sponge (as shown). Prepare the skin before displacing the tissue because it is difficult to maintain the required traction on the tissue for the length of time it takes for the alcohol to dry. Cleanse an area that is at least 10 cm (4 in.) in diameter to ensure that you will have covered the injection site.

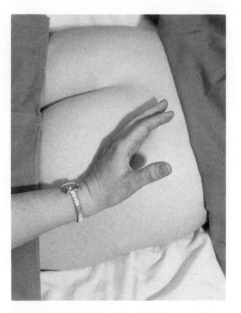

2 After preparing the skin, place the ulnar side of your nondominant hand along the diagonal that extends from the posterior superior iliac spine to the greater trochanter of the femur.

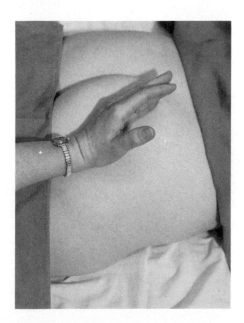

3 Displace the tissue downward and toward the median as far as you can and yet comfortably maintain the traction on the tissue.

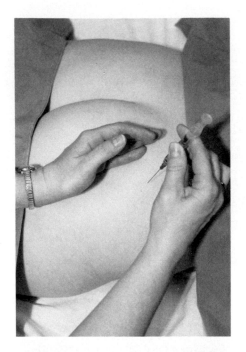

4 Continue to displace the tissue as you insert the needle.

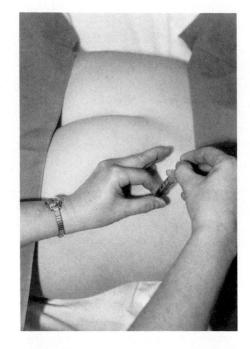

5 Carefully extend the thumb and forefinger of the hand that is displacing the tissue to support the base of the syringe. Aspirate with your other hand. *Do not release the traction on the tissue.*

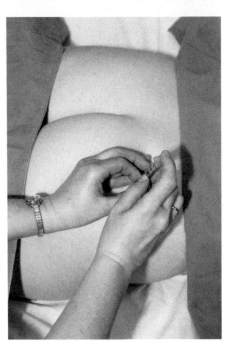

6 Continue to maintain the traction as you slowly inject the medication. When you have completed the injection, wait 10 seconds to provide the necessary time for the medication to disperse into the muscle and to give the muscle time to relax after having been stimulated by the needle and medication.

7 After waiting 10 seconds, remove the needle and immediately lift your other hand to release the tissue. Do not massage the injection site, and advise your client not to exercise or wear tight clothing following the injection. This will minimize the chance for the medication to spread into other layers of tissue.

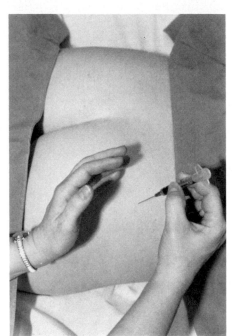

Nursing Guidelines for Managing Insulin Pumps

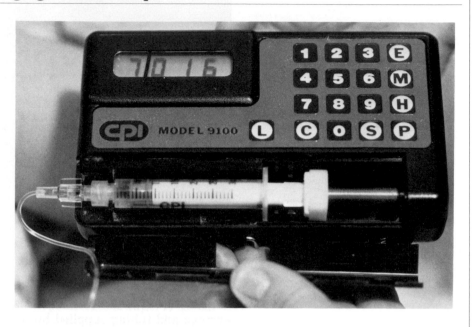

1 *An insulin pump* is a computerized device that delivers a constant insulin infusion throughout the day and night (called the basal delivery), with the capability of administering boluses manually at specified times, for example just prior to meals. Thus, unlike conventional insulin therapy, which relies on single or multiple daily injections, the insulin pump acts more like the client's own pancreas. However, unlike the pancreas, an insulin pump can only respond to the client's programming, based on frequent self-monitoring of blood glucose. There are several pumps available to the diabetic client, and each varies in method of operation and programming. Each pump has rechargeable batteries, a syringe, a programmable computer, and a motor and drive mechanism. Regular (short-acting) insulin is used, and it is contained by the syringe that inserts directly into the pump. A 60–105 cm (24–42 in.) length of plastic tubing attaches on one end to the syringe, and at the other end to a 27-gauge needle that is inserted into the subcutaneous tissue. The client may attach the pump to a leather belt, fabric belt, or shoulder strap or carry it in a purse or pocket.

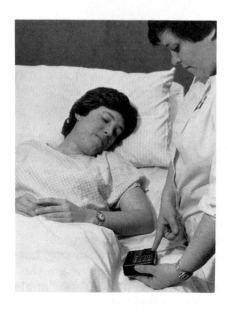

2 *If the physician* decides that your client is a good candidate for insulin-pump therapy, it may be your responsibility to explain the operational principles of the pump (each pump has a detailed manufacturer's manual), to reinforce the client's knowledge about dietary management, and to review self-monitoring of blood glucose (see steps, pp. 152–154). Initially, the basal rate and the meal boluses will be regulated by the physician, based on blood-glucose measurements. Frequent testing of the blood glucose must be performed, and it should become a part of the daily regimen of every client with an insulin pump. It is the client's best assessment tool for measuring the effectiveness of diabetes management.

Administering Intravenous Fluids and Medications

PREPARING THE SOLUTION AND INFUSION SET

Inspecting the Container

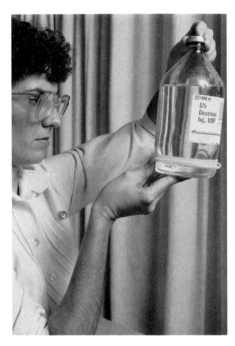

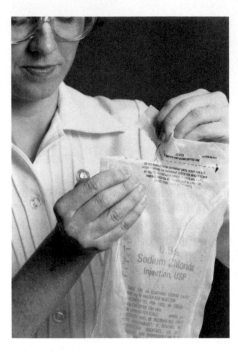

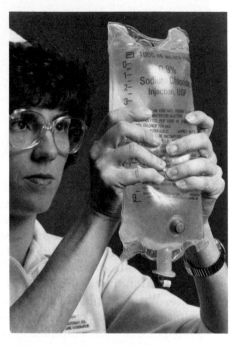

1 Wash your hands and inspect the label to ensure that the solution and amount match the physician's order and that the date for usage has not expired. Hold a glass container against a light source and observe for discoloration, cloudiness, particulate matter, and cracks while you slowly rotate the bottle. Replace the container with a new one if you detect any of these irregularities.

2 Will you administer a solution in a plastic container instead? Remove it from its overwrap after tearing along the broken line.

3 Inspect the plastic container in the same manner you would inspect a glass container, but, in addition, squeeze it gently and observe for leakage. Any irregularity, including leakage, necessitates replacement.

Assembling the Infusion Set

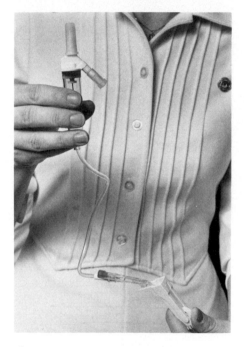

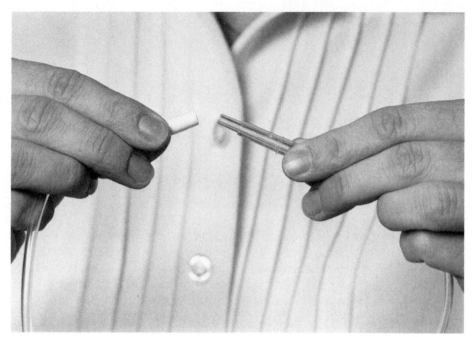

1 Inspect the package that contains the infusion set to ensure that it is intact, and then remove the tubing. If possible, slide the roller clamp directly under the drip chamber. If the tubing has a backcheck valve for the administration of piggyback fluids (as shown), slide the roller clamp up under the backcheck valve. <u>By sliding the clamp up as high as possible, you will have quick access to the clamp for controlling the drip rate</u>, and it will enable you to adjust the rate while closely monitoring the drip chamber. Then close the <u>roller clamp</u>.

2 If you want to allow the client more mobility or to provide extra ports for the administration of medication, you can attach extension tubing to the distal end of the IV tubing. Then close its slide clamp.

Spiking the Container

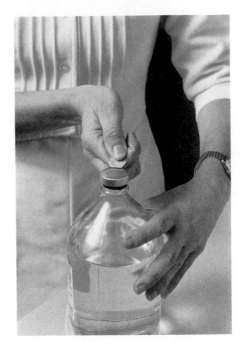
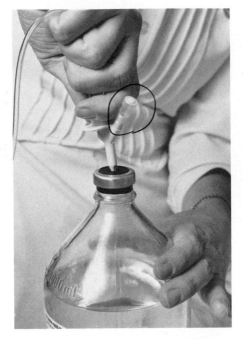
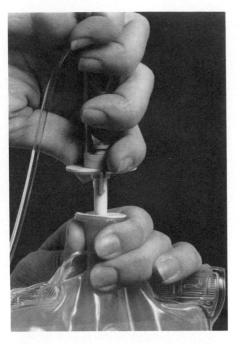

1 To ensure that contaminants have not entered the bottle, inspect the protective metal cap on a glass container to verify that it is intact. Then remove the cap. If the container also has a rubber diaphragm, remove it at this time. You should hear a swoosh of air as you remove it.

2 Place the container on a flat, secure surface. Remove the protective cap from the spike on infusion set, squeeze the drip chamber, and insert the spike into the rubber port of the glass container. Vented tubing, such as this, is more often used with glass containers unless the container itself has a vent.

3 To spike a plastic container, hold the neck securely and remove the protective tab. Then slide the spike through the port. With plastic containers, nonvented tubing is used.

Priming the Infusion Set

1 Hang the solution on an IV pole and, prior to opening the clamps and priming the tubing, squeeze the drip chamber and prime it with solution to the half-fill line. This will minimize the formation of air bubbles in the tubing when you prime the tubing.

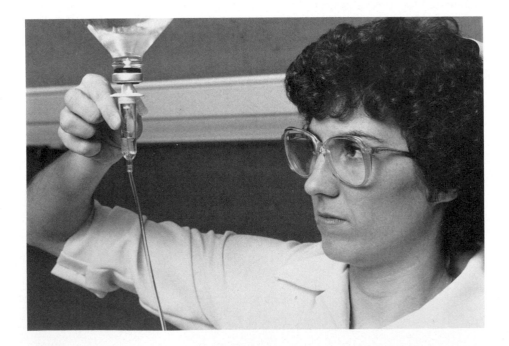

Attaching and Priming a Filter

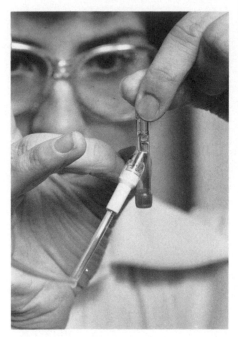

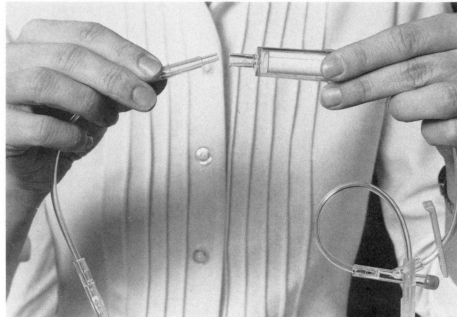

2 Open the clamps and let the solution flow to the end of the tubing to clear it of air. Hold the distal end of the tubing over a waste container or emesis basin as you do this. If the tubing has a backcheck valve (as shown), invert the valve as you prime the tubing and snap it lightly to disintegrate the bubbles. Reclamp the tubing and perform a venipuncture, or attach the primed tubing to the indwelling needle or catheter.

1 Filters are frequently attached to infusion tubing to ensure that particulate matter does not enter the client's bloodstream. Very fine filters (0.22 μ) are the most effective in filtering particulate matter; however, they are so fine that they may become clogged by viscous solutions. Be sure to read the manufacturer's instructions to ensure that your filter is compatible with the prescribed solution. If your infusion set does not have a built-in filter, attach the male end of the infusion set to the female end of the filter. To ensure a secure connection, twist the ends together tightly. Always tape the connection if the solution will be run through a central venous catheter.

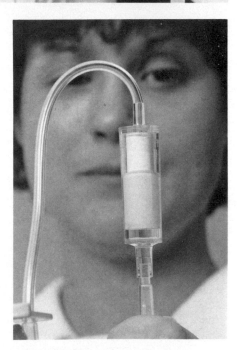

2 Before priming the filter, open the slide clamps on either side. Invert the filter and allow the solution to flow into it from the bottom to the top. Tap it lightly to disintegrate the bubbles.

Labeling the Tubing and Container

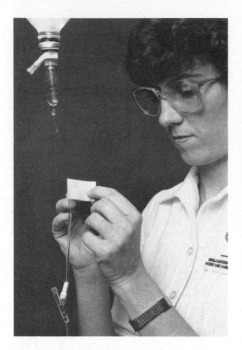

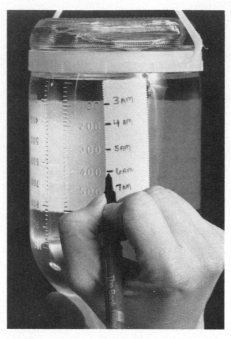

1 Attach a tape tab to the proximal end of the IV tubing, documenting the time and date the solution was hung. Change the tubing at least every 48 hours.

2 If the solution will be run slowly on a "keep vein open" (KVO) basis, label the container with the time and date it was hung. The container should be replaced at least every 24 hours. However, if it will be run more quickly, attach a timing label to enable you to carefully gauge the number of milliliters that must be infused hourly.

PERFORMING A VENIPUNCTURE

Assembling the Materials ⟶

Before selecting the puncture site and assembling the materials, determine whether the client will receive short-term or long-term therapy, and note the viscosity of the prescribed solution. Clients with faster running infusions, viscous solutions, and presurgical and obstetric clients who may require blood transfusions will all necessitate the use of larger needles, and hence, larger veins. Smaller wing-tipped needles are more often used for short-term therapy, for children, for older clients, or for clients with small, fragile veins. To perform a venipuncture, assemble the following materials: sterile gauze pads, tourniquet, air-occlusive 7.5-cm (3-in.) tape, 1.25-cm (½-in.) tape, 2.5-cm (1-in.) tape, bed-saver pad, arm board (optional) and wash cloth padding (optional), antimicrobial ointment such as povidone-iodine, and an antimicrobial skin preparation such as povidone-iodine. For this procedure, we have selected a wing-tipped (butterfly) needle.

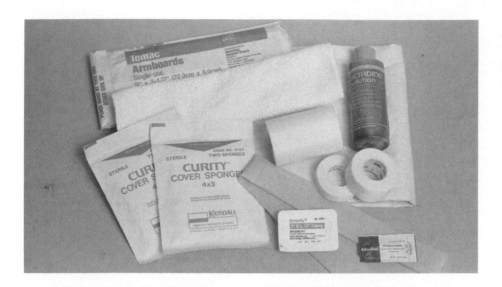

Choosing a Venipuncture Site

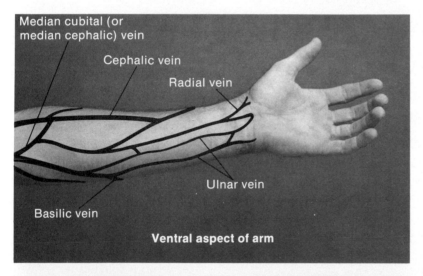

Median cubital (or median cephalic) vein

Cephalic vein

Radial vein

Ulnar vein

Basilic vein

Ventral aspect of arm

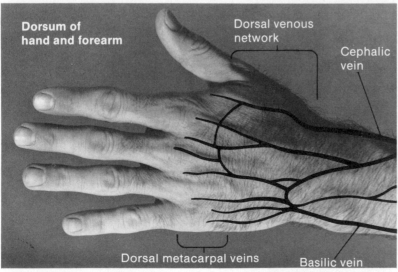

Dorsum of hand and forearm

Dorsal venous network

Cephalic vein

Dorsal metacarpal veins

Basilic vein

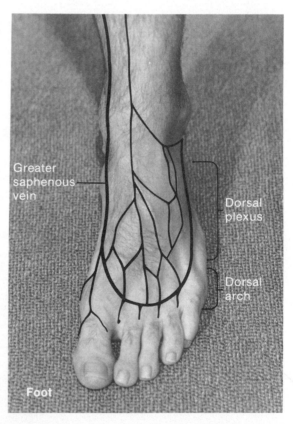

Greater saphenous vein

Dorsal plexus

Dorsal arch

Foot

1 Review these anatomic overlays to assist you in locating the proper sites for a venipuncture.

(Continued on p. 126)

Dilating the Vein

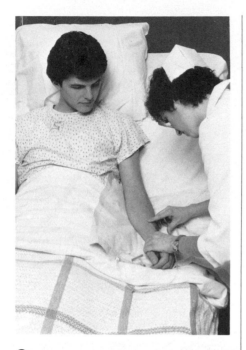

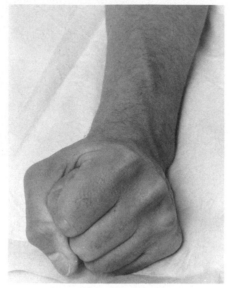

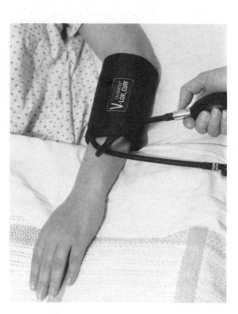

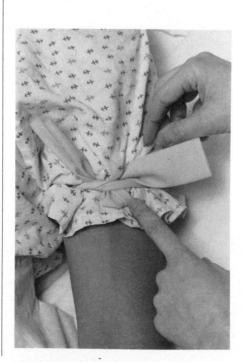

2 Wash your hands and explain the procedure to the client. Plan to use the nondominant arm if your client will have short-term therapy. Never use an arm with an arteriovenous fistula or the involved arm for a client who has had a radical mastectomy. Begin by inspecting the median, distal basilic, and cephalic veins in your client's hand and forearm. Observe for large, superficial, full veins in a site that is neither inflamed nor irritated. Palpate the site to ensure that the vein is soft, unscarred, and relatively straight. Always begin at the distal end of the vein, if possible, to preserve the proximal vein for future IV sites. If you can avoid it, stay away from joints such as the wrist and elbow because needles are easily dislodged in these areas.

1 If the veins are not readily prominent, ask the client to open and close his fist. You may also apply manual pressure by wrapping your hands around the area just proximal to the potential insertion site and squeezing moderately to help dilate the vein. Applying hot, moist towels around the insertion site is also effective for many clients.

2 *Note: If you still have difficulty palpating the veins, wrap a blood pressure cuff below the antecubital fossa and inflate it to just below your client's systolic pressure (usually around 100 mm Hg). Deflate the cuff after palpating the veins. If you plan to use the cuff instead of a tourniquet to dilate the veins, deflate it to 40 mm Hg after having dilated the veins.*

3 When you have selected a viable site, wrap a tourniquet a few inches above it. To prevent pinching the skin, position the tourniquet over an article of clothing such as the sleeve of the hospital gown. The tourniquet should be tight enough to impede venous flow but not so tight that it occludes the arteries. You should still be able to palpate an arterial pulse distal to the tourniquet.

Preparing the Site

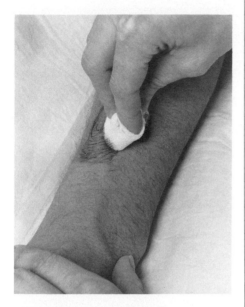

1 Prepare the insertion site by swabbing the skin with an antimicrobial solution such as povidone-iodine. Apply the solution directly to the center of the site with a sterile applicator such as a gauze pad.

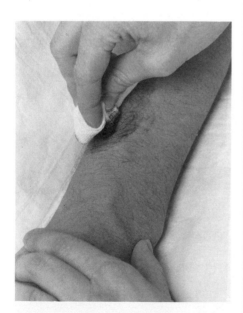

2 Prepare the surrounding skin using a circular motion and working outward to cover an area at least 5 cm (2 in.) in diameter. Repeat the process, using a fresh applicator each time. Allow the solution to dry thoroughly before inserting the needle.

Inserting a Wing-Tipped (Butterfly) Needle

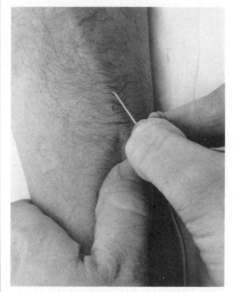

1 With your free thumb, stabilize and anchor the vein distal to the insertion site. Ask the client to sustain a fist if his vein is not prominent. With the needle's bevel up, squeeze the wings together and position the needle at a 30°–45° angle over the vein.

3 In most instances if you have inserted the needle properly, you will see a backflow of blood in the tubing. To prime the needle's tubing, allow the blood to fill its entire length. If the venipuncture has been unsuccessful, withdraw the needle, insert a new, sterile needle, and attempt the venipuncture again proximal to the initial site or in another vein.

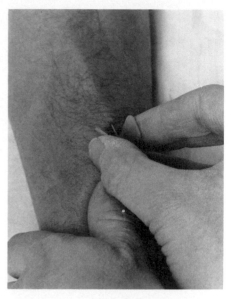

2 <u>As you pierce the skin and enter the vein, decrease the angle to around 15°.</u> Advance the needle into the vein and continue to decrease the angle of the needle until it is parallel to your client's skin. You will feel a release or a gentle pop as the needle enters the vein. Then ask your client to open his fist. Release the tourniquet.

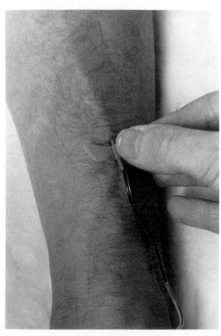

(Continued on p. 128)

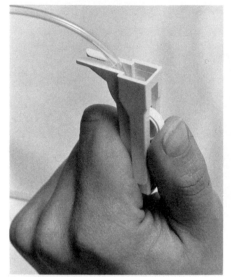

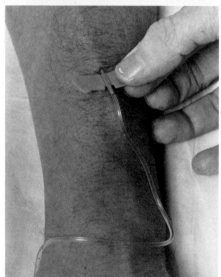

4 If the needle is to be used for the infusion of IV fluids, carefully attach the adaptor of the primed infusion tubing to the needle's connector; slowly open the roller clamp (top) to start the infusion. Observe the drip chamber for an easy flow and inspect the insertion site for the presence of swelling, which would occur if the needle were improperly positioned. When you are certain that the venipuncture has been successful, decrease the flow and prepare to tape the needle and tubing.

Taping the Wing-Tipped Needle

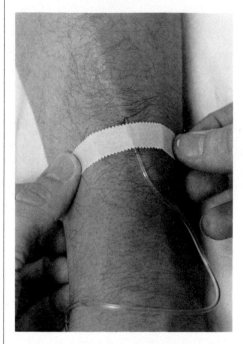

1 We recommend the following method for taping the wing-tipped needle. Cut three 7.5-cm (3-in.) strips of 1.25-cm (½-in.) tape. Place the first strip directly over the wings of the needle.

3 Place the third strip of tape over the looped tubing. Remember to keep the connector hub exposed so that you will have access to it for changing the tubing, for example, or for attaching an adaptor plug.

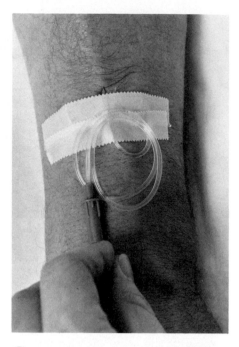

2 Attach the second strip of tape over the distal edge of the first strip. Then loop the tubing.

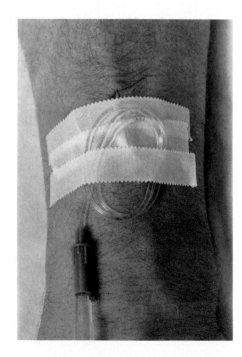

Inserting an Over-the-Needle Catheter (Angiocath)

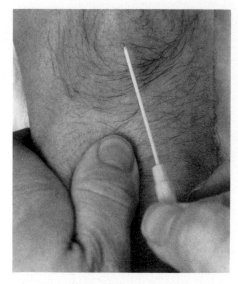

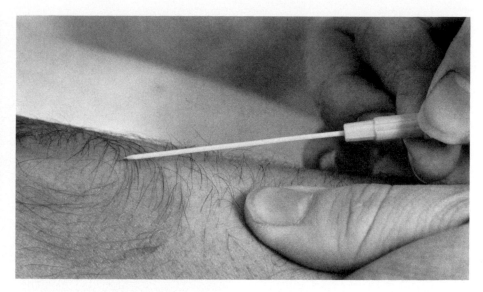

1 Review the preceding steps for preparing the skin and inserting a wing-tipped needle. Position the tip of the over-the-needle catheter

over the selected vein at a 30°–40° angle to the skin. With your free thumb, firmly anchor the vein distal to the insertion site.

As you pierce the skin, reduce the angle of the needle to around 15° (above).

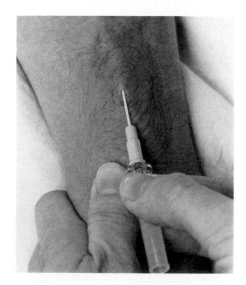

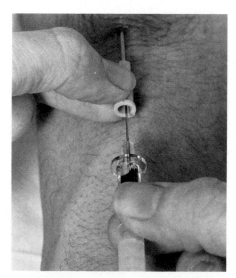

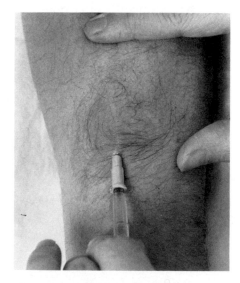

2 Continue to advance the catheter into the vein and decrease the angle as you do until the needle is parallel to the skin. After the catheter has been inserted approximately 2.5 cm (1 in.), release the tourniquet. Remove the protective cap from the distal end of the infusion tubing and hold the tubing carefully between your last two fingers so that you are prepared for the next step.

3 Firmly grasp the catheter hub with your thumb and index finger and withdraw the needle with your free hand. If the catheter has been properly positioned, you should see a backflow of blood in the plastic hub of the needle.

4 After removing the needle, attach the distal end of the primed infusion tubing. Open the roller clamp slowly and observe for an easy flow of solution into the drip chamber. To double check, you can also apply pressure to the vein just proximal to the insertion site (as shown). If the dripping stops in the drip chamber at this time, you can be quite certain that the vein is patent and the needle has been properly positioned.

Taping the Over-the-Needle Catheter

1 An effective way to tape the over-the-needle catheter is to employ the "U" method. To do this, you will need three 7.5-cm (3-in.) strips of 1.25-cm (½-in.) tape. Place the first strip sticky side up under the needle's hub. Fold the end over (as shown) so that the sticky side adheres to the skin.

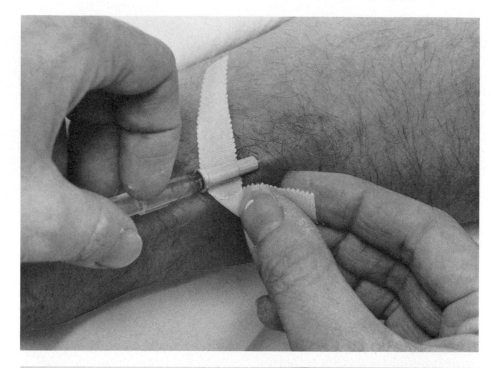

2 Fold the opposite over up in the same manner.

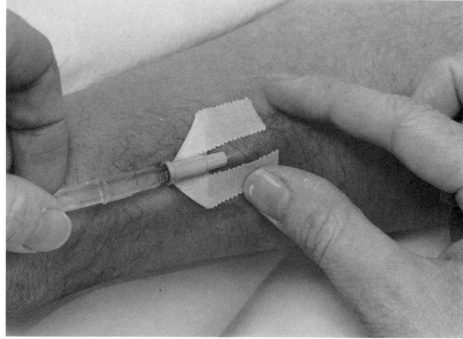

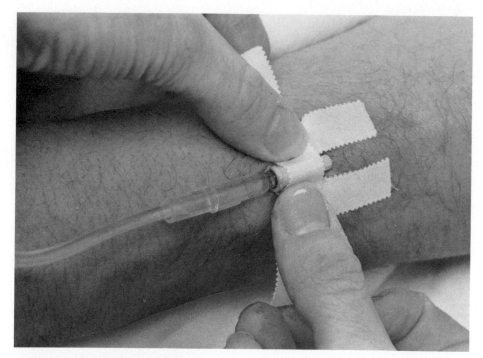

3 Place a second strip of tape sticky side down over the needle's hub.

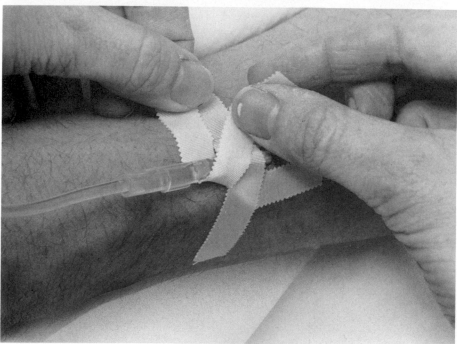

4 Place the third strip of tape sticky side up under the catheter hub and distal to the second strip. Then fold it diagonally across the hub sticky side down (as shown). Do the same for the opposite side of the tape.

Applying the Antimicrobial Ointment and Dressing

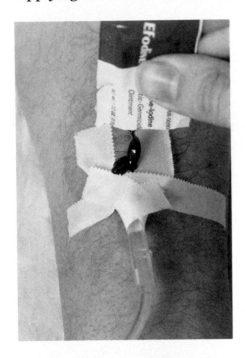

1 Generously apply the antimicrobial ointment directly to the taped insertion site. If possible, always use a single-unit dose to minimize the chance for infection.

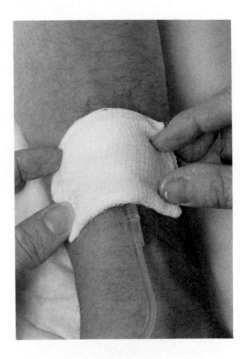

2 Cover the area with a sterile gauze pad. →

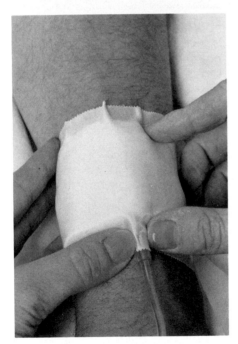

3 Cover the gauze dressing with a 7.5 × 10-cm (3 × 4-in.) strip of tape. *Note: Transparent sterile dressings such as Op-Site are also recommended. These dressings allow close observation of the insertion site without the removal of the dressing.*

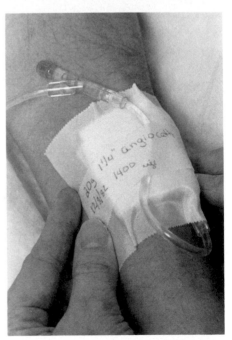

4 Loop the tubing over the tape. → Secure it with a 2.5-cm (1-in.) strip of tape upon which you have written the time and date of insertion, the type and gauge of needle, and your initials. At least daily, gently palpate the insertion site through the dressing to assess for tenderness. If the client has tenderness at the insertion site or an unexplained fever, you must visually inspect the site for redness or discharge. The needle or catheter should be changed every 48–72 hours unless another peripheral insertion site cannot be found at that time.

IMMOBILIZING THE EXTREMITY

Using an Armboard or Splint

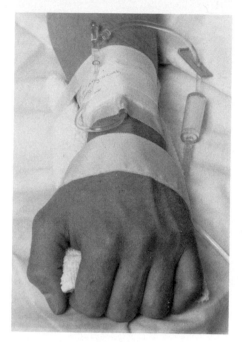

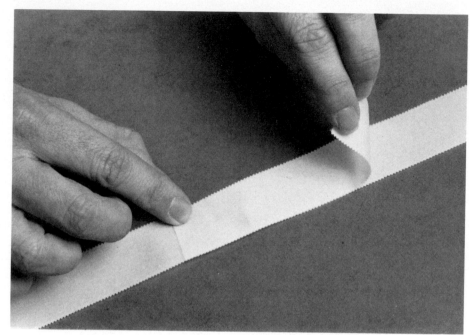

1 To prevent the needle or catheter from dislodging, it will be necessary for you to splint the extremity when a client is disoriented or combative or when the venipuncture site is at or near a joint such as the wrist or elbow. For your client's comfort, be sure to pad the armboard or splint with a small towel or wash cloth. A short splint will usually be adequate if the venipuncture site is in the lower arm or hand, but use a long splint if the site is near the antecubital fossa. The hand should be prone (as shown) and well-supported by the splint if the needle is in the hand or wrist. However, the fingers should be free both to extend and to flex around the armboard.

2 Secure the splint to the arm with two or three tape strips. To make a tape strip, you will need two pieces of tape of equal widths. Tear one piece long enough to encircle the arm and splint. The shorter piece should be just long enough to face the longer piece over the area that would otherwise cover the skin. Place the shorter piece of tape in the center of the longer piece with the sticky surfaces together (as shown). Then wrap the tape strip snugly around the arm and the splint. Be certain, however, that you do not impede circulation. Monitor the client frequently to ensure that color, sensation, and pulses are normal in the hand and arm.

Applying a Commercial Wrist Restraint

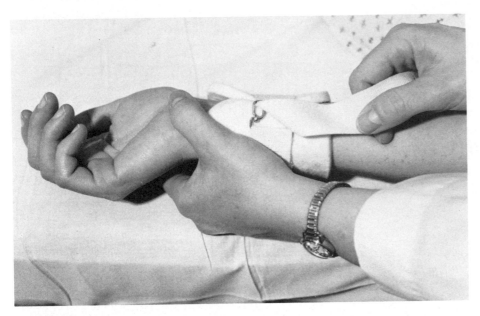

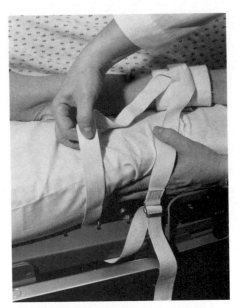

1 If you have a physician's order, you can restrain the wrist of a disoriented or combative client who may potentially dislodge the needle or catheter in the opposite arm. Wrap a commercial restraint snugly (but not tightly) around the wrist to prevent the client from pulling the hand through the opening.

2 Attach the restraint to the bed frame. *Caution: Never attach the restraint to the side rails because this could result in injury to the arm when the side rails are lowered.* Allow enough slack in the restraint to provide the client adequate range of motion yet prevent contact with the opposite arm. Because the restraint will prevent normal movement, it is essential that you remove the restraint and change your client's position every 2 hours. Provide range of motion (ROM) exercises if the client must be restrained on a long-term basis. Also, ensure that color, sensation, and pulses are normal distal to the restraint, and provide skin care such as massages with a moisturizer if the skin under the restraint shows any signs of irritation.

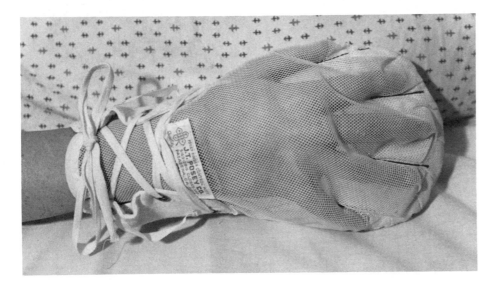

3 As an alternative, a mitt restraint may be applied to prevent the client from removing the needle or catheter in the opposite arm. Ensure that it is tied snugly but not tightly around the wrist and that it is removed at least once per shift (or according to agency protocol) to provide skin care and to perform ROM exercises on the wrist and fingers.

Applying a Gauze Restraint

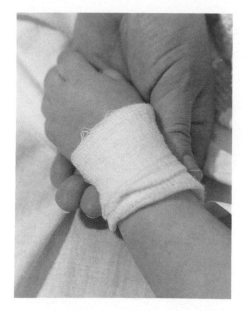

1 If commercially made restraints are unavailable, you can improvise with gauze pads and a strip of gauze roll at least 125 cm (50 in.) in length. First pad around the wrist with a double thickness of gauze padding.

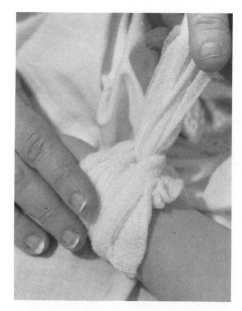

2 Tie the gauze roll around the gauze pad using a knot, such as a slip knot (as shown), that can be readily released in the event of an emergency.

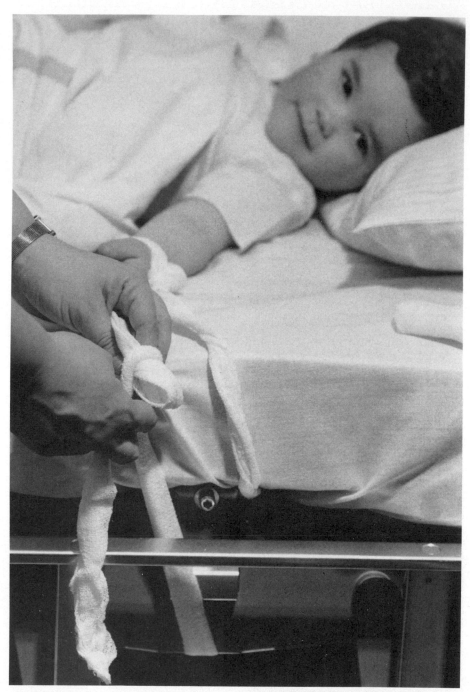

3 Wrap the gauze roll around the bed frame (not the side rails) and tie it in a bow so that you can easily release it in an emergency. When using gauze rather than a commercial restraint, it is especially important that you monitor the client frequently for signs of neurovascular impairment because of the difficulty in controlling the degree of tension on the wrist. Remove the restraint every 2 hours and ensure that color, sensation, and pulse are normal; provide skin care as necessary.

ADMINISTERING INTRAVENOUS (IV) MEDICATIONS

Injecting Medications into Hanging IV Containers

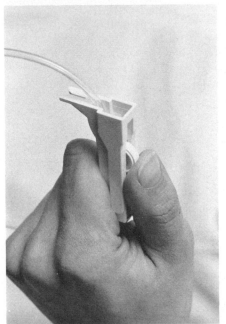

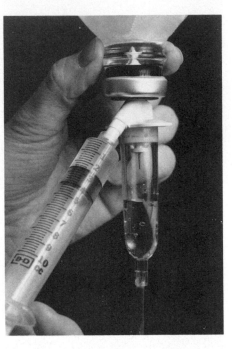

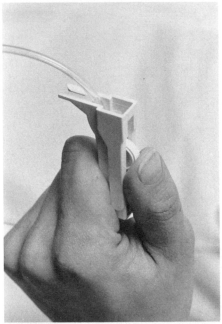

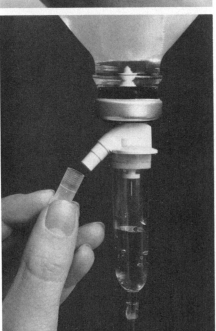

2 Remove the needle from the medication syringe and insert the syringe directly into the air vent. Inject the medication, and then gently rotate the bottle between your hands to mix the medication. Vigorous shaking would produce air bubbles. Open the roller clamp, and adjust the rate of flow to the prescribed amount. Label the bottle with the type and amount of medication, the time and date it was added, and your initials. Document that medication was added to the IV infusion.

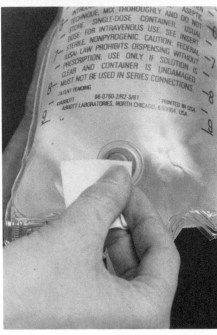

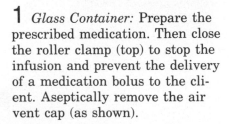

1 *Glass Container:* Prepare the prescribed medication. Then close the roller clamp (top) to stop the infusion and prevent the delivery of a medication bolus to the client. Aseptically remove the air vent cap (as shown).

1 *Plastic Container:* Prepare the prescribed medication, and close the roller clamp (top) to stop the flow of solution. This will prevent the delivery of a medication bolus to your client. Clean the injection port with an alcohol sponge.

Giving Medications by IV Bolus

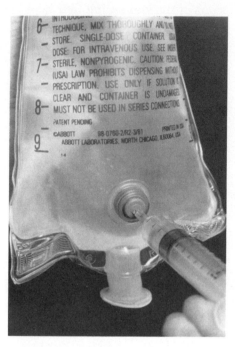

2 Insert the needle into the injection port and inject the medication. Gently rotate the bag between your hands to mix the medication; open the roller clamp to achieve the desired rate of flow. Make a medication label, noting the type and amount of medication, the time and date you added it, and your initials. Attach the label to the IV container, and document the medication.

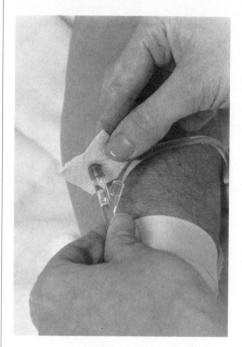

1 *Through a Primary Line:*
After drawing up the prescribed medication, swab the injection port with an alcohol sponge.

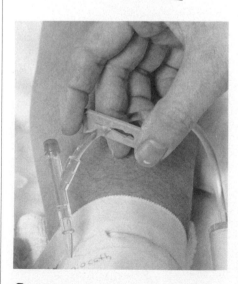

2 Close the roller clamp to stop the flow of the hanging solution; then close the slide clamp on the extension tubing (as shown), to ensure that the medication will be delivered directly into the client's vein.

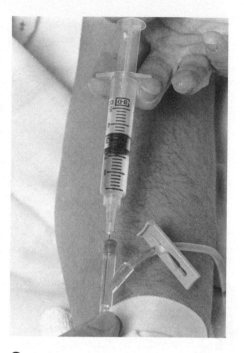

3 If the hanging solution is compatible with the medication, insert the needle of the medication syringe into the injection port. To avoid dislodging the needle or catheter, stabilize the port between the thumb and index finger of your free hand; then aspirate for a blood return to ensure that the needle or catheter is safely in the vein. Inject the medication at the prescribed rate. Stop the infusion immediately if the client exhibits a reaction to the drug. *Note: If the medication is incompatible with the IV solution, flush the tubing before and after the bolus with infusions of normal saline.* Open both clamps, and allow the hanging solution to flow again at the prescribed rate. Document the medication.

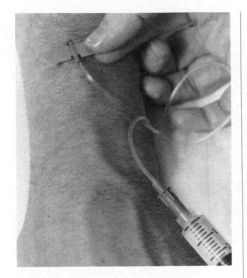

Through a Wing-Tipped (Butterfly) Needle: If an intravenous medication has been prescribed for a client who does not have an indwelling catheter or needle, prepare the medication, and insert a wing-tipped needle (see steps, pp. 127–128). A wing-tipped needle will be more stable than a needle that is attached to a syringe, and it will be less likely to become dislodged and traumatize the client's vein. After inserting the needle, remove the needle from the syringe and attach the syringe to the administration port of the extension tubing. Anchor the wings of the needle with your free thumb and index finger as you aspirate for a backflow of blood. This will not only ensure that the needle is in the vein, it will also fill the extension tubing with blood so that you can inject the medication without forcing air into your client's vein. Then slowly inject the medication at the prescribed rate. This may take anywhere from a minute to several minutes. Stop the infusion immediately if your client shows any signs of an allergic reaction. When the medication has been infused, remove the needle and apply pressure at the insertion site with a sterile gauze pad. Maintain the pressure for a minute, or until the client stops bleeding.

Inserting a Male Adaptor Plug (Heparin Lock) for Intermittent Infusion Therapy

An intermittent infusion set (heparin lock) is an indwelling reservoir in the vein for intermittent infusion therapy when continuous infusion therapy is not indicated. Periodic injections of heparin into the device keep the needle or catheter patent. Be sure to follow your agency's protocol for injections of normal saline and heparin both before and after infusions into the lock. Indications for using either solution will vary from agency to agency.

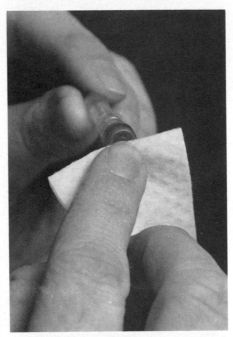

1 When continuous infusion therapy has been discontinued for your client who has an indwelling over-the-needle catheter, you can insert a male adaptor plug (MAP) into the catheter to convert it to a heparin lock. Before inserting the plug, swab the injection port with an alcohol sponge. Maintain asepsis by holding it by its protective cap (as shown).

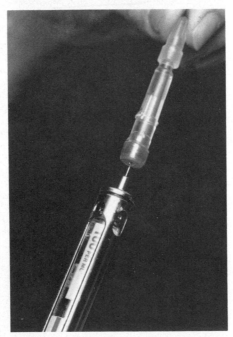

2 Prime the MAP with the prescribed amount of heparinized solution both to keep it patent and to remove air from the chamber. *Note: Normal saline is used to prime the MAP in some agencies.*

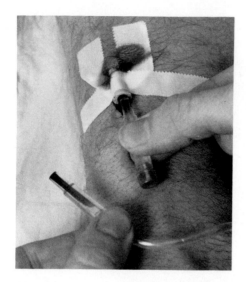

3 Close the roller clamp on the infusion set to stop the infusion, and aseptically remove the protective cap from the MAP. Detach the IV tubing, and insert the primed adaptor plug into the catheter hub. Apply a fresh dressing (see steps, p. 132) being certain to keep the injection port outside the air-occlusive tape for quick access.

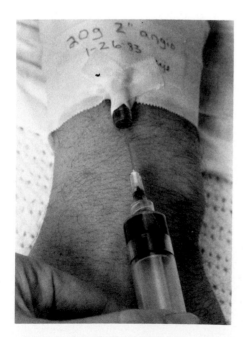

4 To inject medications into the heparin lock, follow this general procedure. Remember to modify it according to your agency's protocol.

a. *In three separate syringes* draw up the prescribed medication: 4 mL normal saline, or the prescribed amount, and 0.5 mL heparinized solution. The syringe needles should be no longer than 2.5 cm (1 in.) and the gauge should be small (25 gauge, for example) to avoid large puncture holes in the injection port.

b. *Swab the injection port* with an alcohol sponge.

c. *Insert the syringe* containing the normal saline and aspirate for a blood return to ensure that the catheter is in the vein.

d. *Inject* 2 mL of normal saline to flush the heparin from the catheter. (Some agencies advocate omitting this step and proceeding to the next step).

e. *Remove the syringe* containing the normal saline, cap it to maintain the needle's asepsis, and attach the medication syringe. Inject the medication slowly, at the prescribed rate of infusion. Observe for adverse reactions to the medication.

f. *Remove the medication* syringe and reattach the syringe containing the normal saline to flush the medication and prepare the lock for the heparin.

g. *Remove the normal saline* syringe and insert the syringe with the heparinized solution to fill the lock and ensure patency for subsequent infusions.

h. *Every 8–12 hours* ensure patency by aspirating and flushing with 2–3 mL of normal saline. Then refill the lock with the heparinized solution. Unless another peripheral insertion site cannot be found, the heparin lock should be changed every 48–72 hours.

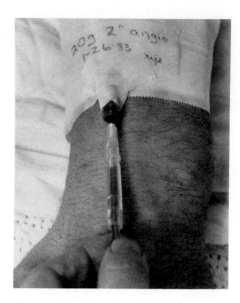

5 To administer intermittent infusions of a hanging solution, attach a 2.5-cm (1-in.) needle to the male end of the infusion tubing. Swab the injection port of the MAP with an alcohol sponge, and insert the infusion tubing (as shown). Adjust the roller clamp to achieve the desired rate of flow.

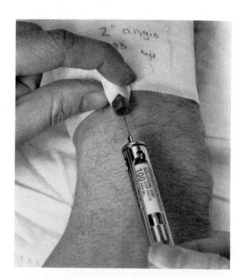

6 After discontinuing the hanging solution, clean the injection port with an alcohol sponge, and inject the prescribed amount of heparinized solution to ensure patency of the lock for subsequent infusions.

Giving Medications via a Partial-Fill (Piggyback) Container

Piggyback medications are administered through an established IV line via a secondary (piggyback) bottle, which attaches to the upper injection port on the primary line. The primary line must have a back-check valve to prevent the tubing from running dry after the piggyback bottle empties. The back-check valve allows the primary solution to run, after the piggyback solution reaches the level of the drip chamber on the primary infusion tubing.

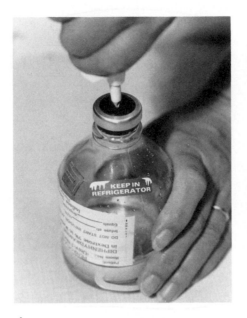

1 The piggyback infusion set can be primed by following the same general steps for priming a primary set (see pp. 122–123). However, the following steps for priming piggyback tubing will ensure that none of the medication is wasted during the priming. This is especially important when minute quantities of medication are to be infused. Close the slide clamp on the piggyback infusion set. On a flat surface, spike the piggyback bottle containing the medication.

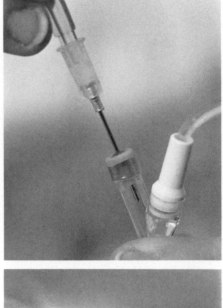

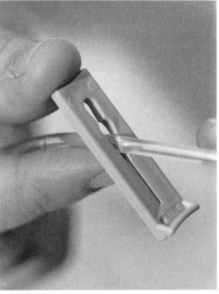

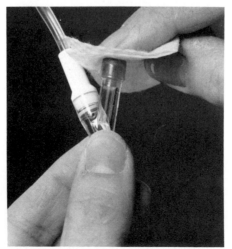

2 Swab the upper injection port on the primary line with an alcohol sponge.

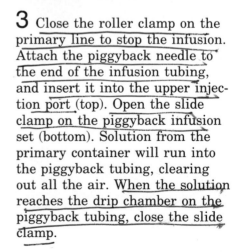

3 Close the roller clamp on the primary line to stop the infusion. Attach the piggyback needle to the end of the infusion tubing, and insert it into the upper injection port (top). Open the slide clamp on the piggyback infusion set (bottom). Solution from the primary container will run into the piggyback tubing, clearing out all the air. When the solution reaches the drip chamber on the piggyback tubing, close the slide clamp.

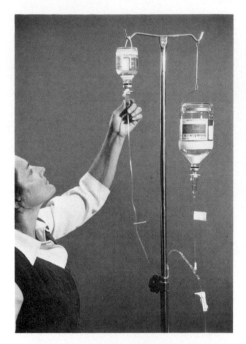

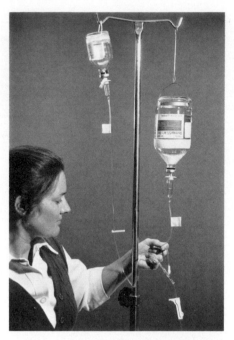

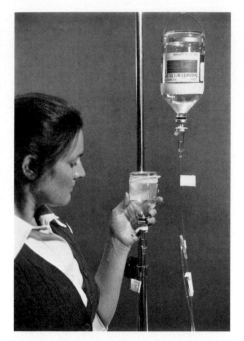

4 Hang the piggyback bottle on the IV pole. You will need an extension hook to rehang the primary set, making it lower than the piggyback container. This will activate the back-check valve. Squeeze the drip chamber on the piggyback tubing and fill the drip chamber to the half-fill mark. Adjust the roller clamp on the primary tubing to regulate the rate of flow. Finally, label the piggyback's infusion tubing with the time and date. Document the medication.

5 *Note: When the piggyback container empties, you can administer the residual medication in the tubing by pinching the primary tubing just above the upper injection port until the fluid level reaches the needle at the upper injection port. When you release the pressure on the tubing, solution from the primary container may move into the piggyback tubing, but the back-check valve will prevent it from entering the piggyback bottle.*

6 If you will need to hang a second piggyback bottle, close the roller clamp on the primary set and lower the empty bottle below the drip chamber on the primary set (as shown). Open the slide clamp on the piggyback tubing and allow the primary solution to fill the piggyback tubing. Close the slide clamp on the piggyback tubing, remove the spike from the empty container, and aseptically insert it into the newly prepared piggyback container. Hang it on the IV pole, open the slide clamp, and adjust the flow rate with the roller clamp on the primary set.

Assembling a Volume-Control IV Set

When it is necessary for you to administer precise doses of dilute medications to a child (or to an adult) over an extended period of time, a volume-control set will make this a safe and effective procedure for your client. Hang it as a primary line for a child. For an adult, it is most often used on a secondary line.

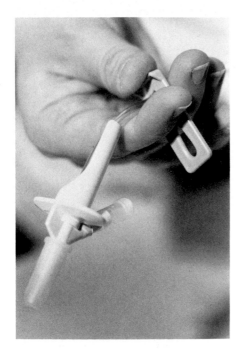

1 Prepare the IV container. Then slide the roller clamp up under the drip chamber and close it off. Close the main slide clamp under the spike (as shown). Remove the spike's protective cover, spike the container, and suspend it on an IV pole.

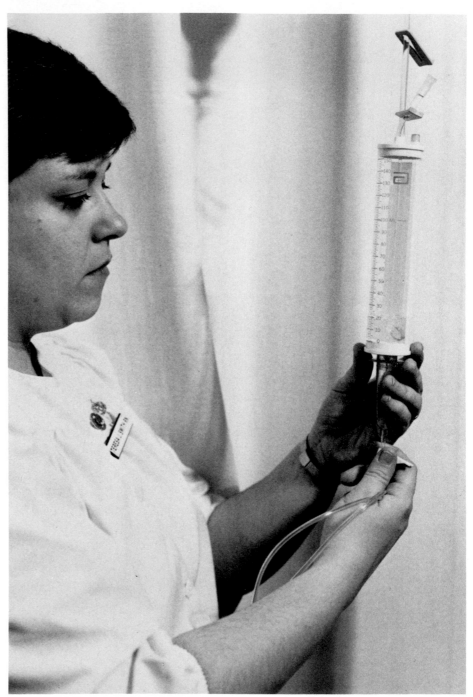

2 Open the main slide clamp and allow 25 mL of the solution to enter the burette (the fluid chamber). Close the main slide clamp.

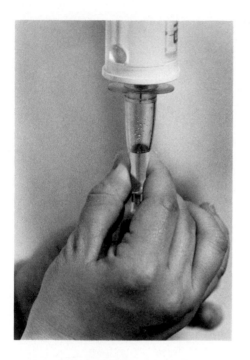

3 Squeeze the drip chamber to fill it to the half-fill line. This should also float the diaphragm at the base of the burette. Then open the roller clamp and allow the solution to flush the air from the tubing. Close the roller clamp. *Note: If the drip chamber becomes overfilled, close all the clamps and invert the burette. Squeeze the drip chamber to expel the excess fluid into the burette.*

4 To add medication to the burette, first ensure that the air filter (on the right in the photo) is open. Then clean the medication port with an alcohol sponge, and inject the prescribed medication (as shown).

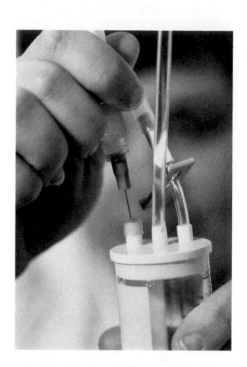

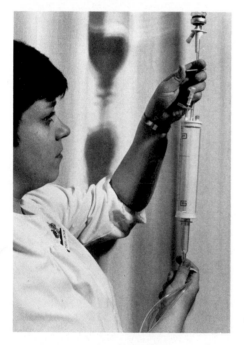

5 If the medication requires diluting, open the main slide clamp to add the desired amount of solution to the burette. Then close the slide clamp.

6 Gently roll the burette between your hands to mix the medication with the solution. Attach the distal end of the tubing either to your client's indwelling needle or catheter, or to the injection port on the primary tubing. Open the roller clamp, and administer the medication at the prescribed rate. The flow will automatically shut off when the burette empties. To refill the burette, repeat steps 2 and 3 above. Be sure to label the burette with the name and dose of the medication and your initials. Document the medication.

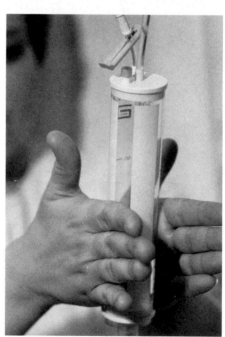

USING INFUSION CONTROLLERS AND PUMPS

Operating the Abbott LifeCare 1000 Controller

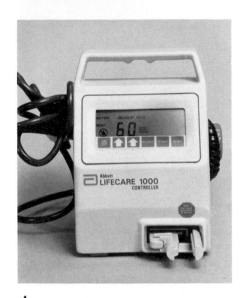

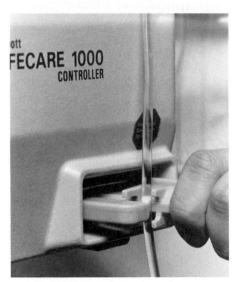

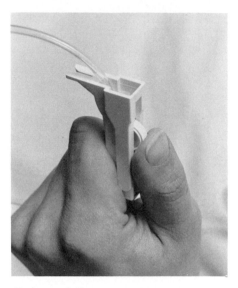

1 Does your agency use infusion controllers to monitor the delivery of IV solutions? These devices control the delivery rate by monitoring and adjusting the drop rate to that of the preset rate. The Abbott Lifecare 1000 Controller (as shown) is used in many agencies. It automatically stops the delivery of the solution and sounds an alarm to alert you when the container is empty, the tubing is kinked or occluded, and in many instances if the solution has infiltrated. It works either on alternating current or battery power, and it attaches to an IV pole. Because it works by gravitational force, rather than by mechanically generated pressure, be sure to hang the IV container at least 1 m (39 in.) above the venipuncture site.

2 Follow the steps, pp. 122–123, to spike the container, prime the infusion tubing, and attach the primed tubing to the indwelling needle. Insert the infusion tubing into the controller's pinch clamp (as shown). Later, when the controller is activated, the pinch clamp will function as a replacement for the roller clamp.

3 Open the roller clamp from its closed position by rolling it all the way up. This will ensure that the only device controlling the rate of flow will be the controller's pinch clamp.

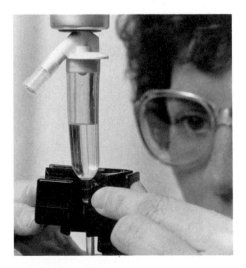

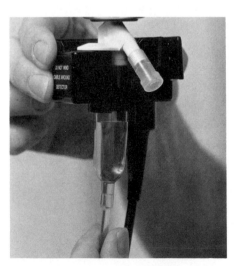

4 Attach the drop detector by inserting it around the infusion tubing just distal to the drip chamber.

5 Slide the device up and over the drip chamber. Snap it into place.

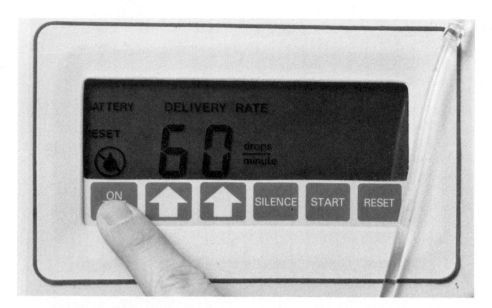

6 To activate the panel, press the "on/off" touchswitch on the far left of the panel.

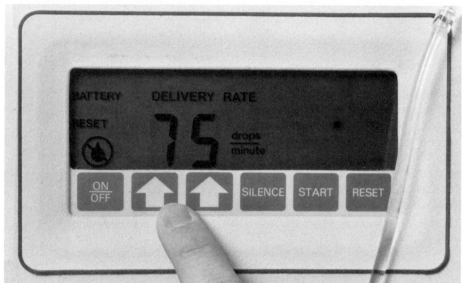

7 Press the touchswitches depicted with arrows until the desired delivery rate has been established. *Note: Refer to the chart on the side panel for milliliters per hour to drops per minute conversion.*

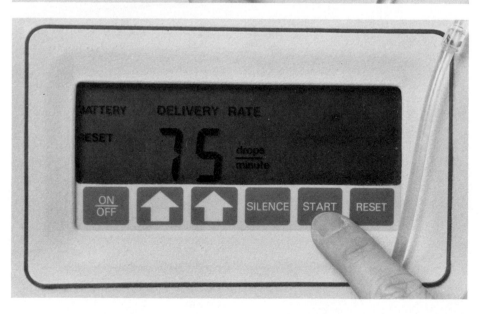

8 Press the start touchswitch to begin operation. A message will appear on the panel telling you the machine is starting up. A drop symbol will then appear and blink on and off once the programmed drop rate has been achieved. Should the alarm sound, press the "silence" touchswitch and read the message panel to determine the problem. Then press the "reset" touchswitch, correct the problem, and push "start" to reoperate.

Using the Abbott LifeCare Model 3 Pump

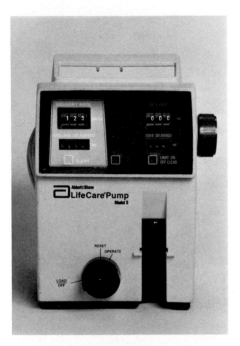

1 Infusion pumps are indicated for clients who need accurate and carefully monitored flow rates, as well as those for whom positive pressure is required for the delivery of highly viscous solutions. The Abbott LifeCare Model 3 Pump is one type of infusion pump that is found in many agencies. It requires the use of special Abbott tubing, which has an inline cassette.

2 Remove the special infusion tubing from its container. Close the slide clamp (as shown) and then close the roller clamp.

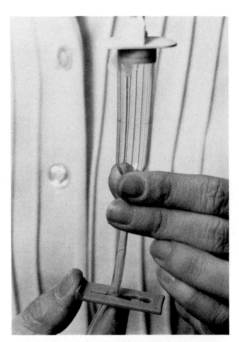

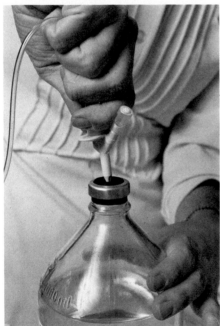

3 Spike the solution container, and suspend the container on an IV pole, making sure the distance from the top of the container to the pump's cassette is around 90 cm (36 in.). Open the slide clamp (bottom) in preparation for priming the tubing. Review the steps, pp. 120–123, to assist you with these steps.

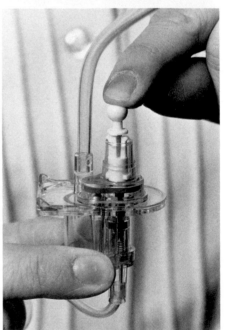

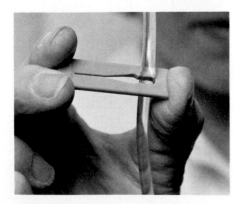

4 Locate the inline cassette, and push down its white plunger (as shown). This will enable the solution to run through the cassette. The cassette is crucial both for the operation of the pump and your client's safety because it maintains the prescribed rate of flow, and it prevents air from entering your client's bloodstream.

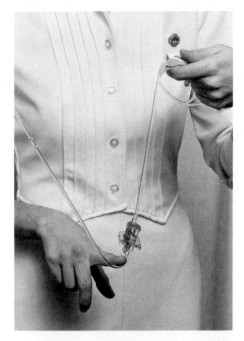

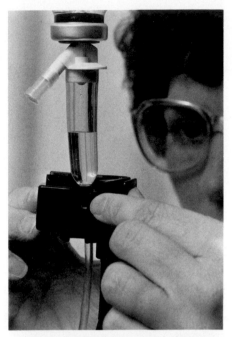

5 Invert the cassette (the white plunger will be lowermost), and completely open the roller clamp to facilitate the rapid flow of solution through the cassette, which will expel air from its chamber. When the solution has passed through the cassette, reduce the flow rate by adjusting the roller clamp; tap the cassette with your fingertips to disintegrate the air bubbles. Run the solution to the end of the tubing, ensuring that you have removed the air bubbles from the entire system. Then close the roller clamp.

6 Attach the drop detector to the →
drip chamber by inserting it around the infusion tubing just distal to the drop chamber (as shown).

7 Then slide it up around the chamber and snap it into place.

8 Set the prescribed delivery →
rate, which is calibrated in milliliters per hour.

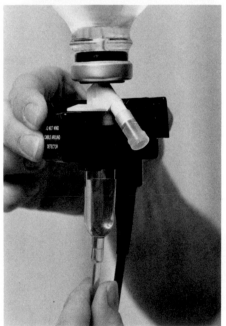

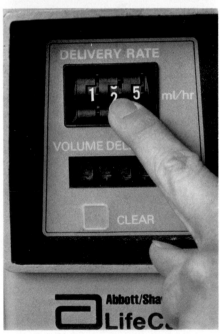

(Continued on p. 148)

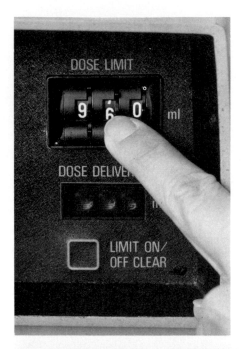

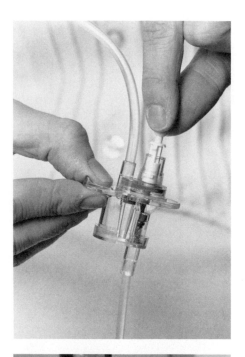

9 You may also set the dose limit (as shown) if you need to administer a specific amount of solution. *Note: After a dose limit has been achieved, an alarm will sound and the solution will continue to infuse at a "keep vein open" (KVO) rate.*

10 Pull up on the white ⟶ plunger on the cassette. This will shut off the solution to gravity flow. To confirm that the flow has ceased, check the drip chamber to ensure that the drops have stopped.

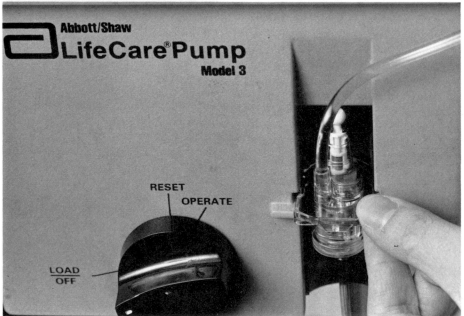

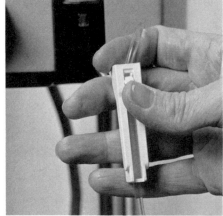

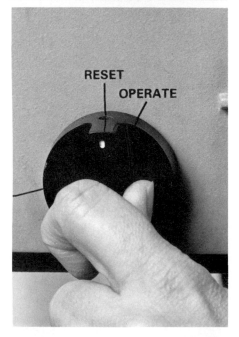

11 Make sure the control switch has been turned to "load/off" and insert the cassette into the pump receptacle with the plunger upright. It will snap into place.

12 Open the roller clamp (right center), and turn the control switch to "reset" (bottom).

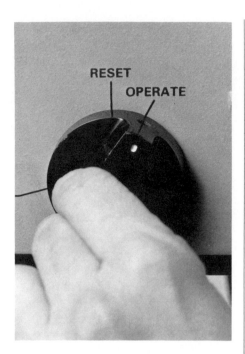

13 After attaching the infusion tubing to your client's venipuncture site, you may then turn the control switch to "operate." Monitor the client frequently, and be alert to the flow alarm, which will sound if the flow rate deviates from the established rate or the container becomes empty. If the alarm does sound, push the silence button and observe the message panel to identify the problem. The pump will have reverted to a KVO rate at this point. Correct the problem and turn the switch to "reset" and then back to "operate" to reactivate the system.

ADMINISTERING IV FAT EMULSIONS

1 Fat emulsions are prescribed for clients who are deficient in essential fatty acids due to disorders such as severe burns, end-stage kidney diseases, ulcerative colitis, or malignancies. They may be administered either via peripheral or central veins, and they are usually delivered along with total parenteral nutrition solutions, which help restore the client's other nutritional deficiencies. It is important that you take the vital signs prior to administering the fat emulsion so that you have a baseline for subsequent assessment during the infusion. If the solution has been refrigerated, let it stand for 30 minutes at room temperature so that the client will be more comfortable during the infusion. Liposyn, however, is stored at room temperature. Inspect the solution for signs of instability, such as discoloration or curdling, and discard the container if you note either of these irregularities. Your agency may specify a certain type of tubing for infusing fat emulsions because some plastic tubings may be incompatible with lipids. If you will deliver the solution via an infusion pump, use the special tubing recommended by the manufacturer of the pump. For gravity infusions, however, a macrodrip tubing will more easily accomodate the fat globules. Spike the container (as shown), and hang it on an IV pole. Then prime the tubing, being certain to flush out all the air. To minimize the formation of air bubbles, prime the tubing more slowly than you would with a less viscous solution.

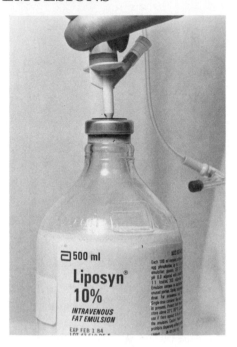

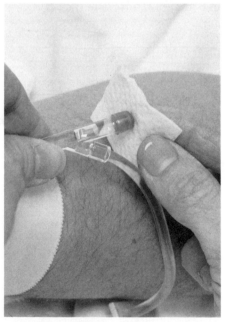

2 With an alcohol swab, clean the injection port that is closest to the insertion site. Using this port rather than others that may be farther up on the infusion tubing will minimize the amount of time during which the fat emulsion will mix with the primary solution and decrease the potential for the emulsion to break down. *(Continued on p. 150)*

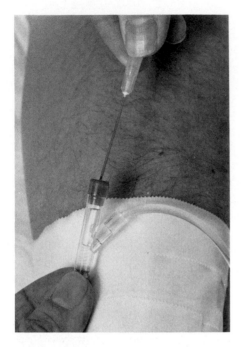

3 Attach a 20-gauge needle to the end of the infusion tubing and insert it into the port. Securely tape the connection. Remember that you must not connect a filter below the insertion of the fat emulsion because the density of the solution would clog the filter.

4 Note that because of its viscosity, the fat emulsion is hung higher than the total parenteral nutrition solution when gravity infusion is used. This prevents the solution from backing up into the infusion tubing. Be sure to label the container with the time and date the solution was hung. To minimize the chance for bacterial growth, the solution should be discarded if it has not infused within 12 hours. To prevent waste, smaller flasks should be hung if the unit of use required over a 12-hour period is considerably less than 500 mL. In most instances, the fat emulsion will be infused slowly at first to test the client's ability to tolerate the lipids. Guidelines for infusion will vary, depending on the manufacturer, the concentration of the fat emulsion, and the route of administration (either peripheral or central vein). Follow physician or agency guidelines carefully to ensure your client's comfort and safety. In many cases, no more than 1 mL/min should be delivered during the first 30 minutes, and vital signs should be taken every 10 minutes. For infants and

children, you may be required to administer as little as 0.1 mL/min. Assess for adverse reactions to the fat emulsion, for example: chilling, fever, headache, nausea, vomiting, dyspnea, and chest pain. If these reactions occur, stop the infusion and notify the physician. If there is no reaction, increase the infusion to the prescribed rate. As a general guideline, the usual adult dosage is 500 mL/day, and it should never be delivered over a period of less than 4–6 hours. A child usually receives 250 mL/day. Continue to assess the client for an adverse reaction during the period of time the fat emulsion is being delivered. In addition, closely monitor the laboratory values for the serum triglycerides and liver function tests, which are indicators of your client's ability to metabolize the lipids. However, blood should not be drawn for 4–6 hours after the fat emulsion has been administered because the lipids would not have left the bloodstream and an incorrect blood value could result.

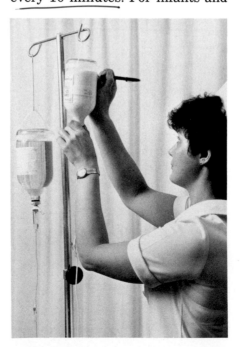

Collecting, Monitoring, and Administering Blood

COLLECTING A BLOOD SAMPLE WITH A VACUTAINER

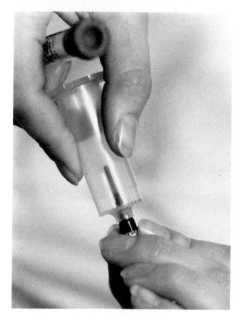

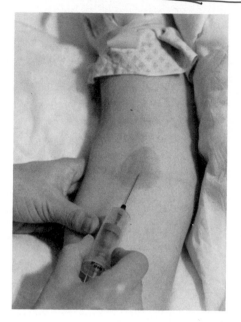

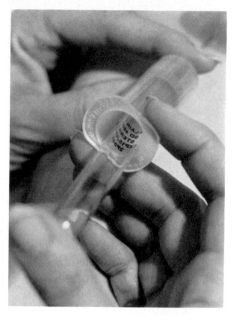

1 Aseptically screw the double-ended needle into the plastic outer container, with the shorter needle positioned inside the outer container (as shown). Then insert the vacuum tube into the outer container with the rubber stopper of the tube resting against the shorter needle.

2 Review the procedures earlier in this chapter for preparing the skin, dilating the vein, and performing a venipuncture, and proceed with the venipuncture at the antecubital space.

3 After puncturing the vein, stabilize the plastic outer container, and gently yet firmly advance the vacuum tube to pierce the rubber stopper with the short needle.

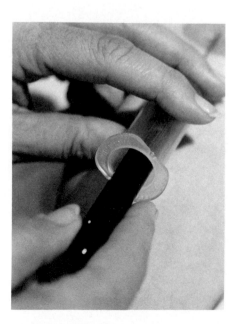

4 Because of the vacuum, blood should immediately begin spurting into the vacuum tube. As soon as it does, release the tourniquet to prevent the blood from seeping into the surrounding tissues. Remove the vacuum tube when it becomes full and set it aside. If required, insert another vacuum tube.

(Continued on p. 152)

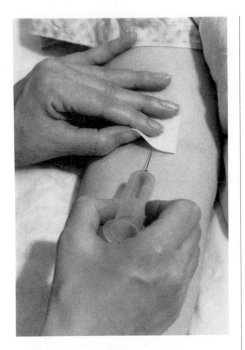

5 For your client's comfort, be sure to remove the vacuum tube, thus preventing vacuum, before you remove the needle from the vein. Then gently remove the needle. Apply a sterile sponge to the site, and ask the client to press on the sponge for 1–3 minutes to stop the bleeding. Once the bleeding has ceased, place a bandage over the puncture site. Arrange for the delivery of the blood to the laboratory, and document the procedure.

TEACHING THE DIABETIC CLIENT SELF-MONITORING OF BLOOD GLUCOSE

Until a few years ago, urine testing was the only method available to the diabetic client for testing of glucose levels at home. Now, however, there are several blood-glucose testing products available, which provide a much more accurate indicator of current glucose levels. In addition, they give greater control over the management of the disease and help in the prevention of acute complications such as hypoglycemia and hyperglycemia as well as chronic complications such as blindness, renal failure, and neuropathies. Of course, the client must continue to test the urine for ketones if he or she is ill or if blood-glucose levels are high. Blood glucose can be monitored both visually and with an electronic meter.

Monitoring Blood Glucose Visually

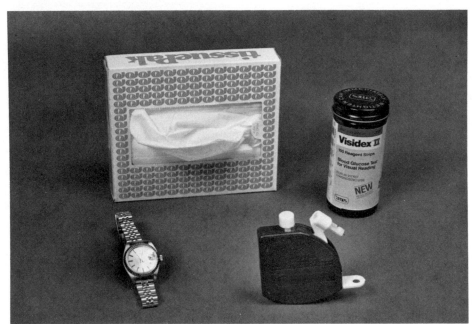

1 For visual monitoring of blood glucose, assemble facial tissue, reagent strips for showing glucose levels, and a watch with a second hand. In addition, you will also need a device for puncturing the skin (usually at the fingertip) to obtain the capillary blood. Either a manual device, such as a needle or lancet, or an automatic device, such as the Autolet (as shown), may be used.

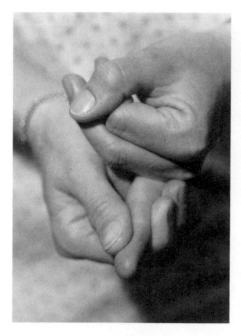

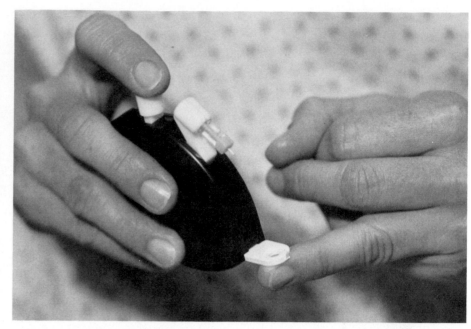

2 Have the client wash both hands with soap and warm water to remove surface bacteria and increase peripheral dilation; the hands then should be dried thoroughly. Instruct the client to squeeze the fingertip while holding the arm below the level of the heart. This will well the blood at the puncture site.

3 The platform of the automatic puncturing device should be placed directly over the puncture site. The periphery of the fingertip should be used because it is less sensitive to pain, and, in many clients, it has fewer cal-

louses than other areas of the finger. To lower the lance and puncture the skin, instruct the client to depress the button (under the client's right index finger).

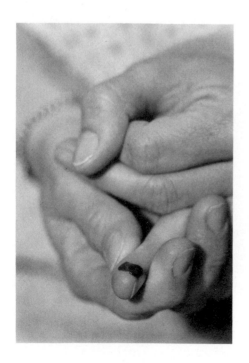

4 The client should then milk the finger by alternately squeezing and releasing the pressure until a drop of blood is produced that is large enough to cover the reagent pad on the test strip.

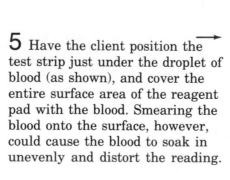

5 Have the client position the test strip just under the droplet of blood (as shown), and cover the entire surface area of the reagent pad with the blood. Smearing the blood onto the surface, however, could cause the blood to soak in unevenly and distort the reading.

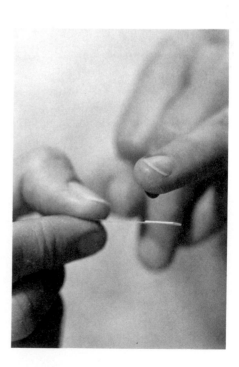

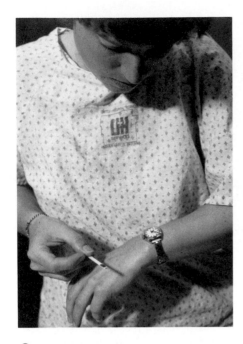

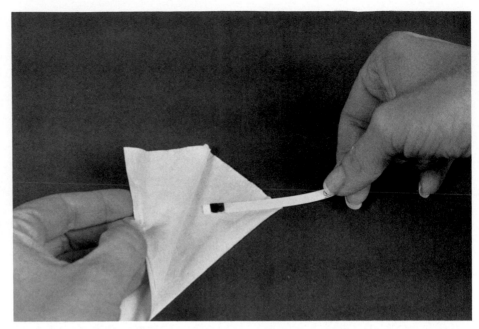

6 The moment the blood touches the strip, the client must begin timing the strip for a period of 30 seconds (or the specified time).

7 When 30 seconds have elapsed, instruct the client to blot the blood gently between the folds of the facial tissue. *Note: This step will vary, depending on* *the manufacturer of the test strip. Follow the instructions for the reagent strips your agency uses.* After blotting the blood, wait 90 seconds (or the specified time).

8 Compare the reagent pad to the colored blocks on the back of the container from which the strip was obtained. If the color of the reagent pad falls between two of the color blocks, instruct the client to take the average of the two values to estimate the glucose level. This is called interpolation. The client should then record the result in a log book, along with the time and date, the time of the last insulin injection (unless a pump is used), and the amount of stress or activity currently being experienced.

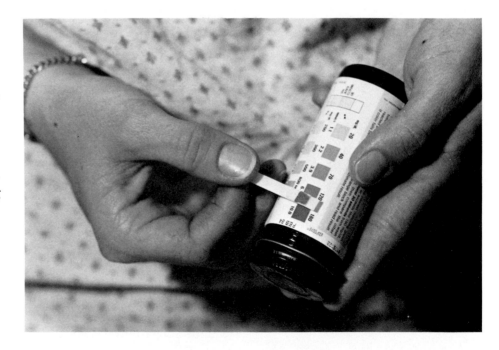

Monitoring Blood Glucose with an Electronic Meter

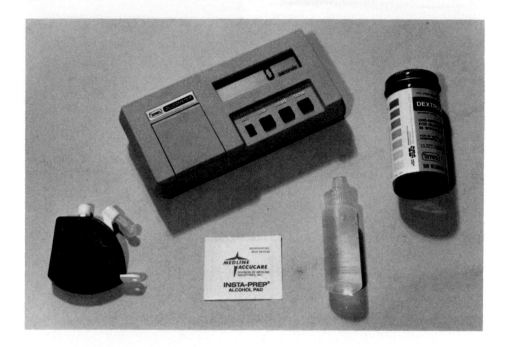

1 Clients who desire a more precise method of blood-glucose monitoring than visual testing may be candidates for an electronic meter. The following is the procedure for using a Glucometer®, a brand of electronic meter. Adapt this procedure for the meter used by your agency or client. In addition to the meter, assemble the following items: a skin-puncturing device, an alcohol sponge for the skin preparation (optional, the client may instead wash both hands with soap and water), a squeeze bottle filled with tap water, the reagent strip required by the manufacturer of the meter, and a lint-free paper towel.

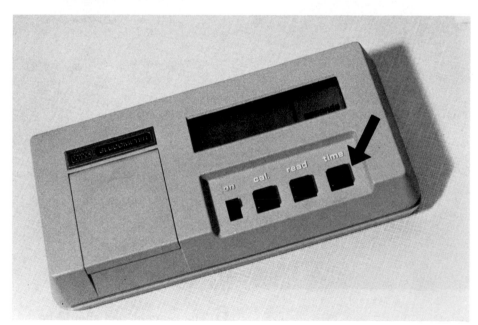

2 Review steps 2–4, p. 153, for preparing and puncturing the skin and obtaining a large drop of blood. Prior to puncturing the skin, turn the meter on. Once the blood droplet has been obtained, instruct the client to press the "time" button. Approximately 4 seconds will pass before the first buzzer sounds.

(Continued on p. 156)

INITIATING AND MONITORING BLOOD TRANSFUSIONS

Nursing Guidelines for the Safe Administration of Blood

- To ensure its viability, a blood infusion should be started within 30 minutes after it has been issued from the blood bank.
- For normal, healthy adults, use an 18–19-gauge needle or catheter to enhance the flow rate and to prevent injury to the red cells (hemolysis). Children and clients with small or thin-walled veins may require needles as small as 23 gauge: Monitor these clients carefully for adverse reactions and expect a much slower infusion rate.
- Use a special blood administration set with a filter specified by your agency for filtering out clots and broken-down blood cells.
- Hang only 0.9% normal saline with the blood. Dextrose, Ringer's solution, medications and other additives, and hyperalimentation solutions are incompatible and may result in hemolysis or clumping.
- To prevent incompatibilities with a primary solution, and for a more secure insertion site, avoid piggybacking the blood into the injection port of an existing primary line. Perform a venipuncture at a different site or (with a physician's order) remove the infusion set from an existing indwelling 18–19-gauge needle and attach the primed blood infusion set directly to the indwelling needle.
- Remember to flush an existing needle with 50 mL of 0.9% normal saline before infusing the blood.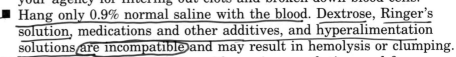
- Hang the blood and normal saline approximately 1 m (3–4 ft) above the client's heart for an optimal flow rate.
- Administer the blood at the rate of flow prescribed by the physician. Obtain an order for the administration rate if one has not been written.
- The maximum time for infusing a unit of blood is 4–6 hours, as recommended by the American Association of Blood Banks (Widmann, 1981:218). There is an increased potential for bacterial growth in blood that is allowed to hang for a longer period of time.
- To prevent circulatory overload for clients with cardiac disorders, administer the transfusion more slowly than you would normally and monitor the client closely for an adverse reaction.
- Blood should be warmed *only* when large amounts are infused rapidly and could otherwise cause hypothermia and arrhythmias. Rapid infusions more typically occur in the operating room, emergency room, or in the critical care setting.

Administering Blood or Blood Components
Assessing and Planning

1 Prior to administering the blood, carefully compare the data on the crossmatch report and requisition form to the blood unit information. Check the following data with another health care professional: the client's name and hospital number, the blood unit number, blood expiration date, blood group, and blood type. Inspect the blood for abnormalities such as gas bubbles or black sediment, which are indicative of bacterial growth and necessitate returning the blood to the blood bank.

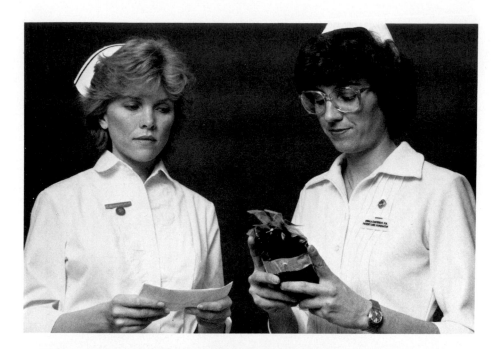

2 Explain the procedure to the client. Both you and a co-worker should then compare the blood unit information to the data on the client's wristband. Ensure that the client's name and hospital number positively match the data on the blood unit; then sign the blood transfusion form according to agency policy. Reconfirm data from the client history regarding known allergies or previous adverse reactions to blood transfusions. Be sure to take and record the vital signs to provide a baseline for subsequent assessments during the transfusion.

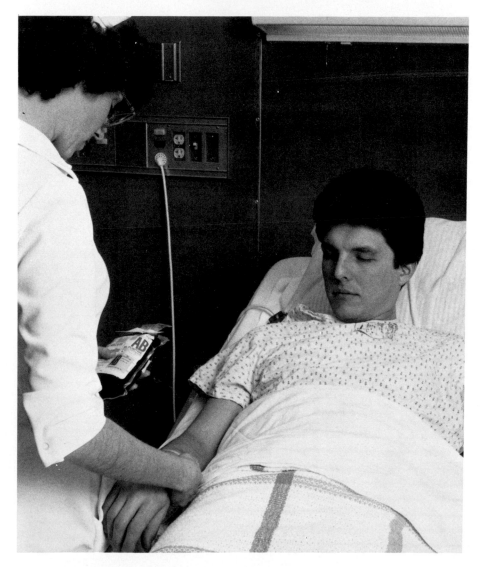

(Continued on p. 160)

Implementing

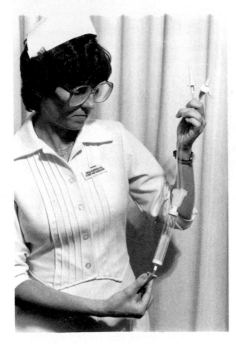

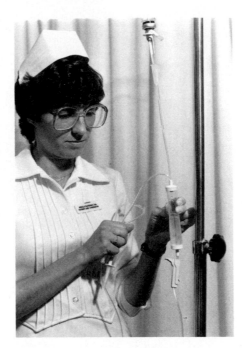

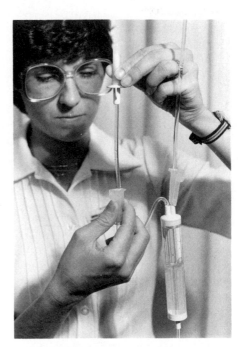

3 Review the procedures earlier in this chapter for performing a venipuncture and spiking and priming infusion sets. Obtain a "Y" infusion set for the administration of blood, as specified by your agency. Ensure that the attached blood filter is appropriate for the whole blood or blood components that will be transfused. Close all the clamps on the "Y" set (as shown) and spike a container of 0.9% normal saline with one of the "Y" spikes. Hang the container.

4 Open the clamp on the normal saline line and squeeze the drip chamber to prime the upper line and blood filter. Tap the chamber to remove any residual air.

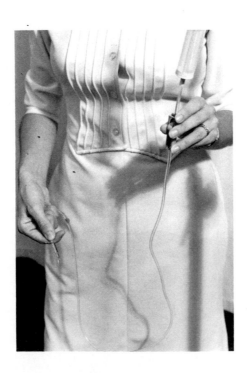

5 Open the clamp on the empty line on which you will eventually hang the blood. The normal saline line will flow up the blood line to prime that part of the "Y." Then close the clamp on the blood line, leaving the clamp on the normal saline line open.

6 Open the main roller clamp to prime the lower infusion tubing and flush out the air. Close the main roller clamp.

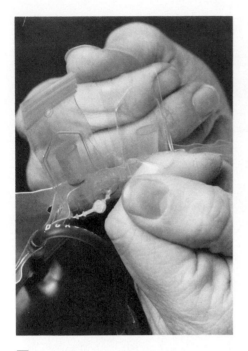

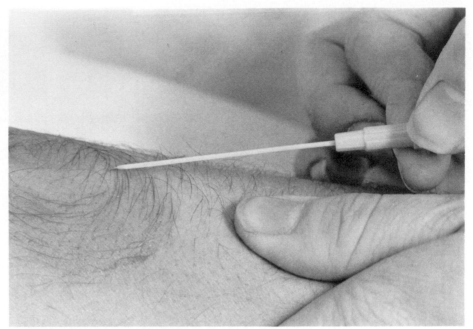

7 Aseptically pull apart the plastic tabs on the blood container (as shown) to expose the blood port.

9 Perform a venipuncture with an 18–19-gauge needle or catheter, or, if the physician has ordered its discontinuation, remove the infusion tubing from an indwelling 18–19-gauge needle. Attach the primed infusion set to the needle, tape it securely, and, if necessary, secure a splint or armboard to the client's arm to ensure the needle's stability. If appropriate, run in 50 mL of the normal saline to flush a preexisting needle of an incompatible solution. Otherwise, close the upper roller clamp on the normal saline and open the clamp to the blood. Adjust the main roller clamp to deliver approximately 10–25 mL over the next 15 minutes.

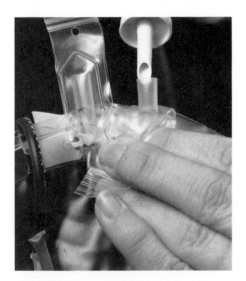

8 Insert the remaining "Y" spike into the blood port, and hang the blood at the same level (1 m) as the normal saline.

(Continued on p. 162)

Evaluating

10 Assess the client frequently over the next 15–30 minutes and monitor him for signs of an adverse reaction to the transfusion (Table 3–1). After the first 15 minutes of the transfusion, take the vital signs again and compare them to the baseline. Be especially alert to a sudden decrease in blood pressure or a rise in temperature. If the vital signs are stable, gradually increase the rate of flow to the prescribed rate. Continue to monitor the client and document the vital signs at least hourly, or more frequently, depending on agency guidelines. If your client has a cardiac disorder, or if large amounts of blood are being infused over a short period of time, auscultate the lung bases for adventitious breath sounds such as crackles (rales) that could indicate circulatory overload. When the blood has been infused, flush the tubing and filter with 20–50 mL of the normal saline to deliver the residual blood. Then either run the normal saline at a KVO rate or hang another solution as prescribed. Maintain the venipuncture site in case the client develops a delayed reaction to the blood. Document the procedure.

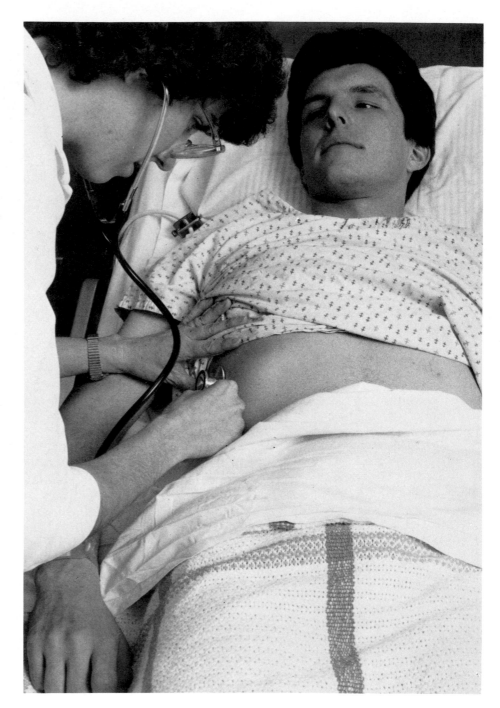

Table 3–1   Recognizing Transfusion Reactions

Reaction type	Clinical indications	Nursing interventions
Allergic: caused from a sensitivity to a plasma protein in the donor blood	*Mild:* rash, hives, itching *Severe:* wheezing, laryngeal edema, bronchial spasm, anaphylactic reaction	For a mild reaction: slow down infusion rate, monitor client carefully, notify physician, and administer prescribed injections of antihistimines. For severe symptoms: stop transfusion; keep vein open with a slow infusion normal saline; notify physician; administer prescribed injections of antihistimines, or if more serious, epinephrine or corticosteroids; stay with client and monitor for potential anaphylaxis.
Febrile or Septic: caused from bacterial contamination, improper storage or refrigeration of the blood, and other unknown factors	Chills, increased temperature, headache, hypotension, lumbar or leg pain, nausea, and vomiting	Maintain venipuncture site, but stop transfusion immediately; change infusion set as soon as possible; notify physician and blood bank; send used infusion set to lab for culturing; administer prescribed antibiotics, antipyretics, vasopressors, or steroids; stay with client; monitor vital signs; observe for anaphylaxis.
Hemolytic: caused from incompatibility of donor blood with recipient blood, improper storage or refrigeration, improper infusion with dextrose or any other additive or solution other than 0.9% normal saline	Anxiety, restlessness, chills, increase in temperature, chest pain, cyanosis, hematuria, hypotension, tachycardia, and tachypnea. If untreated, shock and anuria ensue.	Discontinue transfusion, maintain venipuncture site, change infusion set and keep vein open with normal saline or prescribed solution, notify physician, administer oxygen, obtain blood and urine samples and send them to blood bank with the suspect unit of blood, administer prescribed diuretic or vasopressor, stay with client and monitor vital signs and intake and output.
Circulatory Overload: caused from excessive infusion amounts or too rapid an infusion rate	Chest or lumbar pain, cyanosis, dyspnea, moist productive cough, crackles (rales) in lung bases, distended neck veins, increase in central venous pressure	Discontinue infusion, but keep vein open with dextrose, or as prescribed; raise head of bed and deliver oxygen; notify physician; administer diuretics and aminophylline as prescribed; stay with client and monitor vital signs; prepare for a phlebotomy if symptoms are severe.

References

Brunner, L. S., and Suddarth, D. S. 1982. *The Lippincott manual of nursing practice,* 3rd ed. Philadelphia: J.B. Lippincott.

Button, G. R. Oct. 1982. Tips on avoiding sluggish transfusions. *RN* 45:125.

Centers for Disease Control. 1981–1984. *Guidelines for the prevention and control of nosocomial infections.* Atlanta, Ga: U.S. Department of Health and Human Services.

Fredholm, N. A. 1981. The insulin pump: a new method of insulin delivery. *AJN* 81:2024–2026.

Friedman, F. B. Jan. 1983. Restraints: when all else fails, there still are alternatives. *RN* 46:79–88.

Gever, L. N. March 1982. Administering drugs through the skin. *Nursing '82* 12:88.

Hutchinson, M. M. 1982. Administration of fat emulsions. *AJN* 82:275–277.

Intramuscular injections. March 1979. Philadelphia: Wyeth Laboratories.

Joyce, M. A., et al. April 1983. Those new blood glucose tests. *RN* 46:46–52.

Kirilloff, L. H., and Tibbals, S. C. 1983. Drugs for asthma: a complete guide. *AJN* 83:55–61.

Kirkis, J., and Ettorre, D. April 1983. Seven sticky problems (and their solutions) in blood transfusions. *RN* 46:59–63, 94.

Kozier, B., and Erb, G. 1983. *Fundamentals of nursing,* 2nd ed. Menlo Park, Calif.: Addison-Wesley Publishing.

Krueger, E. A., and Jaeckels, D. L. 1972. *Parenteral medication: teachers' guide.* Philadelphia: J.B. Lippincott.

McConnell, E. Feb. 1982. The subtle art of giving *really* good injections. *RN* 45:25–35.

Nemchik, R. May 1983. The new insulin pumps: tight control—at a price. *RN* 46:52–59.

Nursing '82 Books. 1982. *500 Nursing tips and timesavers.* Springhouse, Pa.: Intermed Communications.

Nursing Photobook. 1981. *Giving medications.* Horsham, Pa.: Intermed Communications.

Nursing Photobook. 1982. *Managing IV therapy.* Springhouse, Pa.: Intermed Communications.

Rettig, R. M., and Southby, J. July/Aug. 1982. Using different body postures to reduce discomfort from dorsogluteal injections. *Nurs Res* 31:219.

Setting the record straight: IV therapy and the issue of pressure. June 1981. North Chicago: Abbott Laboratories.

Smith, S. F., and Duell, D. 1982. *Nursing skills and evaluation.* Los Altos, Calif.: National Nursing Review.

Sorensen, K. C., and Luckmann, J. 1979. *Basic nursing: a psychophysiologic approach.* Philadelphia: W.B. Saunders Co.

Stevens, A. D. 1981. Monitoring blood glucose at home: who should do it. *AJN* 81:2026–2027.

Surr, C. W. 1983. Teaching patients to use the new blood-glucose monitoring products, part I. *Nursing '83* 13:42–45.

Surr, C. W. 1983. Teaching patients to use the new blood-glucose monitoring products, part II. *Nursing '83* 13:58–62.

Todd, B. Jan./Feb. 1983. Using eye drops and ointments safely. *Geriatric Nurs* 53:56–57.

Trifiletti, P. E. Sept./Oct. 1982. Nitroglycerin ointment: application and use. *Crit Car Nurse* 46–48.

Widmann, F. K., et al. 1981. *The technical manual of the American Association of Blood Banks,* 8th ed. Washington, D.C.: American Association of Blood Banks.

Unit II

Performing
Specialized
Nursing
Procedures

NURSING ASSESSMENT GUIDELINE

Prior to teaching the examination, gather subjective data from the client. A comprehensive client history should include a complete evaluation for the following factors:

Risk factors: client history of breast surgery, cancer, or fibrocystic disease; family history of cancer, fibroids, mother's taking of diethylstilbestrol (DES); history of smoking and/or exposure to carcinogens; history of obesity, diabetes mellitus, or hypertension; history of chronic psychological stress; use of estrogens; dietary intake high in animal fats.

Personal factors: client's age—risk increases steadily after age 35, with the greatest risk occurring in clients over age 85; ages at which menstruation and menopause began—clients with early menstruation (11 years or younger) or late menopause (after 52 years) are at greater risk; age at first full-term pregnancy—clients over 30 years and nulliparous clients are at higher risk, clients having their first child at age 20 or younger have decreased risk; discharge or secretions in nipples—color, amount, frequency; changes in breasts since adulthood—size, shape, color; mammography history and results; knowledge of breast self-examination, frequency of performance, and time of month it is performed.

TEACHING BREAST SELF-EXAMINATION

Assessing and Planning

The most common site for cancer in the adult woman is the breast, and the single most effective means for improving survival rates in breast cancer is early detection of breast tumors using breast self-examination. This important procedure should be incorporated into the discharge planning for *all* your adult female clients.

1 Provide a warm and private environment for your client, and arrange for her to sit facing away from the door. Explain that she should routinely perform breast self-examination about a week after her menstrual period has begun because at that time her breasts will have been the least swollen and a lump will be more readily detected. To ensure consistency, menopausal clients or those who have had hysterectomies or oophorectomies should perform the examination at the same time every month, for example on the first day of the month.

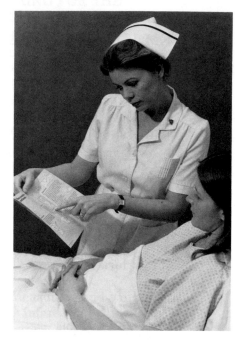

Take your time, encourage questions, and give the client literature on breast self-examination, such as the free pamphlets provided by the American Cancer Society. The goal of this procedure is to familiarize your client with the way her breasts normally look and feel. Optimally, the examination will give her confidence in her knowledge base and skill in assessing abnormalities so that should cancer be detected, she will have found it at its earliest, most treatable stage. In addition, teaching your client breast self-examination will enable you to assess for abnormalities at the same time.

Implementing

2 The assessment consists of both inspection and palpation. To begin the inspection segment of the examination, instruct the client to sit on the side of the bed and to lower her gown to the waist. Explain that she should relax her arms in her lap and inspect her breasts in a large mirror. If a mirror is unavailable, she should pretend that you are a mirror so that she can follow each step without losing the continuity of the examination. As she looks in the mirror, explain that each breast may normally deviate slightly from the other in size and symmetry, but she should be alert to any monthly *changes* in contour and appearance. Instruct her to look for swelling, puckering, dimpling of the skin, changes in texture and color, as well as a change in a mole. Striae (stretch marks) are normal, and symmetrical venous patterns are fairly common in fair-complexioned women. Explain, however, that diffuse, blue casts, suggestive of an increased blood supply to an area, should be followed up with a physician's examination. The areolae may also vary slightly in size and shape from one another, but differences in color, rashes, scaling, or ulcerations should be noted. Discharge from the nipple is usually abnormal in the mature, nonlactating woman; an inverted nipple can also signal a problem, especially if it was recently everted. Explain also that an inverted nipple that becomes everted during movement can occur with an underlying pathology. *Note: At this time, you should also be alert to* peau d'orange, *skin that is large-pored and edematous caused by a tumor obstructing the lymph glands. This is an advanced sign of breast cancer, and generally not necessary to include for client education.*

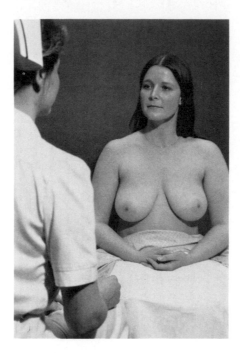

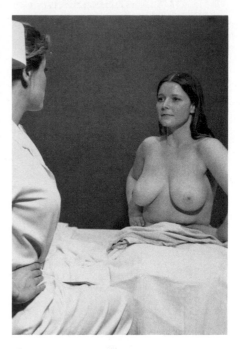

4 While continuing to squeeze her waist, she should turn from side to side so that she can view all of the breast tissue.

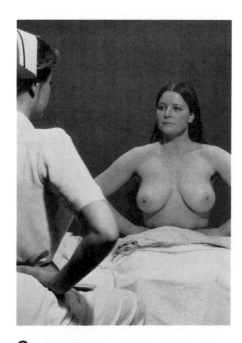

3 Instruct the client to tense her pectoral muscles by squeezing her waist. She should look again for asymmetry in size and contour, dimpling, puckering, or retractions of the skin.

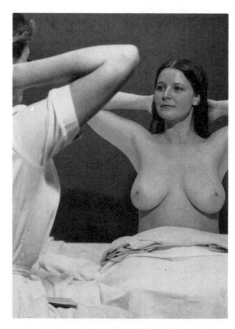

5 Demonstrate raising the arms by placing them behind the head. This will enable the client to look for unilateral changes in symmetry and contour of each breast.

(Continued on p. 172)

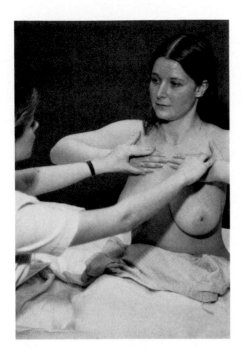

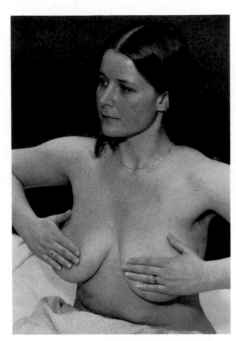

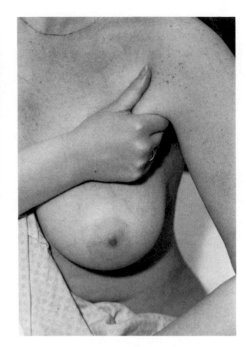

6 To begin the palpation segment of the examination, wash your hands; and then show your client how to sweep her breasts bilaterally. Explain that this is done to assess for lumps in the upper breast tissue, which begins just under the clavicles. Show her how to position her hands at the clavicles (as shown) and to sweep them downward onto the nipples (above center). Occasionally, a hardened area will be palpated, and most often it is a rib. To ensure that it is, the client should be shown how to palpate across the area to feel for the underlying rib. If the hardened area is not contiguous, she should see a physician. This segment of the examination can be facilitated if it is performed in the shower. The wet skin will enhance the sensitivity of the fingertips.

7 Show the client how to assess the muscle and lymph tissue at the axillae. To relax the muscle, she should rest an arm in her lap, with the elbow slightly flexed. She should then grasp the tissue between the thumb and fingers of her opposite hand and gently squeeze the tissue in a rolling motion to palpate for lumps or swollen lymph glands.

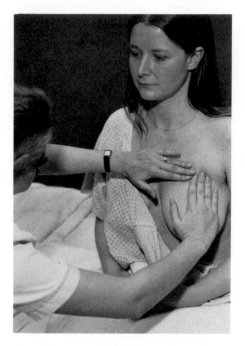

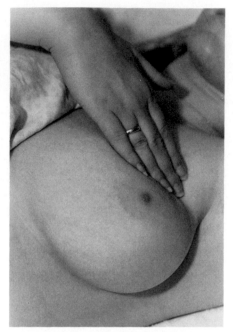

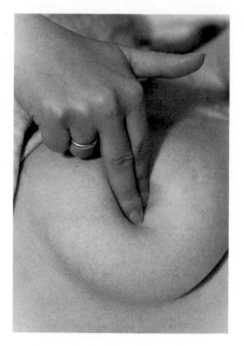

8 While she is sitting, teach her the procedure for palpating each breast in concentric circles. This is the portion of the examination that the woman will regularly perform in a supine position. Show her how to find the 12:00 position at the periphery of the breast tissue, the uppermost and outermost section. Explain that she should palpate around the breast in a circular fashion, using flattened fingers, until she returns to 12:00. In this photo, the nurse is showing her client how to palpate with the right hand and guide the movement with the left hand. Explain that a ridge of firm tissue at the curve of the lower breast is normal. However, she should see a physician if she detects lumps, knots, or thickened tissue. Typically, a malignancy is painless, attached to underlying tissue, and it occurs most often in the upper outer quadrant.

9 For self-examination, the client should lie down, and while supine, apply the above technique. To examine the left breast (as shown), a towel or a small pillow should be placed under the left side and shoulder, and her left hand should be positioned behind her head. This position will more evenly distribute the breast tissue over the chest wall. Explain that she can facilitate the gliding motion and increase the sensitivity of her fingertips by generously applying lotion to her fingertips. After palpating in a complete circle around the outer breast tissue, she should advance an inch toward the nipple and repeat the process until the *entire breast* has been examined in this manner.

10 After the client has examined the breast, she should next examine the nipple. She should depress the nipple with her index and middle fingers to palpate the area underneath, which is referred to as the *well*. This is a common location for tumors, and it is all too often missed during a cursory examination.

(Continued on p. 174)

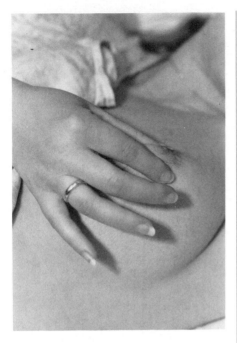

11 Instruct her to gently squeeze and milk the nipple to assess for discharge. Any new discharge in an adult nonlactating female is significant, and it should be referred to a physician.

Evaluating

12 After completing the assessment of the left breast, the client should repeat the examination in the right breast while you observe and answer any questions she may have.

When the assessment has been completed, compare your observations with those of the client. Arrange for a physician referral if you have detected any abnormalities. Reassure her that most lumps and abnormalities (eight out of ten) are benign, but that only a physician can make a diagnosis and arrange for the appropriate treatment. For women with fibrocystic breasts, suggest that a graph be made, noting areas of lumps and thickened tissue. This will provide a comparison so they can quickly determine whether the lumps are preexisting or indicative of change.

ASSISTING THE CLIENT WITH POSTSURGICAL MASTECTOMY EXERCISES

Postsurgical arm and shoulder exercises are crucial to the full recovery of your clients who have had mastectomies because they help to maintain circulation in the involved arm, reduce edema, and promote maximum function. If your client is scheduled for a mastectomy, consult with her physician prior to the surgery to determine the type of mastectomy anticipated so that you can develop an individualized exercise plan that can be implemented as soon as the client arrives in the recovery room. In addition, with physician approval, you can arrange for a visit by a member of the American Cancer Society's "Reach to Recovery" support group or other similar groups in your community for the postsurgical period. To ensure that your client's progress warrants the increased range of movement, check with her physician prior to initiating each new exercise. The movements depicted in the following photographs range from the simple to the advanced.

The Exercises

1 Passive range of motion (ROM) exercises can be initiated as soon as the client arrives in the recovery room; once she has returned to her room you can begin assisted ROM exercises on her involved shoulder (as shown). Review the procedures in Chapter 2 to assist you with the movements involved. Because the client may have both discomfort and apprehension about stretching the incisional site, be sure to explain the reason for the exercises and reassure her that the movements will be adapted to her level of tolerance. For maximal joint mobility, these exercises should be performed in sets of ten, three times a day.

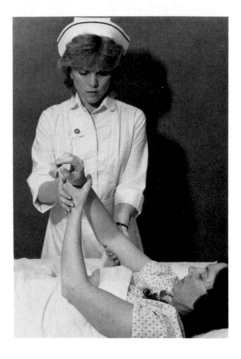

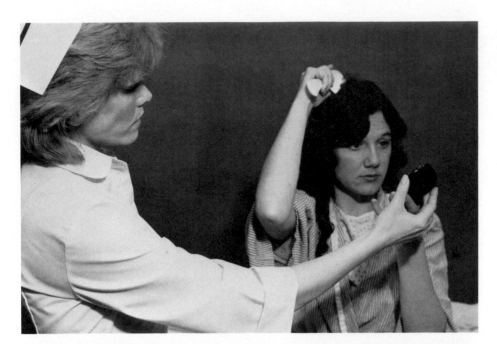

2 By the second postoperative day, activities of self-care using the involved arm should be encouraged as much as possible. For example, combing the hair, putting on makeup, or washing the face are all activities that will exercise the involved arm.

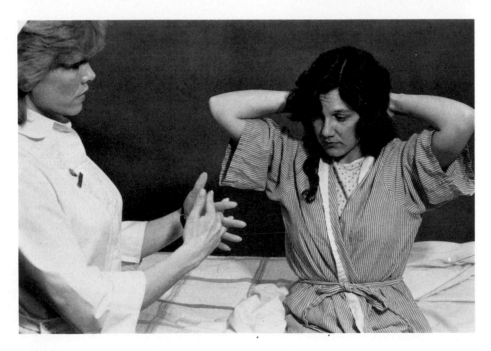

3 When your client is able to actively lift her involved arm without assistance, instruct her to clasp her hands behind her head (as shown).

(Continued on p. 176)

4 She should then attempt to touch her elbows together, or to bring them as close together as possible. This movement will flex, externally rotate, and adduct the involved shoulder.

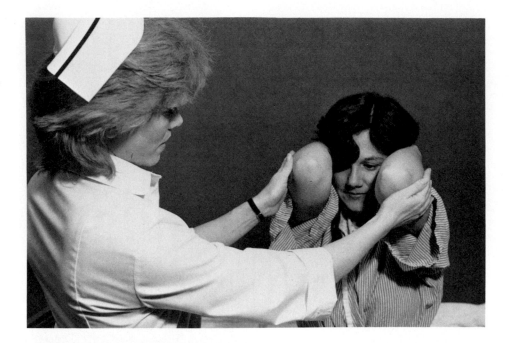

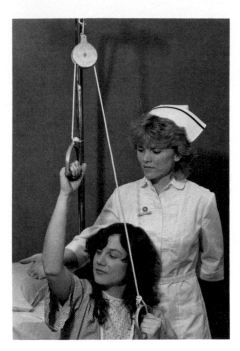

5 You can also use assistive devices to achieve shoulder flexion. With physician approval, assemble a rope and pulley system onto an overhead trapeze bar. The client should grasp the hand grips and begin the exercise with the involved arm in the lower position. Instruct her to pull down gently with the hand of the uninvolved arm, allowing the involved arm to be raised gradually (as shown). Explain to the client that some discomfort and a sensation of stretching the incision is normal, but that to achieve maximum shoulder range, she should flex the shoulder as much as possible. *Note: The client may adapt this exercise at home by placing a rope over a stable shower curtain rod or over a wall hook.*

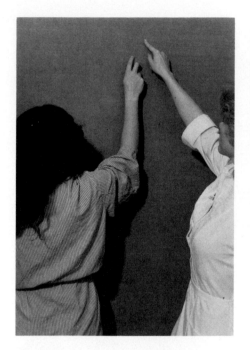

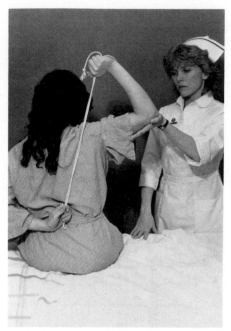

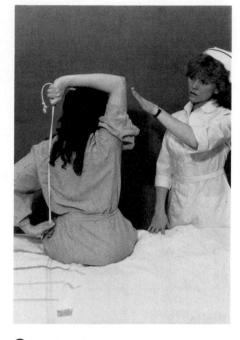

6 You can also teach the client how to "climb a wall," which will promote shoulder flexion without the use of an assistive device. The client should face the wall and position her involved arm at shoulder level. Gradually she will scale the wall by "walking" her fingertips upward (as shown). Encourage her to achieve maximum shoulder ROM. *Note: Place a tape marker on the wall to indicate her progress after each exercise. This will give her a goal to strive for with each new attempt.*

7 Around the second postoperative week, usually after the sutures have been removed, the client can begin exercises that will maximize external rotation and abduction of the shoulder. A 75-cm (30-in.) rope can be used to assist the client in achieving maximum range. Instruct her to grasp the rope, holding the lower end in her uninvolved hand in the back at the level of her waistline. The top of the rope should be held in the hand of her involved arm at about the level of her head.

8 She should very gently pull down on the rope with the hand of her uninvolved arm, guiding the involved arm through abduction and external rotation. This exercise should be performed at least three times daily in sets of ten each.

9 Just prior to discharge, show the client how to achieve maximum shoulder flexion by touching her fingertips behind her back with the involved arm uppermost. This exercise simulates the range required for zipping back zippers and fastening brassieres.

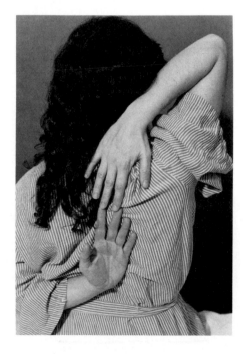

PROVIDING PERINEAL CARE

Using a Squeeze Bottle

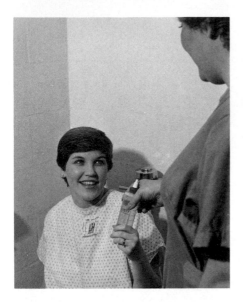

1 A very simple method for providing perineal care is the use of a squeeze bottle filled with tap water warmed to approximately 100 F. A postpartum client can use this method after every voiding to cleanse her perineum.

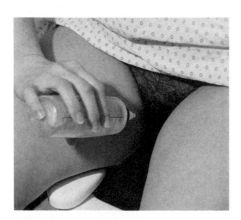

2 Instruct the client to insert the nozzle of the bottle between her legs and to squirt the bottle so that it sprays onto the perineum. Explain to the client that it will take several squirts to thoroughly cleanse the area. She should then blot her perineum from front to back when she has finished with the squeeze bottle, using either toilet paper or clean wipes provided by your agency.

Preparing a Sitz Bath

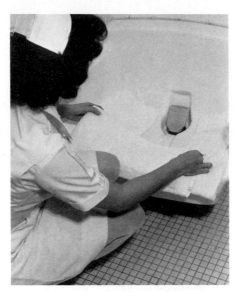

1 A sitz bath is prepared for clients who have vulvar pain and swelling and who require warmth to heal the perineal area, for example after vaginal hysterectomies, vulvectomies, childbirth, or hemorrhoidectomies. Ensure that the basin has been thoroughly scrubbed with a disinfectant cleaning agent. Place towels around the seat to pad the area where the client will sit. This will not only promote comfort but it will also prevent the client from slipping on the wet, slick surface of the tub. Padding the basin prior to running the water will prevent the towels from floating out of place.

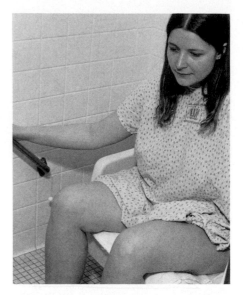

2 Adjust the temperature of the sitz bath so that it is in the range of 100–105 F. If the system does not have a built-in thermometer, use a bath thermometer to verify the temperature. The bath should fill from a third to a half of its capacity, and many models will continuously drain to provide a source of fresh water for the client. Assist the client into the sitting position. If you cannot stay with her during the prescribed treatment time, make sure the emergency call light is within her reach. Because of the warmth of the water, the client must be monitored periodically for potential fainting.

Using a Surgi-gator

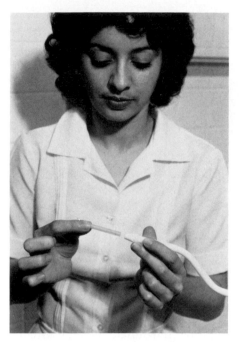

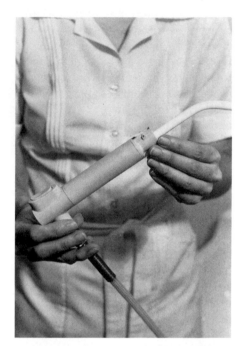

1 If your agency has a Surgi-gator perineal care system for cleansing and providing warmth to the perineum, you can teach your client how to use the system on her own for the times in which it is prescribed, as well as during the times she experiences perineal discomfort.

Every client is issued her own applicator. Explain to the client that she must first insert the soap cartridge into the proximal end of the applicator.

2 The proximal end is then inserted and snapped into the dispensing handle that connects to the wall-mounted unit. Explain that depressing the control button on the dispensing handle delivers both the cleansing cycle and the rinse cycle. Make sure the temperature is set at approximately 100 F.

3 Instruct the client to sit on the toilet, spread her legs apart, and insert the Surgi-gator applicator between her legs so that it is just distal to her perineum.

4 After depressing the control button, she can adjust the distance of the applicator to her perineum to achieve the desired force of spray. Remind her to return the applicator to the bedside for subsequent use.

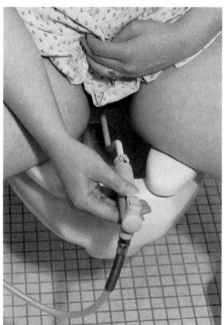

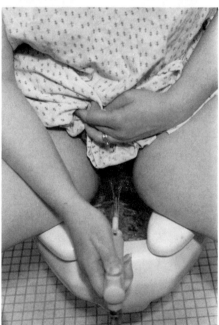

Performing Prenatal Techniques

ASSESSING THE PRENATAL ABDOMEN

Measuring Fundal Height

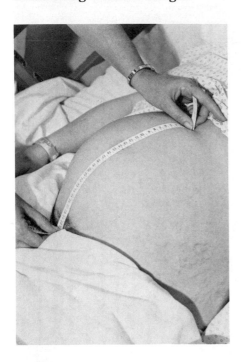

Assessing uterine size by measuring fundal height is often initiated in the client's second trimester. It is continued into the third trimester as a routine assessment tool for monitoring fetal growth. Although it is not a precise indicator of fetal development, it will alert you to sudden growth spurts found, for example, in multiple gestations, or to a lag in progression indicating intrauterine growth retardation. To measure the fundal height, obtain a nonstretchable tape measure; position one end at the fundus and measure the distance to the symphysis pubis in centimeters. Up until the third trimester, the measurement will, on average, correlate with the gestational age. For example, at 24-weeks'

gestation, the fundus measures around 24 cm for the average woman, and it will normally be at the level of the umbilicus.

Using McDonald's Rule

When the client is in her third trimester, apply McDonald's rule to estimate gestational age. For example, if your client measures 28 cm from the fundus to the symphysis pubis, you can estimate gestational age in lunar months by calculating in the following manner:

$$\frac{\text{Fundal height in cm}}{3.5} =$$

Gestational age in lunar months

$$\frac{28 \text{ cm}}{3.5} = 8 \text{ lunar months}$$

Inspecting and Palpating Fetal Parts

Palpate and locate fetal parts prior to auscultating for fetal heart tones (FHTs). Once you have identified the fetal back, you can readily elicit heart sounds because there is less bone and tissue through which to auscultate. Provide warmth and privacy for your client; for her comfort and to relax the abdominal wall, make sure she has recently voided. After explaining the procedure, elevate her head slightly and ask her to flex her knees, which will further relax the abdomen. Expose the abdomen from the xiphoid process to the symphysis pubis, and then inspect it to help you assess the position of the fetus. Does it appear to lie up and down in a longitudinal position or left and right in a transverse position?

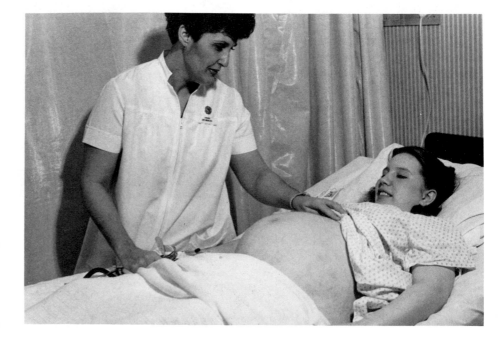

Performing Leopold's Maneuvers

Leopold's maneuvers are performed to determine fetal position. Make sure your hands are warm, and perform the assessment between contractions, whether Braxton Hicks or labor contractions.

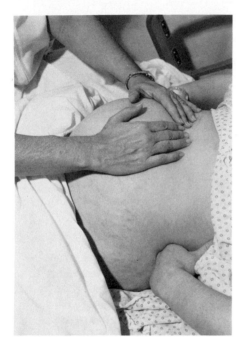

First Maneuver: Face the client and bilaterally palpate the upper abdomen. This will help you determine which of the fetal parts is in the uterine fundus. The breech is large, soft, and asymmetrical; the head is round, hard, and it moves more freely.

Second Maneuver: Continue facing the client, and place each hand along the sides of the abdomen. Gently but firmly palpate with your palms and fingers. Assess one side and then the other to determine the side on which the fetal back lies. One side should feel smooth and quite firm—the fetal back; the other side should be indentable and less resistant—the extremities on the opposite uterine wall. ⟶

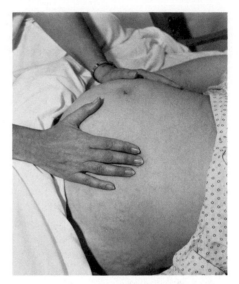

Third Maneuver: While still facing the client, position your dominant hand over the lower abdomen just proximal to the symphysis pubis, and firmly palpate with your thumb and index finger. Explain to the client that this maneuver may be uncomfortable. This maneuver helps to confirm the data gathered in the first maneuver. Again, the head will be round, hard, and ballotable (moveable) if it has not already engaged. The breech will feel soft and asymmetrical. (This assessment will be much more difficult if the presenting part has already engaged.) ⟶

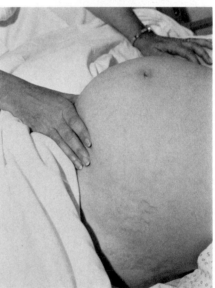

Fourth Maneuver: Face the client's feet and position your hands on both sides of the abdomen with your fingers curving downward toward, and immediately above, the pubis. This maneuver will help you locate the cephalic prominence, which is the most prominent portion of the fetal head. Press deeply with your fingertips because you will need to palpate through several layers of tissue, muscle, and fluid. The cephalic prominence is located on the side in which your fingers meet the greatest resistance. If it is located on the side opposite the back, the head is flexed and a normal delivery will probably ensue. If it is located on the same side as the back, the head is extended and the face or brow will probably present. Again, the greater the engagement, the more difficult the assessment. ⟶

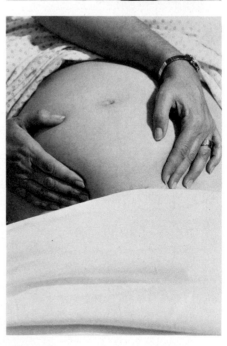

Auscultating Fetal Heart Tones

Once you have located the fetal back using Leopold's maneuvers, you can readily auscultate FHTs. This assessment will also reconfirm your assessment of the location of the fetal parts. However, in an emergency, auscultate in the midline between the umbilicus and symphysis pubis, the site in which FHTs are the loudest in the more typical cephalic presentation. With a fetoscope, the FHTs will be inaudible until weeks 18–20 of gestation, and at that time the point of maximum intensity is just above the pubis. Thereafter, the point of maximum intensity varies depending on the fetal position and presentation. Most often it can be best heard over the fetal back.

Using a Fetoscope

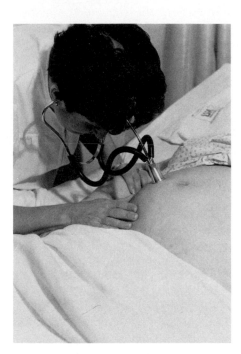 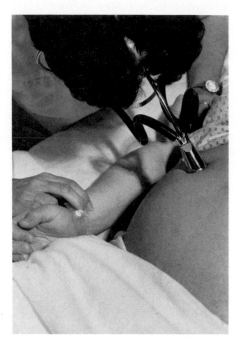

1 Position the warmed fetoscope over the palpated fetal back. Move the fetoscope around until you locate the point of maximum intensity. Generally, with cephalic presentations, the FHTs can be heard in the lower quadrant, toward the mother's flank. In breech presentations they can be heard closer to the midline around the level of the umbilicus. Apply slight pressure with the fetoscope bell to elicit the sounds.

2 When the heart tones are at their loudest, palpate the mother's radial pulse as you count the FHTs. This will ensure that you have not confused the mother's *souffle* with the fetal heart tones. This *souffle* is a soft, rushing sound produced by blood moving through the uterine arteries, and it is synchronous with the maternal heart rate. Count the FHTs for one full minute. They should normally range from 120–160 beats/minute.

Using Ultrasonic (Doppler) Auscultation

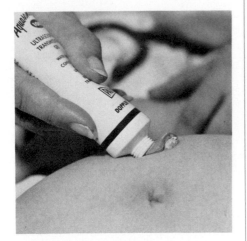

1 Review the procedure, p. 389, for a description of the Doppler. An ultrasonic transducer has the advantage of detecting FHTs by the twelfth week, and occasionally as early as the ninth or tenth week. Lubricate an area over the fetal back using a thin layer of conducting jelly.

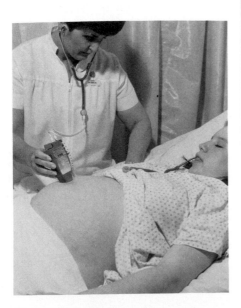

2 Position the transducer over the lubricated area. If the Doppler has an extra head set, allow the mother to listen simultaneously. Count the beats for a minute. You may also elicit a *bruit,* a hissing sound produced by blood moving through the umbilical arteries and other fetal vessels, as well as a *souffle.*

USING NITRAZINE TAPE TO ASSESS FOR AMNIOTIC FLUID

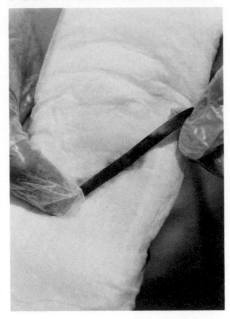

1 When assessing for the possibility that your client's amniotic membranes have ruptured, you can perform the nitrazine test to determine the pH of the expelled fluid. Place a nitrazine test strip over the peri pad or over the garment on which you or your client have detected the fluid.

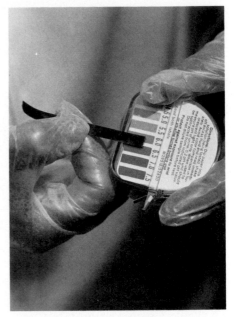

2 Compare the results to the color chart on the nitrazine container. Amniotic fluid is alkaline, at a 7.2 pH, and the darker the test strip, the more likely it is that the membranes have ruptured. *Note: A false positive may result if a recent vaginal examination was performed using a water-soluble lubricant, or if the fluid contains blood.*

If your assessment reveals that the membranes might have ruptured, determine the time of rupture and the characteristic of the fluid, for example, color, consistency, and odor. Inspect the perineum and introitus for the presence of a prolapsed cord. Auscultate FHTs. A lowered rate of 100 beats/minute or less and/or the presence of the cord necessitates positioning the client in deep Trendelenburg or in a knee-chest position, which will either allow gravity to remove the presenting part from the cord or minimize cord compression. Notify the attending physician *immediately* for further intervention.

PROVIDING COMFORT MEASURES

Applying Counterpressure to Relieve Leg Cramps

Applying Pressure to Relieve Back Pain

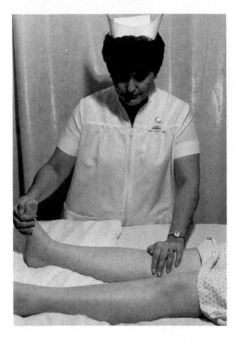

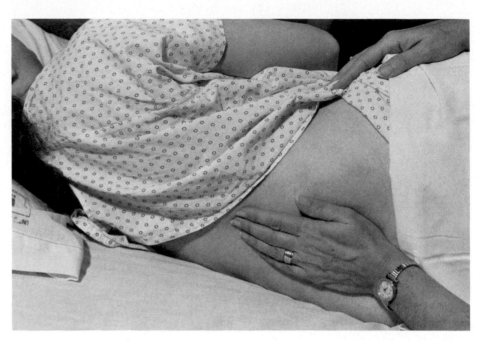

Your pregnant client may experience painful muscle spasms in her legs, especially during the third trimester when circulation is impaired in the lower extremities and the weighty uterus presses on the nerves in her legs. These cramps are often precipitated when the client is recumbant and extends her feet. They can be relieved by straightening the leg with one hand as you dorsiflex the foot with the other hand. Be sure to teach this technique to your client's partner.

If your client experiences back pain, which may be caused from increasing curvature of the back or a relaxation of the pelvic joints, assist her onto her side and apply firm pressure with the heel of your hand to the sacrococcygeal area. Continue the even pressure until the discomfort is diminished or relieved.

Performing Postpartum Techniques

ASSESSING THE MOTHER

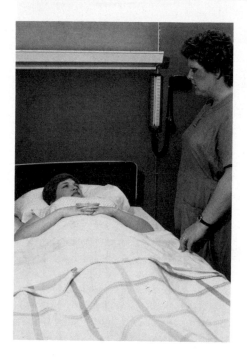

Wash your hands and explain the procedure to your client. Be sure to provide privacy. To make the process as comfortable as possible, ensure that the client has recently voided. Begin the assessment by taking vital signs to ensure that they are within normal limits when compared to the baseline. Frequent assessment is essential, especially during the first 24 hours when the client is at the greatest risk for postpartum hemorrhage.

Palpating the Fundus and Bladder

The fundus should be assessed for location and tone at frequent intervals, according to agency protocol, until around the tenth day postpartum when it is usually no longer palpable. Because most clients are discharged much earlier than this, instruct the client in self-examination so that she can be alert to changes in her uterus. To assess the fundus and bladder, lower the head of the bed so that the abdomen will be relaxed. Ensure that the client has recently voided, because a full bladder will displace the fundus. Fundal height is measured in relationship to its distance in finger breadths from the umbilicus. To measure the distance, position your ring finger directly over the umbilicus so that your small finger is closest to the client's head. Using your ring finger as a fulcrum, roll your hand back and forth gently. If the fundus is more than a finger's breadth (FB) above the umbilicus (U) or more than two below, reposition your fingers in the appropriate direction. Document the measurement accordingly, for example: 1 FB ↑ U; or 1 FB ↓ U; or @U. At the same time, note the fundal relationship to the midline. Displacement to either side of the midline is usually caused by a distended bladder. Normally the fundus will be at the midline. If it is displaced, palpate the bladder gently, following the procedure, p. 434. Also, describe the uterine tone. Optimally, it will feel firm and well-contracted; it should not be excessively tender to the touch.

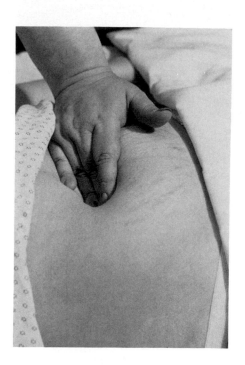

Evaluating the Lochia

Inspecting the Perineum

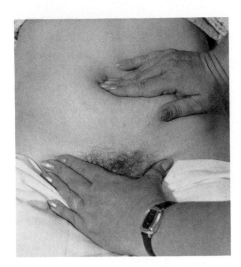

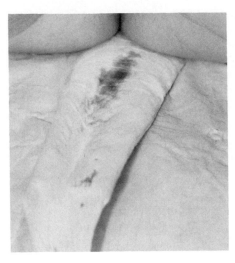

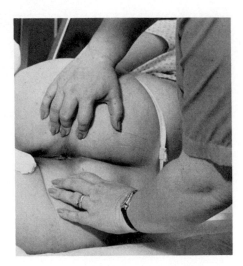

Performing Fundal Massage: If the uterus feels soft and boggy, perform a light massage in an attempt to contract and harden it. Ask the client to flex her knees to relax her abdomen, and to release the peri pad so that you can clearly assess the amount, color, and consistency of the lochia expelled during the massage. Place the flattened fingertips of your dominant hand at the client's fundus. To prevent uterine prolapse, provide support with your other hand (as shown). Lightly massage the fundus in a circular motion. If the uterus does not respond to a light massage, repeat with more vigorous movements. If the client's uterus is nonresponsive and remains soft and boggy, and if this is accompanied by copious bleeding, contact the physician for immediate intervention. *Caution: Never massage a well-contracted uterus. Overstimulation can result in muscle fatigue and uterine relaxation.*

To assess the lochia, detach the peri pad from the client's sanitary belt. Be sure to remove it from the front to the back to minimize the risk of contaminating the vagina with rectal discharge. Note the amount, character, and odor of the discharge. During the first few days, the lochia should resemble menstrual blood in that it should be dark and red (lochia rubra). After the third day it should appear more serous and brown in color (lochia serosa). Clots are usually abnormal and could mean that the client has retained placental tissue. If clots are found, further investigation is indicated and a referral may be necessary. Be sure to ask the client about her evaluation of the bleeding and the number of pads she has saturated. Four to eight saturated pads may be considered normal over a 24-hour period. However, if your client has had a cesarean delivery, that amount would be excessive. Also, foul-smelling lochia on a fresh pad could be indicative of an infection. Document the amount and character of the lochia, for example: lochia rubra, moderate amount with a few small clots; or lochia serosa, scant.

To inspect the perineum, instruct the client to assume a side-lying (Sim's) position. It is important that she flex the top leg to minimize the strain on the episiotomy. Gently separate the buttocks, which will enable you to fully inspect the perineum. Assess the area for stage of healing, presence of edema, bruising, dehiscence, and signs of infection, as well as for hemorrhoids. Document your observations. If indicated, apply ice packs to the perineum for the first 12 hours to minimize edema. After the first 12 hours, apply heat, such as chemical heat packs or perilights, or encourage the use of a sitz bath. If your client has had a cesarean delivery, it is still important to assess the perianal area for the presence of hemorrhoids.

Inspecting and Palpating the Breasts

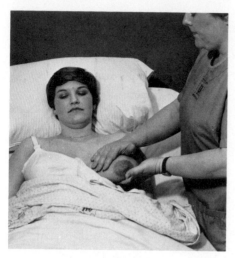

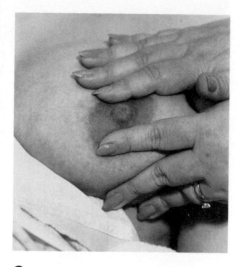

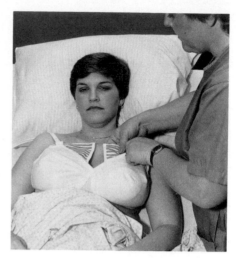

1 Raise the head of the bed, wash your hands, and ask your client to lower her gown so that you can examine her breasts. Inspect each breast, noting reddened areas or any irregularities such as asymmetry; and if present, assess the degree of engorgement. Palpate each breast, assessing for heat or nodules caused by occluded milk ducts. These occur most frequently in the upper outer quadrants.

2 Inspect and palpate the areolae and nipples. Gently spread the areola between your fingers, noting cracks, fissures, tenderness, blood, or a buildup of secretions. Also assess for erectility of the nipple by rolling the nipple between your thumb and index finger. If cracks or fissures are noted, encourage the client to keep the flaps of her bra unhooked and down to enhance air drying. Creams or ointments should be used only in instances of severe irritation because most require removal prior to breast feeding, resulting in increased irritation to the area. It is acceptable to use pure hydrous lanolin, however, because it is more readily absorbed into the skin and does not require removal prior to breast feeding.

3 For engorgement in breast-feeding mothers, which usually lasts from 36–48 hours or until the true milk comes in, apply chemical heat packs prior to breast feeding, or encourage a hot shower, which will aid in the letdown reflex. If your client is a nonnursing mother, she may also experience breast discomfort until her milk dries up. Ensure that her bra fits well and that it provides the necessary support for her breasts. Chemical ice packs may also be inserted into each cup (as shown) to help minimize the engorgement. If you apply nonchemical ice packs, be sure to wrap them with cloths prior to inserting them into the bra. Remember that heat, massage, and the expression of breast milk will increase the production of milk, and they should be avoided in the nonnursing mother.

ASSISTING WITH INFANT FEEDING

Provide time for the mother to prepare for infant feeding. For example, she may wish to void, and she should wash her hands and get into a comfortable position. To provide her with privacy, draw the curtain around her bed and shut her door. Be sure to verify that the infant's name and identification numbers match those of the mother.

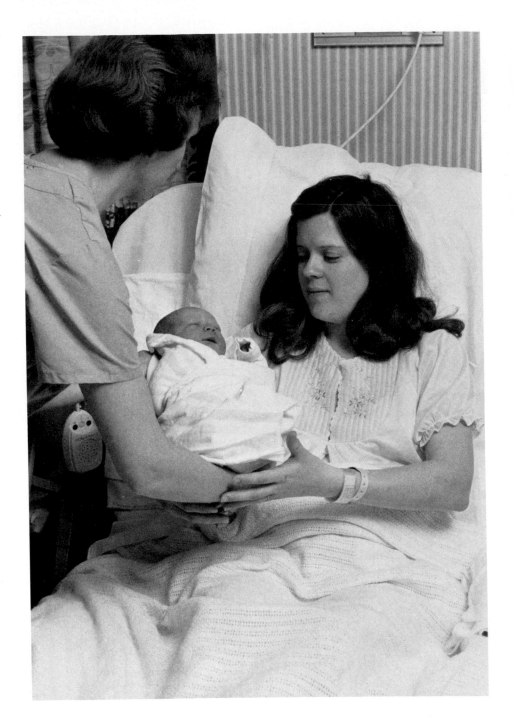

Positioning the Infant

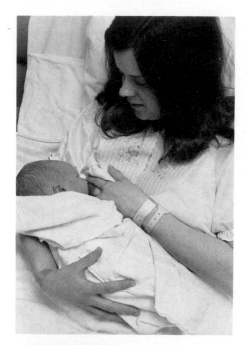

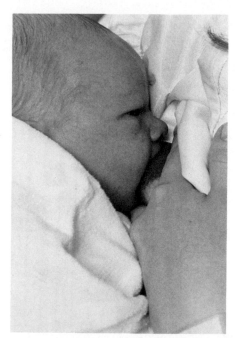

1 *The Cradle Hold:* A commonly used position for breast feeding is the cradle hold in which the mother is sitting upright, with the infant's head held in the crook of her arm and its buttocks cradled in her hand.

2 Note that the mother positions her index and middle fingers on both sides of the areola, squeezing gently. This encourages the infant to place his mouth around as much of the areola as possible, which in turn stimulates the milk ducts underneath the areola. This hand position also prevents the breast from obstructing the infant's nose.

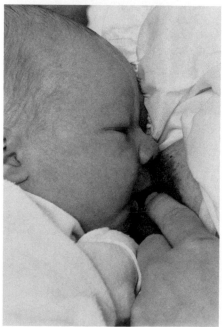

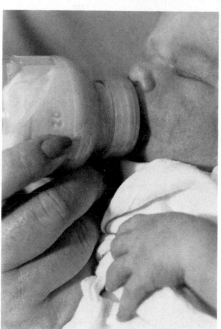

3 When the mother desires to remove the infant from her breast, instruct her to break the suction by inserting her finger between the areola and the infant's mouth (as shown) or to gently insert a finger into the infant's mouth. To protect her nipples, remind her to always break the suction prior to removing the infant from the breast. To help prevent sore nipples, encourage the mother to switch to her other breast after 3 minutes on the first day, and to increase the time by a minute a day to a maximum of 10 minutes per breast, or to the standard advocated by your agency.

4 Bottle-fed infants are positioned in the cradle hold position because it enhances the warmth and physical closeness that occur with breast feeding. The bottle should *always* be held rather than propped up, and the nipple must be full of milk to avoid introducing air into the infant's stomach.

(Continued on p. 192)

5 *Football Hold:* This position is recommended for mothers who have had a cesarean delivery, because it enables them to support the infant's weight off their abdomens. The infant is held supine along the forearm with the head supported by the mother's hand. The infant's weight can be supported by a pillow.

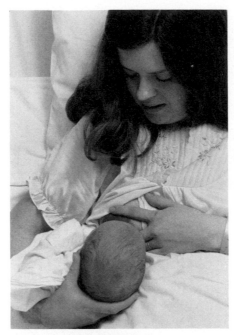

6 *Side-Lying:* When the mother wishes to rest, a side-lying position will enable her to lie down with the infant at her side rather than in her arms. The infant can be supported in the side-lying position by placing a rolled blanket or towel behind his back. This position is also excellent after cesarean deliveries.

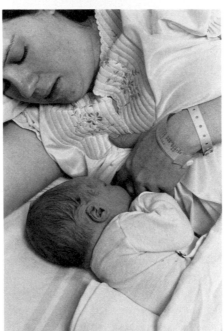

Burping the Infant

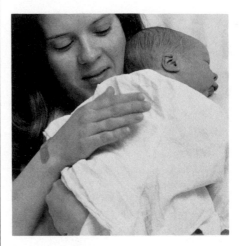

1 After feeding the infant at each breast, the mother should gently burp him by patting or rubbing his back to expel the air bubbles. She can hold the infant over her shoulder (as shown) with a diaper or towel placed under his mouth to absorb any fluid that may potentially be expelled.

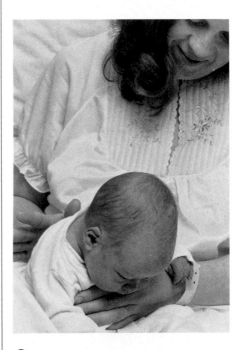

2 In another burping position, the infant sits with his head flexed forward. The mother supports his chest and head with one hand and pats or rubs his back with the other.

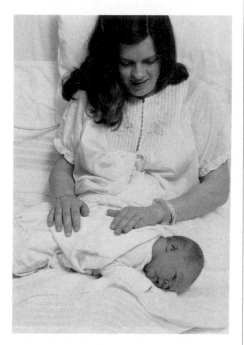

3 The infant can also be burped in a prone position over the mother's thighs. Positions 2 and 3 are recommended for newborns because either position allows the mother to see the infant's face, which will alert her to potential choking and aspiration.

Massaging the Breasts for Manual Expression of Breast Milk

Teach your breast-feeding client how to massage her breasts to facilitate the manual expression of breast milk. This will enable her to produce a small amount of milk or colostrum, which will help entice a disinterested infant to eat. It will also allow her to relieve breast engorgement and to store milk for future feedings in her absence.

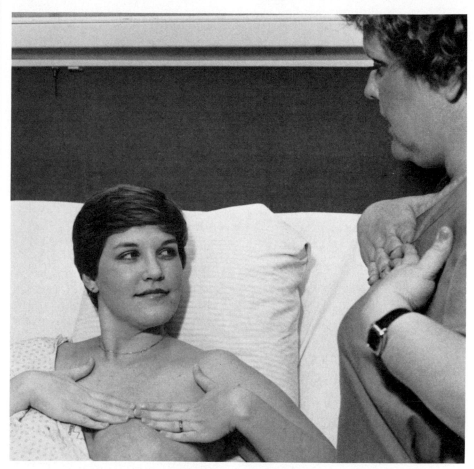

1 The mother should first wash her hands. Explain that breast massage will enhance the flow of milk through all the milk ducts. Show her how to sweep her fingers from the chest wall onto the upper surface of the breast.

(Continued on p. 194)

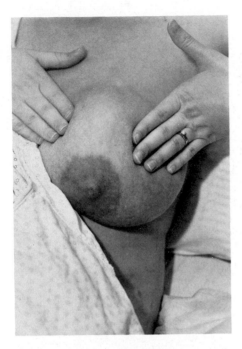

2 Next, she should slide her fingers down both sides of the breast.

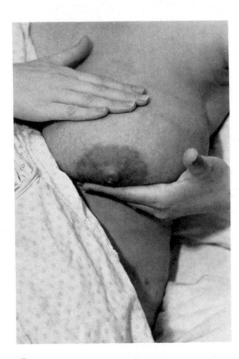

3 Her hands should then be positioned on the top side and under side of the breast, sweeping toward the areola.

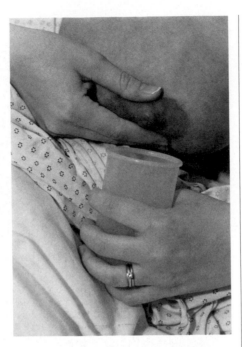

4 She can manually express the milk by grasping the areola between her thumb and index finger. As she presses the thumb and index finger together, the breast should be held against the chest wall to express the milk. She should then repeat the nipple compression as she repositions her thumb and index finger in a circular fashion around the breast. Instruct her to alternate the massage with the manual expression to facilitate the complete emptying of each breast. Ensure that the expressed milk does not run over her fingers but, rather, directly into the sterile container.

USING BREAST PUMPS

Breast pumps are used to express milk for the relief of breast engorgement in the nursing mother, as a means of maintaining lactation, or as a method for milk storage when the mother must be absent from feedings. In the hospital, aseptic technique is used; after she is discharged, the mother can use clean technique.

Managing Hand Pumps

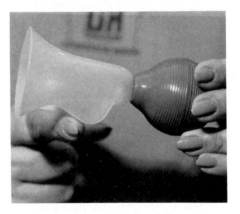

1 The bell pump is an inexpensive and simple method for obtaining breast milk on a short-term basis, for example, for the maintenance of lactation for an occasional missed feeding. Explain to the mother that she should hold the pump so that the reservoir is lowermost (as shown).

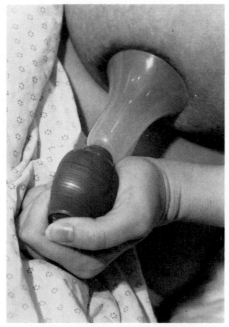

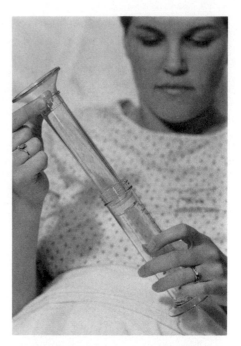

2 After washing her hands and performing breast massage, instruct the mother to squeeze the bulb and then center the breast shield over her nipple. She should then release and compress the bulb to pump each breast. When the reservoir becomes full, she should pour the milk into a sterile plastic bottle or into a plastic liner from a commercial nurser if she wishes to store the milk for her baby. Glass containers should be avoided because leukocytes in breast milk have a tendency to adhere to the sides of these containers (Paxson, 1979:61–64).

3 The Marshall Kaneson pump is a popular brand of hand pump that can be used routinely for milk storage. Instruct your client to aseptically insert the inner cylinder into the outer cylinder (as shown).

4 She can then select and attach the flange that will more closely accomodate her nipple and breast size. The flange will screw into the inner cylinder.

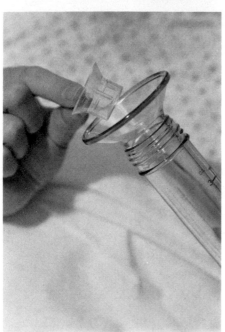

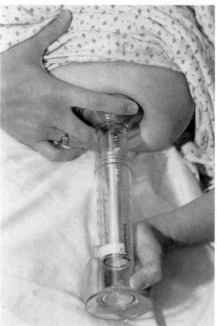

5 Instruct the client to center the flange of the inner cylinder directly over her nipple. To pump the breast, she must slide the outer cylinder in and out in a piston-like movement. After pumping each breast, she should then pour the milk into a plastic container, as described in step 2. After each use the breast pump should be thoroughly cleansed according to agency protocol, dried, and stored in a closed container at the bedside. After discharge from the hospital, the client may either boil the apparatus or wash it in an automatic dishwasher that reaches 180 F.

Assisting with Automatic Pumps

Automatic pumps such as the Medela are an efficient and time-saving method of obtaining breast milk on a long-term basis. Adapt the following procedure when using the automatic pump employed by your agency.

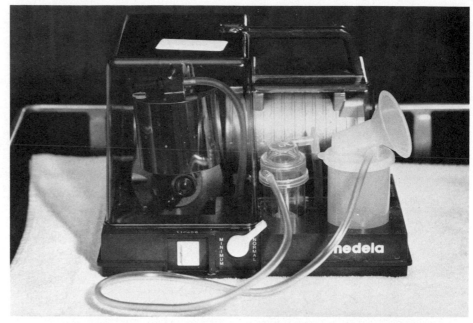

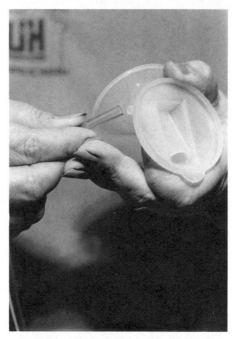

1 To assemble the equipment, begin by attaching the hose to the breast shield.

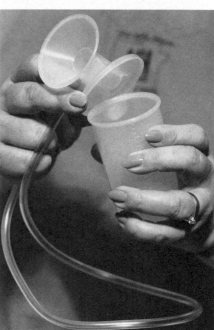

2 Snap the breast shield onto the plastic container.

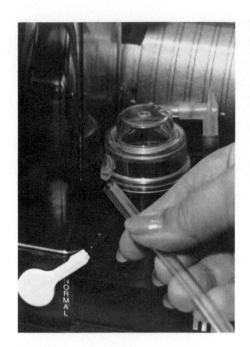

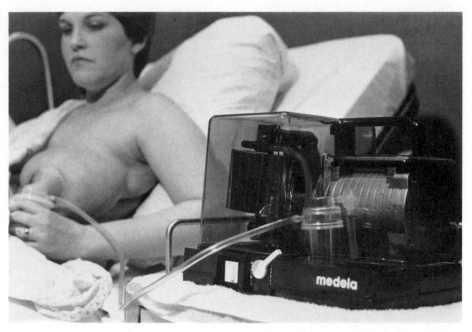

3 Attach the distal end of the hose to the container on the pump.

4 Instruct the mother to position the breast shield so that it is centered over her nipple.

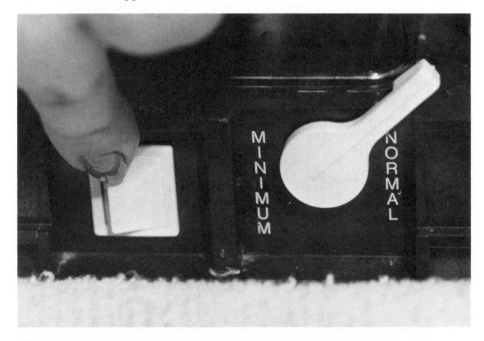

5 She can then adjust the control lever on the pump to the desired amount of suction. The pump works best on the "normal" setting, but "minimal" should be used if her nipples are sore or cracked. Store the milk and cleanse the equipment according to the procedure for using hand pumps.

Caring for the Newborn

ADMITTING THE NEONATE TO THE NURSERY

Obtaining Footprints

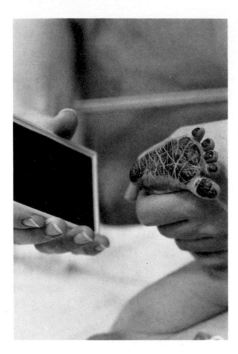

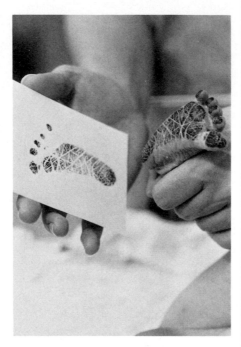

1 If your agency requires footprints and/or palm prints as a part of the permanent birth record, recording them may be the responsibility of the nurse who admits the newborn to the nursery. To obtain the footprints wipe any vernix off the sole of the foot and position the carbon plate over the entire length of the newborn's foot. Use moderate pressure as you ink the sole because too much ink can obscure the lines and creases.

2 After inking the foot, press the footprint sheet onto the inked sole. To stimulate the newborn to spread his toes, press the footprint sheet from the heel to the toes. Repeat the process on the other foot, and then file the prints in the infant's chart. After obtaining the footprints, rub the soles of the feet with baby oil and wipe the feet with a towel or cloth diaper to remove the ink. Your agency may also file the mother's fingerprint along with her newborn's footprints.

Instilling Silver Nitrate

The instillation of either a 1% silver nitrate solution or an antibiotic ophthalmic solution such as erythromycin is a procedure mandated by most states as a prophylaxis for gonococcal ophthalmia neonatorum. Although many agencies require the immediate instillation in the delivery room, others delay the process until the neonate's admission into the nursery to facilitate the newborn's bonding with the parents.

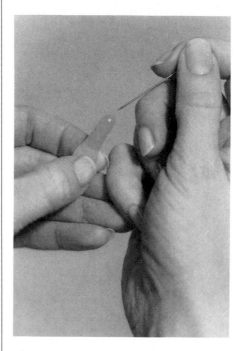

1 To administer the silver nitrate solution, pierce the wax ampul with the needle that is usually provided with the ampuls.

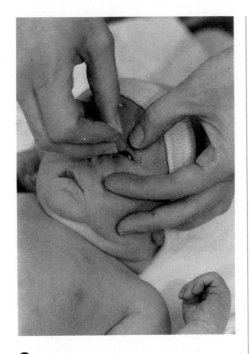

2 Lightly touch the upper lid, which will cause the neonate to open the eye, and then apply gentle pressure on the lower lid to expose the lower conjunctival sac. Instill one or two drops (according to agency guidelines) into the sac. Avoid instilling the medication directly onto the cornea because this could cause corneal irritation. Allow the eye to close so that the medication can be spread over the surface of the eye. Repeat the procedure in the other eye. If you are administering an antibiotic ointment, instill the ointment into the conjunctival sac from the inner to outer canthus (review procedure, p. 93). Because either medication could result in a mild conjunctivitis, be sure to explain to the parents that this is a temporary condition.

Administering a Vitamin K Injection

A vitamin K injection is administered as a prophylaxis for transient coagulation deficiency in the neonate. If prescribed, it is usually given on the day of birth because the coagulation disorder would potentially appear between the second and fifth day after birth.

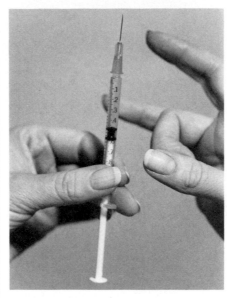

1 Wash your hands and draw up the prescribed dose of the medication into a tuberculin syringe that has a 25-gauge needle. Usually, 0.5–1 mg is administered.

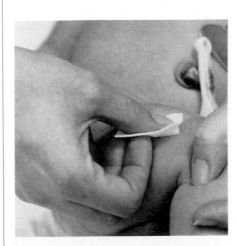

2 Swab the anterolateral segment of the upper thigh (the vastus lateralis muscle) with an alcohol sponge. Allow the alcohol to dry.

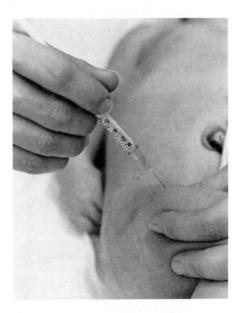

3 Bunch the tissue between your thumb and index finger, and quickly insert the needle at a 90° angle to the thigh. Aspirate to check for a blood return. When you are certain you are in a non-vascular area, slowly inject the solution so that you will evenly distribute the medication and minimize the newborn's discomfort. Remove the needle and massage the site with an alcohol sponge. Document the administration of the medication.

Obtaining a Blood Sample

Blood samples are obtained during the first few hours of birth as an assessment for hypoglycemia. Those at especially high risk include the following: infants of diabetic mothers, premature infants, infants small or large for gestational age, infants who are ill, and infants of prolonged or very stressful labor.

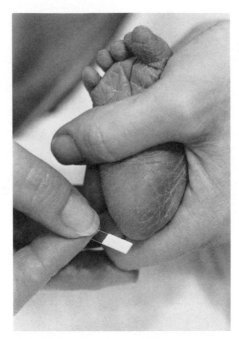

2 Position the pad of a reagent strip directly under the puncture site and collect a large droplet of blood onto the pad without smearing the blood. Review the steps, pp. 152–154, for visually monitoring blood glucose.

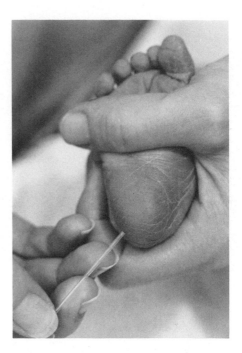

3 When a hematocrit has been ordered for evaluation of blood volume, prepare the heel and pierce the skin, according to step 1. Warming the heel prior to making the puncture will improve both blood flow and the accuracy of the test. Place the capillary tube at the puncture site and allow it to become at least half full of blood.

4 After obtaining the blood, place one end of the capillary tube into Critoseal to prevent specimen loss. Follow agency guidelines for spinning the tube in a centrifuge and reading the value.

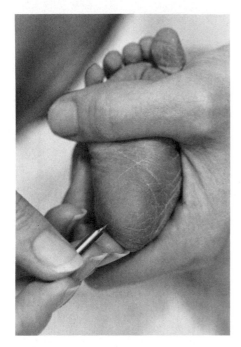

1 To obtain the blood sample, dorsiflex the foot and prepare the lateral aspect of the heel with an alcohol sponge. When the alcohol has dried, firmly pierce the skin with the lancet, just deeply enough to elicit a large droplet of blood.

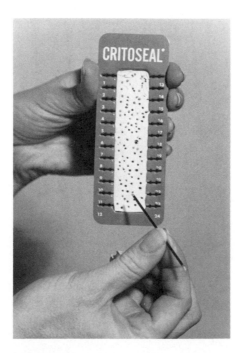

ASSESSING THE NEONATE

Performing a General Inspection

Wash your hands with an antimicrobial soap, and prepare to assess the infant in a warm environment such as the radiant warmer or at the mother's bedside. Remove the diaper and shirt, but keep the infant's stockinette cap on for as long as possible to minimize the heat loss through his head. The heart-shaped foam pad worn by the infant in these photos is holding a temperature probe in place.

Observe the resting posture. A normal-term infant's posture is flexed even when he is asleep. Also, note the color. In white infants, the color is normally ruddy or pink tinged. Darker-skinned infants can be assessed by inspecting the lips and mucous membranes, which are normally pink. A yellow cast may indicate jaundice; a blue tint at the feet, hands, and mouth is often indicative of sluggish peripheral circulation. This is usually transient, clearing in several hours. However, cyanosis, along with restlessness and choking, requires immediate suctioning to remove esophageal mucus. Count the respirations for a full minute and note their quality. Normally, they should range between 40–60 breaths per minute. Because neonates are diaphragmatic breathers, observe the abdomen rather than the chest for respirations. Respirations greater than 60 and less than 30 per minute, as well as substernal and subcostal retractions, are abnormal. With cyanosis, they could be indicative of aspiration or of disorders such as respiratory distress, transient tachypnea, or congenital heart disease. These infants should be referred to the attending physician immediately.

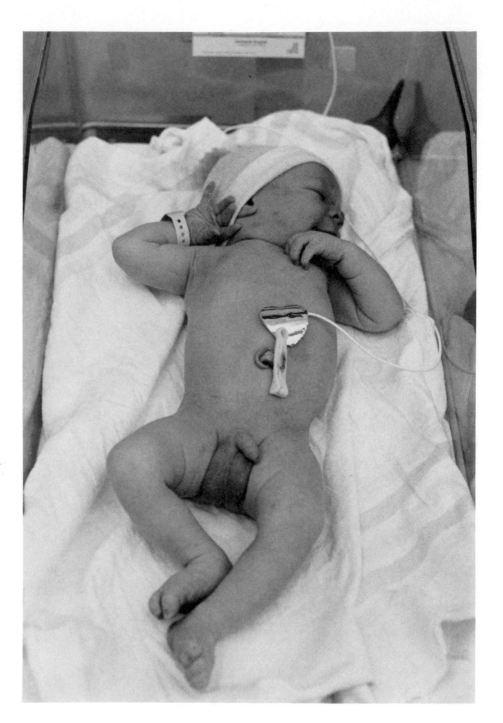

Auscultating

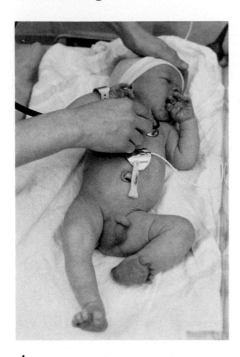 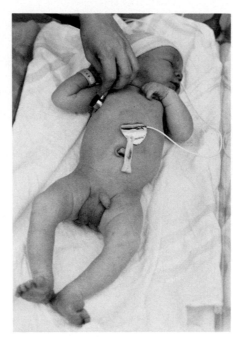 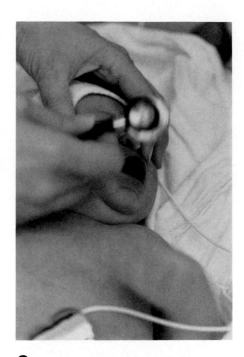

1 Auscultation, especially for heart sounds, should be performed when the infant is quiet. It is usually a good idea, therefore, to auscultate before initiating the hands-on assessment. Auscultate over the precordium for a full minute to assess apical pulse. Note the rate, rhythm, and intensity of the pulse. It should normally range from 130–160 beats/minute. However, the pulse may be as low as 90 at rest or as high as 200 when the infant cries. Be alert to irregularities such as arrhythmias or murmurs, which are heard as slurs or clicks between lub and dub.

2 Auscultate over the lung fields to assess breath sounds. Review Chapter 6 to assist you with auscultation sites and breath sounds. The latter, however, are not readily detected and identified in the newborn. Be alert to diminished breath sounds when comparing one side to the other, as well as to crackles, wheezes, and rhonchi.

3 Assess the patency of the nares by alternately obstructing each naris with an index finger. Listen with the stethoscope over the open naris to assess airflow. If the airflow is abnormal, either suction with a bulb syringe or attempt to pass a sterile catheter gently down the naris. Notify the physician if one or both nares are obstructed.

Taking an Axillary Temperature

While the infant is quiet, insert a thermometer into the axillary area; hold it in place for 3–5 minutes. An axillary temperature is often preferable to a rectal temperature because the rectum maintains the core temperature longer than the skin. Therefore, the axillary temperature will more readily alert you to rapid temperature changes that frequently occur in the newborn. The axillary temperature should normally register around 35.9 C.

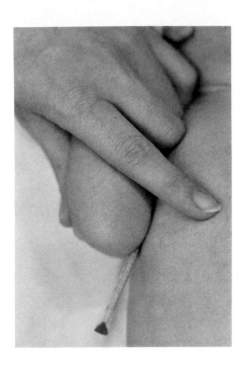

Palpating

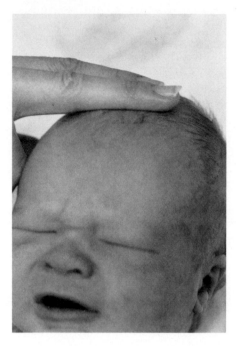

1 Begin your hands-on assessment of the neonate at the head by palpating the fontanelles (soft spots), both the anterior fontanelle (as shown) and the posterior fontanelle at the occiput. It is a good idea to measure your own fingers in centimeters to give yourself a built-in tape measure. The anterior fontanelle is normally 2–3 cm in width, 3–4 cm in length, and diamondlike in shape. It can be described as soft, which is normal, or full or bulging, which could be indicative of increased intracranial pressure. Conversely, a depressed fontanelle could mean that the neonate is dehydrated. The posterior fontanelle is smaller, triangular in shape, and it closes within 6–12 weeks, or it may be closed at birth. The anterior fontanelle usually closes within 12–18 months.

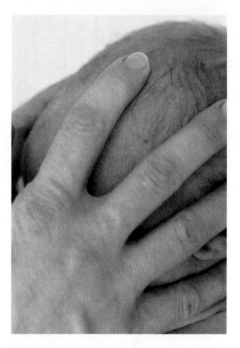

2 Palpate the sutures, which are the junctions of the cranial bones and are normally moveable. Overriding sutures are normal in the first week of life secondary to the molding of the head during birth. Fixed sutures are abnormal and should be called to the physician's attention.

(Continued on p. 204)

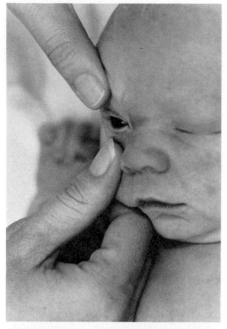

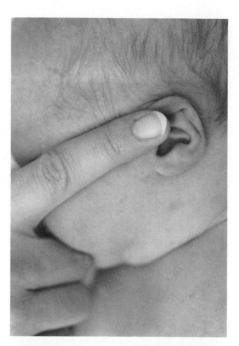

3 Inspect the eyes by gently separating the lids. Assess the pupillary reflex with an ophthalmoscope or penlight to ensure that the pupils react equally to light. Also observe for the equality of pupil size. Unequal pupils could suggest birth trauma. Note whether the corneas appear cloudy, which is indicative of a congenital infection, or hemorrhagic, which is usually transient and caused from pressure during delivery.

4 Assess the infant for low-set ears, which may be indicative of chromosomal abnormalities and are often associated with genitourinary disorders. Normally, the pinna of the ear is in a straight line with the outer canthus of the eye.

5 Assess the development of the ear cartilage next. If the auricle stays in the position in which it is pressed, or returns to its original position slowly, it usually means that the gestational age is less than 38 weeks. Also, inspect for preauricular skin tags, which are usually normal and are often removed for cosmetic reasons.

6 To assess the rooting reflex, lightly stimulate the cheek by stroking from the outer corner of the mouth toward the ear on the same side. The infant should turn toward the finger in an attempt to suck. Teach this technique to the breast-feeding mother.

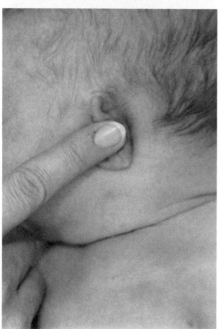

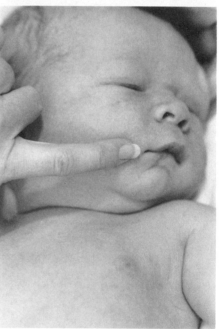

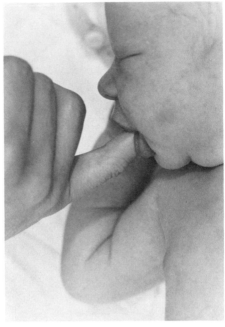

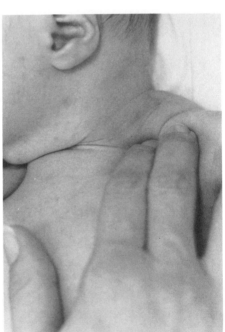

7 Assess the sucking reflex by placing a finger in the neonate's mouth. In addition, inspect and palpate the hard and soft palates to assess for clefts as well as for Epstein's pearls, which are white specks occasionally found on the gums and hard palate and may be palpated as hardened areas. These are normal and usually disappear after several days. You might also palpate neonatal teeth on the gum line. Because there is a potential for aspiration, notify the physician that you have found them in the event that removal is indicated. Deciduous teeth, however, are not removed.

8 Bilaterally palpate the neck to assess for masses, trachial deviation, an enlarged thyroid, or swollen lymph glands. Although the trachea normally is slightly at the right of the midline, the other findings are abnormal and should be referred to the physician. Also, assess the sternocleidomastoid muscles for symmetry and the shoulder joints for full range of motion.

9 Palpate the clavicles to ensure that they are symmetric and contiguous. A lump along one of the clavicles could be a fracture site caused from a traumatic delivery.

10 Elicit the startle reflex with a loud noise, for example, by clapping your hands together. Normally, the newborn will abduct and extend his arms. The fingers will extend and then flex into a "C." An asymmetric response suggests a fractured clavicle or an injury to the brachial plexus. Lack of a response is indicative of a hearing loss or brain damage.

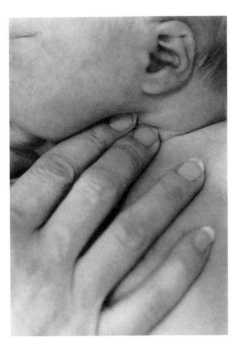

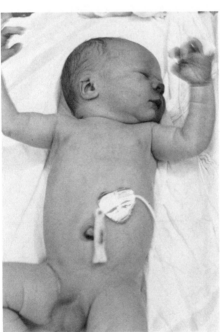

(Continued on p. 206)

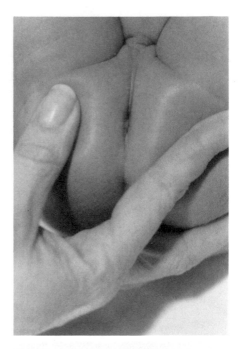

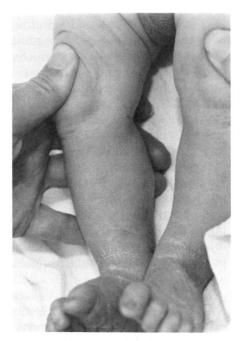

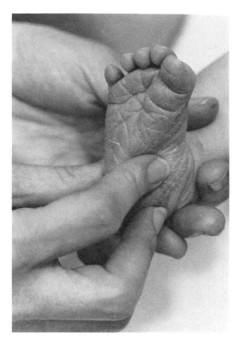

18 Spread the buttocks and assess the anus for patency and placement. If the anus appears to be either anteriorally or posteriorally positioned, the physician should be notified. In females, a rectal-vaginal fistula could be present, or this could represent a blind pouch with the true rectum correctly positioned but not patent. Patency is confirmed by the passage of the first meconium stool.

19 Continue to palpate the lower extremities for range of motion and bilateral symmetry of bones, muscles, and movement.

20 Inspect each foot to assess for clubfoot. Normally the foot is positioned at the midline of the tibia. A foot that is both inverted and plantarflexed and cannot be manipulated to midline requires a referral to the physician for further assessment. Also, inspect the soles of the feet for creases. If the creases do not cover the sole, the infant is probably less than 38 weeks gestational age.

21 To assess for congenital hip dislocation, perform the Ortolani click test. Position your middle fingers over the greater trochanters and your thumbs along the medial thighs. Then flex the hips and knees.

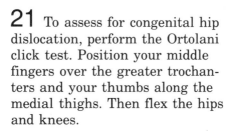

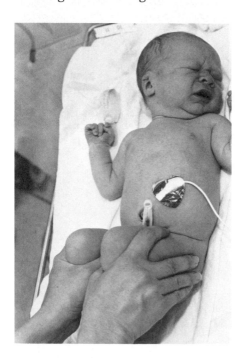

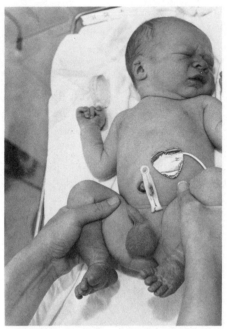

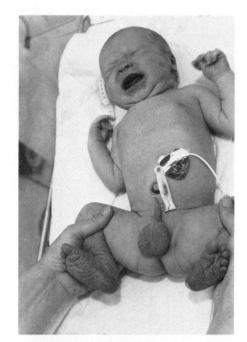

22 Gently abduct the hips and flex them to an even greater degree.

23 Externally rotate the hips. ⟶ Unilateral or bilateral limitations in mobility, along with audible clicking, occurs with hip dislocation or subluxation. Notify the physician for further evaluation.

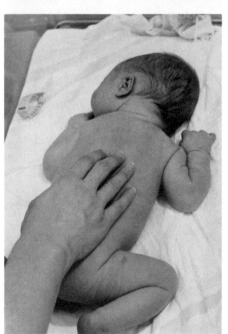

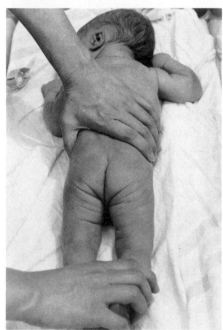

24 Place the neonate in a prone position and inspect and palpate the spine to assess for missing vertebrae and defects. Assess for dimples, sinuses, and tufts of hair, especially in the sacrococcygeal area, where a nevus pilosus (hairy nerve) is often indicative of spina bifida. Mongolian spots may also be present on the buttocks and in the dorsal lumbar area. These are bluish areas found usually in dark-skinned ethnic and racial groups. Be sure to explain to the parents that these spots are normal and that most fade within the first or second year.

25 Straighten the legs and observe for symmetry in the creases of the buttocks and legs. Asymmetry could suggest a congenital hip dislocation.

Taking an Arterial Blood Pressure

Measuring and Weighing the Infant

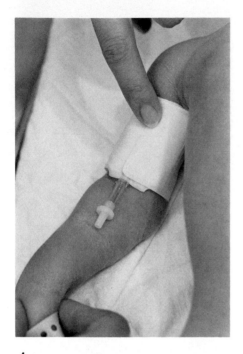

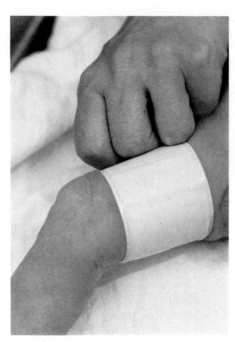

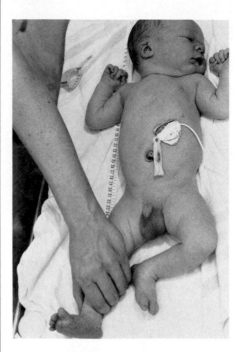

1 If your agency requires blood pressure monitoring for the neonate, you will probably use an ultrasonic device such as the Doppler. Wrap a blood pressure cuff of the appropriate size around the newborn's upper arm (see procedure guidelines, Chapter 7). Attach the cuff to the Doppler device and obtain the pressure reading according to manufacturer's instructions. A diastolic pressure less than 40 and a systolic pressure greater than 100 require further investigation. If the newborn is crying, the reading may be falsely elevated.

2 If the femoral pulses are weak or absent, suggesting coarctation of the aorta, assess the blood pressure in the leg. Wrap the cuff around the upper thigh and obtain the pressure reading. The reading should be slightly higher in the leg than in the arm. A vast difference between the two, however, helps to confirm coarctation of the aorta, and you should obtain a pressure reading in all four extremities.

1 To measure the infant's length, place him in a supine position and extend one of his legs. The tape measure is then positioned from the top of the head to the heel.

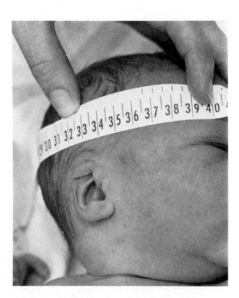

2 The head circumference is measured along the broadest part of the occiput with the tape positioned just slightly above the eyebrows. If the head is severely molded from the delivery, repeat the measurement daily.

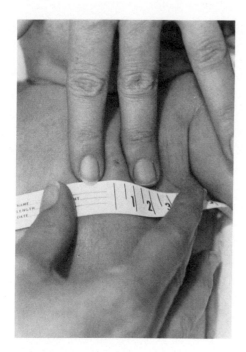

3 You may also measure the breast tissue to further evaluate gestational age. Compress the tissue between your thumb and index finger and measure the tissue in centimeters. At a normal gestational age, the tissue should measure between 0.5–1 cm. An absence of or decreased breast tissue is often indicative of prematurity or a newborn who is small for gestational age. Also observe for supernumerary nipples, which are not harmful and may be removed at a later date. Both female and male infants may have breast engorgement with actual milk production caused by the presence of hormones. Be sure to explain to the parents that this is normal.

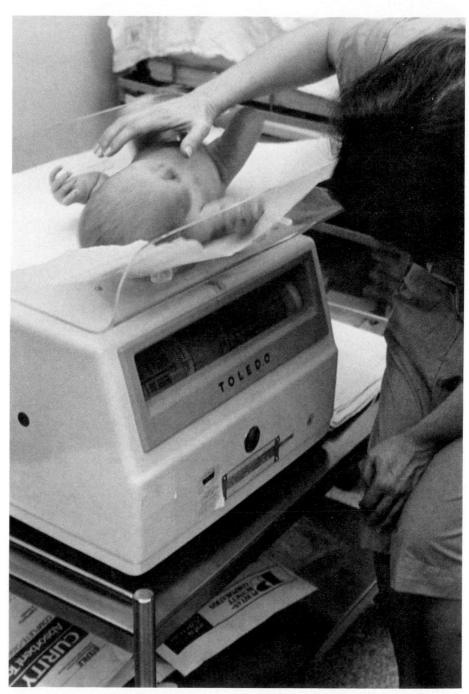

4 The neonate may lose 5%–10% of his body weight over the first 3–5 days because of normal fluid loss and low intake. Therefore, you must weigh the infant daily to monitor weight loss or gain. The scale should be balanced at least every shift and covered with a fresh paper or pad before weighing each infant to prevent cross contamination and to minimize heat loss. Always place your hand above the infant to prevent her or him from falling off the scale.

PROVIDING NEONATAL CARE

Giving Umbilical Cord Care

Suctioning

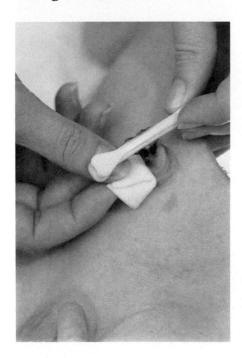
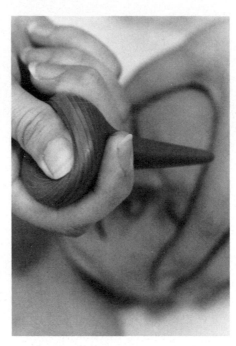
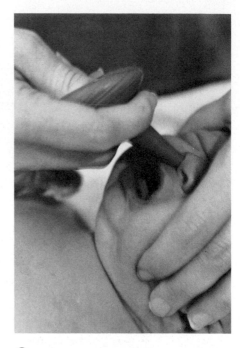

To help prevent infection and to promote drying of the umbilical cord, cleanse the cord daily with alcohol, povidone-iodine, or antibiotic ointment, according to agency guidelines. Be sure to swab around the entire surface of the cord base. The cord will usually fall off on its own after 7–10 days. Observe for redness or discharge, which are signs of infection, and be certain to keep the diaper below the cord. Instruct the parents in cord care.

1 *Using a Bulb Syringe:* A bulb syringe is kept in the newborn's crib for removing secretions in the nose and mouth. To correctly use the bulb syringe, first depress the bulb with your thumb.

2 Insert the tip of the nozzle into each naris and allow the bulb to slowly expand. Be sure to stabilize the infant's head with your free hand to minimize the risk of injuring the nasal mucosa. If indicated, suction the mouth as well. To remove the drainage from the bulb syringe, compress the bulb and point the nozzle over a tissue. Be sure to instruct the parents in the proper use of the bulb syringe.

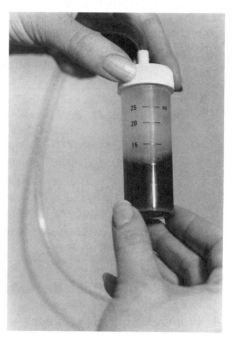

head with your free hand as you pass the catheter into the pharynx. When you enter the pharynx, begin sucking on the suction tubing as you withdraw the catheter. The secretions will collect in the mucous trap (see above). Observe the neonate for color changes because suctioning can stimulate a vagal response with bradycardia. Remember that "gently but thoroughly" is the rule of thumb with neonates.

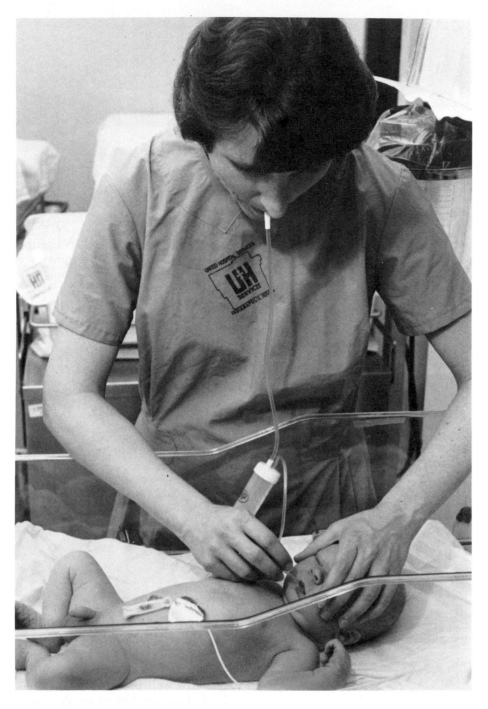

DeLee Mucous Trap: A DeLee mucous trap is used when congestion is deeper than the nose and mouth, and the secretions may potentially block the airway. The suction catheter is inserted through the infant's mouth or nose into the pharynx, and the suction tubing is inserted into your mouth so that you can aspirate the secretions into the collection trap. Stabilize the newborn's

(Continued on p. 214)

CHAPTER OUTLINE

Assessing the Gastrointestinal System

THE GASTROINTESTINAL SYSTEM

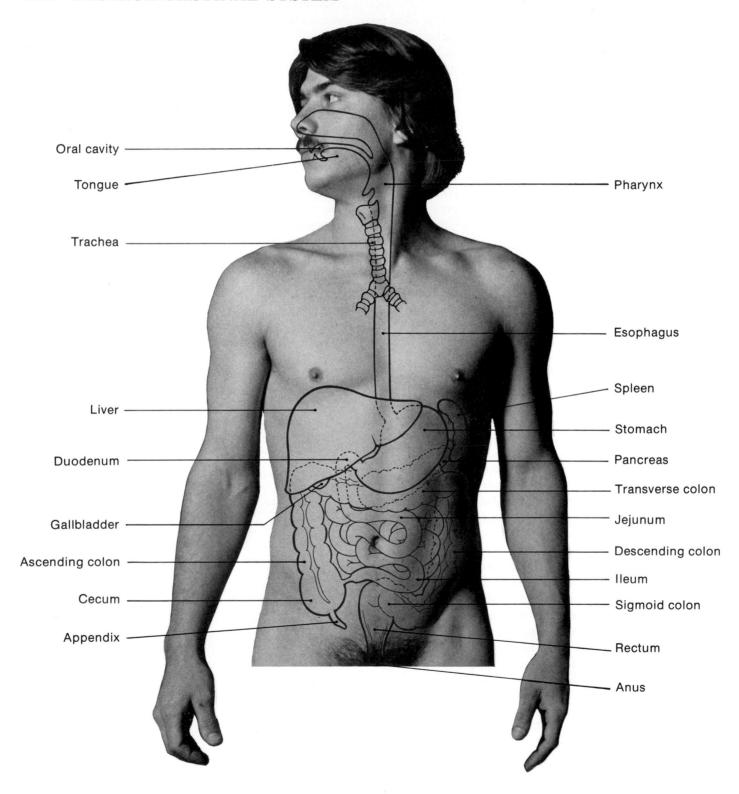

Oral cavity

Tongue

Trachea

Liver

Duodenum

Gallbladder

Ascending colon

Cecum

Appendix

Pharynx

Esophagus

Spleen

Stomach

Pancreas

Transverse colon

Jejunum

Descending colon

Ileum

Sigmoid colon

Rectum

Anus

EXAMINING THE ABDOMEN

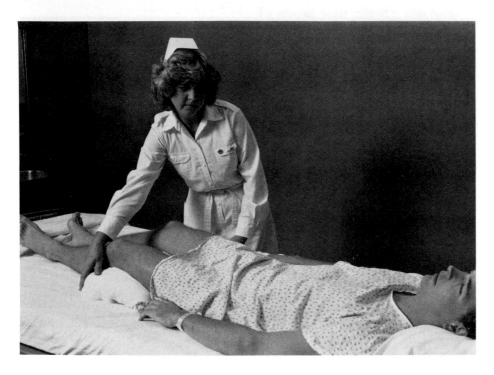

To examine the client's abdomen, you should provide a quiet, warm, and private environment. Explain the assessment procedure, and ensure that the client has recently voided. Assist the client into a supine position, and place pillows under his head and knees to help relax the abdominal muscles. As you are preparing the client, observe his body alignment and facial expression for objective indicators of discomfort, such as grimacing or flexing the legs, which often occurs with acute appendicitis or peritonitis. Remember that your examination should begin with a visual inspection of the abdomen, followed by auscultation, and finally percussion and palpation. Because touching and temperature variations stimulate both peristalsis and muscle guarding, these reactions would alter the frequency and character of bowel sounds.

Inspecting the Abdomen

Expose the abdomen from the sternum to the pubis. Note the contour of the abdomen, which can be described as rounded, flat, or scaphoid (concave). Observe for distention; asymmetry, which could indicate the presence of a mass; or peristaltic waves, which although not often seen, are indicative of intestinal obstruction in the adult or pyloric stenosis in the infant. Also observe for unusual pigmentation; striae, which occur after a pregnancy or weight gain; and loose skin folds, which can occur with weight loss. Assess the umbilicus for inversion, or for eversion in clients with umbilical hernias or extreme ascites, and make a note of any abdominal scars. Also, observe the epigastrium for the presence of pulsations. Mild pulsations may normally be seen in very thin clients; however, vigorous pulsations occur in clients with right ventricular hypertrophy or with masses anterior to the aorta. Be alert to a pronounced venous network in the abdominal area. This is seen in adults with hepatic obstruction, portal hypertension, or ascites. However, it may normally be seen in infants and children. Note the presence of any ostomies, the color and character of the stoma, the appearance of the peristomal skin, and the amount and character of the effluent (fecal drainage) in the pouch.

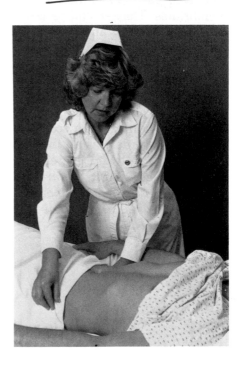

→

Auscultating the Abdomen

Review this anatomic overlay to assist you in dividing your client's abdomen into quadrants. The epigastric, umbilical, and hypogastric areas are further delineated. For auscultation, palpation, and percussion, you should develop your own pattern of assessment—for example, a clockwise examination of each of the four quadrants—and follow the same pattern consistently.

To auscultate the abdomen, warm the diaphragm of the stethoscope and then place it in the center of each of the four quadrants, counting the frequency and character of the bowel sounds for a full minute. Move the stethoscope to various areas within the quadrant if you are unable to elicit sounds in the center. Generally, you will be able to hear 5–34 bowel sounds per minute. With hyperperistalsis you will hear more frequent, high-pitched gurgling. These sounds will occur with diarrhea, gastroenteritis, or intestinal hemorrhage. In a late obstructive process, paralytic ileus, or peritonitis, bowel sounds are typically absent. However, with a developing obstruction, bowel sounds may be absent in the quadrant in which the obstruction occurs, yet increase in frequency proximal to the point of obstruction.

During auscultation you should be alert to circulatory sounds such as bruits. These are swishing sounds, which may be heard in the midepigastric area in clients with diseased aortas. Venous hums are softer and more continuous than bruits and may be heard in the upper epigastric area and over the liver in clients with advanced cirrhosis. Friction rubs sound like sand paper rubbing together, and they are heard best with the client taking deep respirations. They may be heard over diseased livers, spleens, and gall bladders.

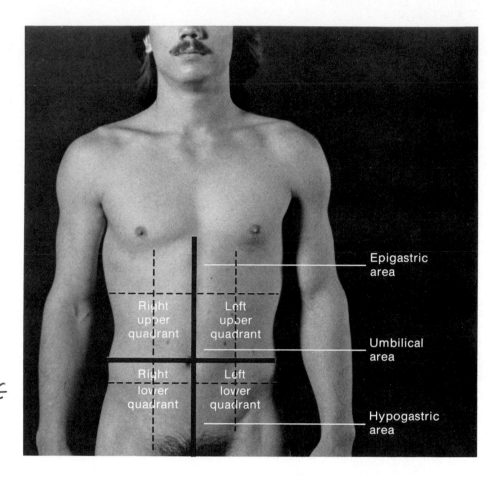

Epigastric
area

Right upper quadrant

Left upper quadrant

Umbilical
area

Right lower quadrant

Left lower quadrant

Hypogastric
area

Percussing the Abdomen

To percuss the abdomen, place your middle or index finger on the client's skin, and then strike that finger with the same finger on your opposite hand to elicit sounds. This assessment technique will reveal the density of the underlying structures. Hollow cavities, such as the empty intestine, will elicit high, tympanic sounds. Dull, flat sounds are heard over a distended bladder or over an organ, such as the liver in the right upper quadrant or the spleen in the left upper quadrant. You may also hear dullness while percussing the left lower quadrant over the sigmoid colon prior to the client's defecation. Dull sounds in other locations may be indicative of an abnormality such as a mass.

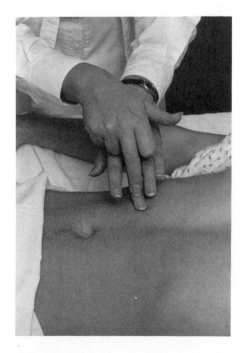

Palpating the Abdomen

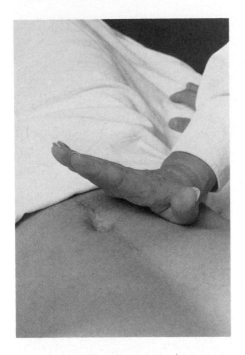 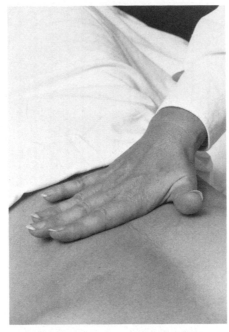 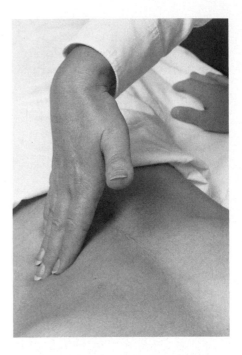

Lightly palpate the abdomen to determine muscle tone, tenderness, distention, organ size, pulsations, or the presence of a mass. You might use your entire hand not only because it is more comfortable for the client and the process will produce less muscle guarding, but also because you will have a larger surface area from which to assess abnormalities. Roll the hand over an abdominal area starting with the heel of the hand, progressing to the palm, and finishing at the fingertips. If you prefer, palpate with flattened fingertips, as in the center photo. A healthy abdomen should feel soft and supple, but you will feel resistance with a distended abdomen, and it will be less pliant. *Note: Clients with peritonitis, who have board-like abdomens, will find even light palpation extremely uncomfortable.*

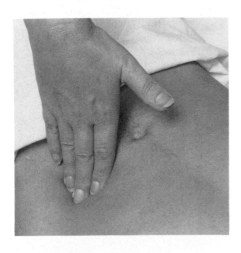

Deep Palpation: Deep palpation is employed after light palpation to assess for enlarged organs or for the presence of masses. In addition, if your client feels discomfort over a particular area during light palpation, you can use this technique to assess for rebound tenderness. This is found in clients with peritoneal inflammation or appendicitis. Gently and slowly press your flattened fingertips approximately 6–8 cm into the quadrant *opposite* that in which you elicited pain; then quickly release the pressure. Your client will feel a sudden, sharp pain over the original area of discomfort if rebound tenderness is present. *Caution: Never deeply palpate the right lower quadrant if appendicitis is suspected. Deep palpation is also contraindicated in clients with rigid abdomens, or in those who may have pancreatitis or ectopic pregnancy because the procedure can be very painful and it could also cause serious injury to the client.*

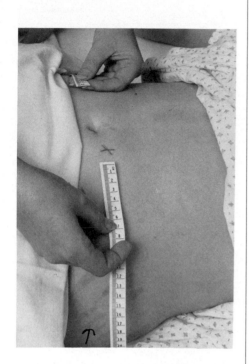

Measuring Abdominal Girth: To assess for increasing degrees of distention, including ascites, you will need to measure the abdominal girth daily and at the same time of day—for example, before breakfast. Mark a spot on the abdomen with indelible ink to ensure that you measure around the same circumferential site with each measurement. Measure the girth of the abdomen, using a nonstretchable tape measure, and record the result. Daily increases in girth are significant and should be reported to the attending physician. (Note the presence of striae on this client.)

EXAMINING THE RECTUM

Inspecting the Rectum

Before inspecting the rectum, provide your client with privacy, explain the procedure, and assist her into Sim's position. Expose the buttocks, and inspect the rectal and sacral areas for the presence of external hemorrhoids, alterations in the integrity of the skin, pilonidal cysts, and fissures.

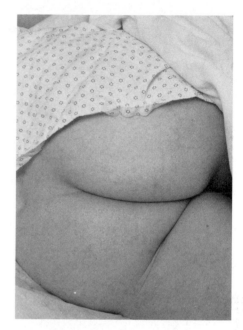

Palpating the Rectum

Put on a disposable examination glove, and lubricate your index finger with water soluble lubricant. Ask the client to breathe deeply and to bear down. Gently and slowly insert your index finger 5–10 cm (2–4 in.) into the rectum, past the external and internal sphincters. Palpate along the circumference of the rectal wall to assess for the presence of masses, fistulae, or stool. Use special care if the client has external or internal hemorrhoids. Assess sphincter tone by asking the client to tighten the sphincter around your finger. After removing your finger, inspect the glove for the presence of stool, blood or mucus. →

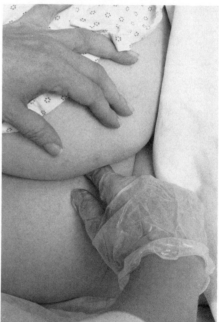

Managing Gastric Tubes

Nursing Guidelines for Managing Gastric Tubes

Single-Lumen Tubes

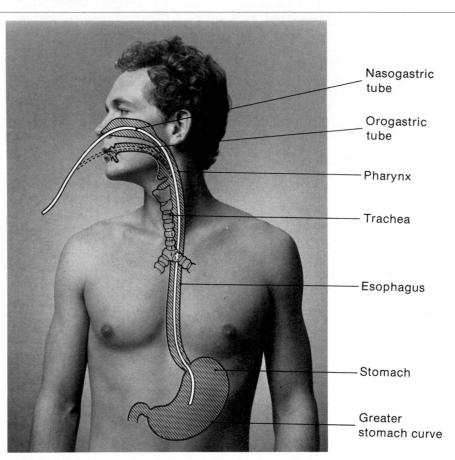

- Nasogastric tube
- Orogastric tube
- Pharynx
- Trachea
- Esophagus
- Stomach
- Greater stomach curve

Description	76–125 cm (30–50 in.) in length, rubber or plastic material, may have radiopaque tips for X-ray film detection, smaller-lumen tubes may have insertion guides.

Levin-type tubes: 12–18 French (F) for adults
                                  8–12F for children
                                  5–8F for infants
Pediatric feeders: 8F
Oral tubes: 30–40F

Uses	Gavage, administration of medications, lavage, diagnostic evaluation, decompression
Nursing Considerations	■ Chill rubber tubes in icy water prior to insertion, if desired. ■ Warm plastic tubes in hot water prior to insertion, if desired. ■ Most tubes are inserted through the nose unless the nasal route is contraindicated. ■ Larger-lumen tubes cause more irritation to the stomach, esophagus, and nose.

- For decompression, the tube should be connected to intermittent suction.
- Smaller tubes (8F) may require insertion guides for easier intubation.
- Check tube placement in stomach before *any* instillation.
- Provide oral and nasal hygiene at least three to four times a day.

Double-Lumen Tubes

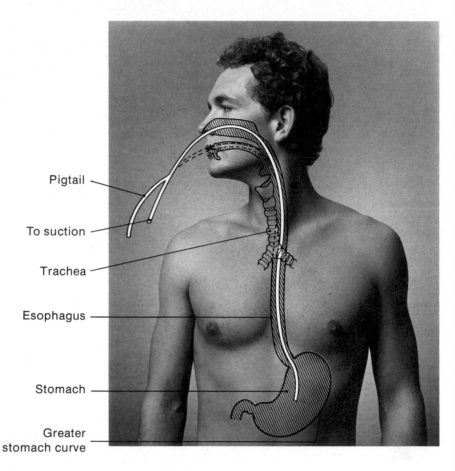

Pigtail

To suction

Trachea

Esophagus

Stomach

Greater
stomach curve

Description

85–125 cm (35–50 in.) in length, plastic or rubber material, may have radiopaque tips for X-ray film detection and mercury-weighted tips to facilitate movement to the stomach.

12–18F for adults
  8–12F for children
  5–8F for infants

Oral tubes: 30–40F

Uses

Decompression, lavage, gavage

Nursing Considerations

- Irrigate sump tubes through large port only.
- Inject *only* air into pigtail port of sump tubes, after reconnecting the large port to suction.
- For decompression, sump tubes work best when connected to continuous suction at 30 mm Hg.
- Check for correct stomach placement before *any* instillation
- Provide oral and nasal hygiene at least three to four times daily.

(Continued on p. 228)

- When client is restricted to nothing by mouth, monitor gastric pH every 4 hours to assess for acidity; if acidic, obtain an order for an antacid.
- Remove tube only after an assessment that reveals active bowel sounds, the passing of flatus, and an undistended or minimally distended abdomen.

Triple-Lumen Esophageal-Nasogastric (Blakemore) Tubes

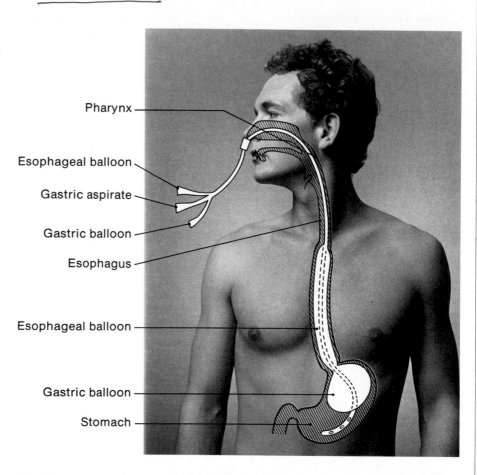

Pharynx

Esophageal balloon

Gastric aspirate

Gastric balloon

Esophagus

Esophageal balloon

Gastric balloon

Stomach

Description

86–98 cm (36–39 in.) in length; X-ray film opaque; latex rubber; has ports for gastric balloon, esophageal balloon, and gastric aspiration.
16–20F for adults
12F for children

Uses

Compression, as a tamponade for control of esophageal bleeding; decompression; lavage

Nursing Considerations

- The tube is usually inserted by a physician.
- The client requires constant observation while the balloons are inflated.
- A Levin or sump tube is sometimes inserted into the opposite naris for aspiration of the esophagus.
- Provide comfort measures while the tube is in place: blankets during lavage, backrubs and skin care, oral and nasal hygiene.
- A football helmet may be positioned on client's head so that exterior traction on the tube can be achieved by taping the tube to the face guard.

■ The esophageal balloon is deflated for 5 minutes every 8–12 hours to prevent erosion to the esophagus.
■ Tape scissors to the head of the client's bed for emergency tube cutting (deflating both balloons) in the event of acute respiratory distress.

Four-Lumen (Minnesota Sump) Tubes

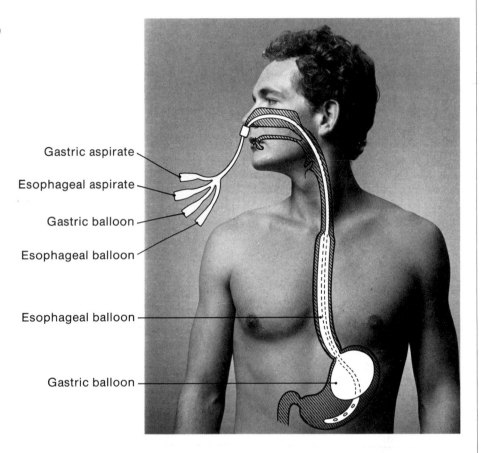

Gastric aspirate

Esophageal aspirate

Gastric balloon

Esophageal balloon

Esophageal balloon

Gastric balloon

Description	Has a fourth port for esophageal aspiration; thus, the need for a Levin or sump tube is eliminated.
Uses	See Blakemore tube, opposite page.
Nursing Considerations	See Blakemore tube, opposite page and above.

(Continued on p. 230)

Implementing

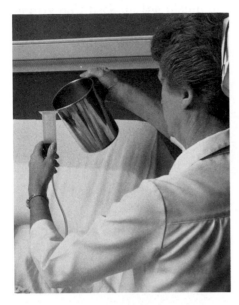 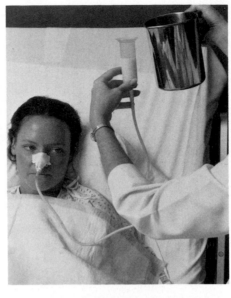 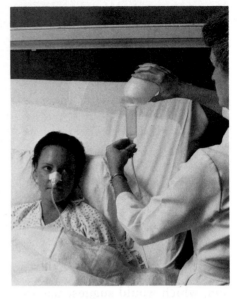

4 Remove the bulb or piston, and reinstill the measured aspirate via the syringe barrel to prevent loss of electrolytes and gastric juices. For effective gravity flow, hold the syringe 30–45 cm (12–18 in.) above the client's abdomen. To make this feeding as pleasant as possible, try to avoid instilling the gastric contents directly in front of the client.

5 Before the aspirate drains from the neck of the syringe, begin pouring the feeding solution into the syringe barrel. This will prevent the instillation of air into the client's stomach. Raise or lower the syringe if you need to adjust the flow to ensure a slow instillation of the feeding.

6 When the desired amount of feeding has been poured, flush the tubing with 30–50 mL of water, unless contraindicated. Be sure to add the water before the feeding solution has drained from the neck of the syringe. Clamp the tube before removing the syringe to prevent reflux of the feeding. Secure the tube to the client's gown.

7 For better absorption, have your client remain in Fowler's position for 45–60 minutes after the solution has been infused. If this is uncomfortable, she may be positioned in a slightly elevated right side-lying position (as shown) so that the solution can flow by gravity from the greater stomach curve to the pylorus. Wash and dry the syringe and the other feeding containers, and return them to the bedside stand. Document the feeding in the chart and on the intake and output record.

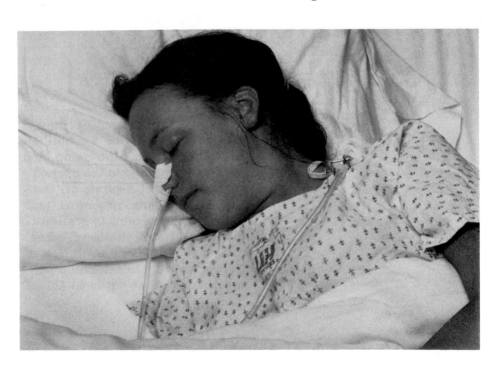

Evaluating

8 Assess for alterations in fluid volume, nutrition, and bowel elimination. If these occur, the rate of infusion or the concentration of the feeding solution may need altering. Monitor the fluid and electrolyte status by checking laboratory values and assess the client's vital signs, skin turgor, intake and output balance, and mucous membranes. Query the client about the presence of thirst, the primary indicator of dehydration. Unless contraindicated, periodically instill water into the nasogastric tube if the need has been determined by your assessment. Perform urine glucose tests every 6–8 hours to assess for glycosuria, which can be caused by the high osmolarity of the feeding solution. Administer nasal and oral hygiene after each feeding, and weigh the client daily, if prescribed.

Giving a Continuous-Drip Tube Feeding

Note: Review the guidelines for giving an intermittent tube feeding, and make the following variations.

Planning

There are several ways to administer a continuous-drip tube feeding. One simple method is to obtain the commercial screw-on drip chamber and tubing apparatus available for your client's bottled feeding solution.

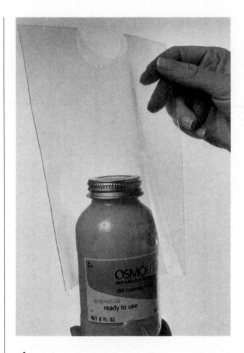

1 Place the plastic bag over the bottle containing the feeding solution so that the hole in the bag is centered over the bottle's neck.

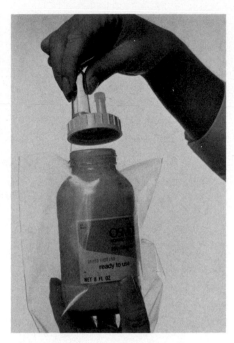

2 Remove the bottle cap and screw on the drip chamber and tubing apparatus.

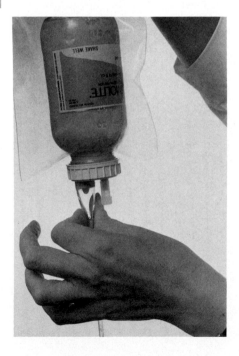

3 Turn the bottle upside down and squeeze the drip chamber to fill it to one-third to one-half of its capacity. Then allow the solution to flow to the end of the tubing, and clamp it off.

(Continued on p. 244)

Implementing

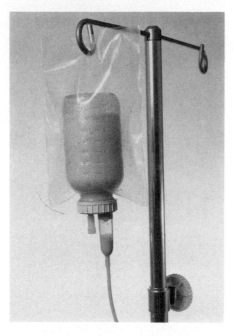

4 Hang the solution on an IV pole that has been adjusted to 30–45 cm (12–18 in.) above the client's abdomen. After you have aspirated and measured residual gastric contents, connect the feeding tube to the gastric tube, and reinforce the connection with a piece of tape. Adjust the drip rate to deliver the feeding over the desired length of time.

Managing Infusion Pumps

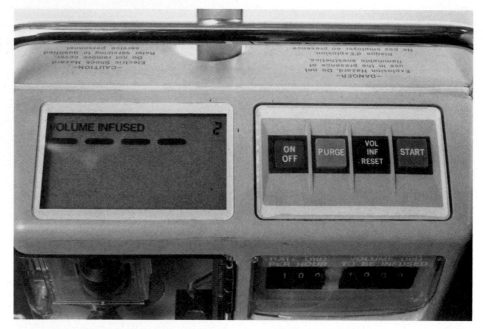

5 Infusion pumps are often used to feed clients who have either smaller-bore gastric tubes or intestinal tubes for which gravity flow or drip-regulated methods of infusion are inadequate. Pumps are also indicated for clients who require careful monitoring of their intake or who need a spe-

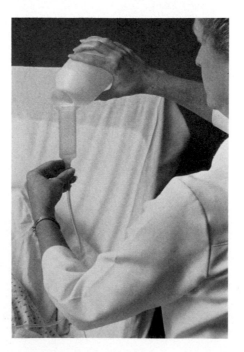

cific amount of formula infused over a specified period of time. Familiarize yourself with the types of infusion pumps your agency uses and follow the operating instructions for those pumps. See guidelines for operating the Abbott LifeCare pump, Chapter 3.

Evaluating

6 To ensure adequate absorption of any continuous-drip feeding and to verify correct stomach placement, discontinue the feedings every 6 hours, or as indicated, and aspirate and measure gastric contents. Then, flush the tubing with 30–50 mL of water to ensure patency as well as to increase fluid intake. *Note: To prevent spoilage, the same solution should not be hung for longer than 3–4 hours at a time (or the manufacturer's recommended time).*

ADMINISTERING AN ICED GASTRIC LAVAGE

Assessing and Planning

1 Take the client's vital signs to establish a baseline for subsequent assessment, and inspect and palpate the abdomen to assess the degree of distention. Explain the procedure, tell the client why it is being done, and reassure her or him. Insert a nasogastric tube if one is not already in place (see steps, pp. 231–236).

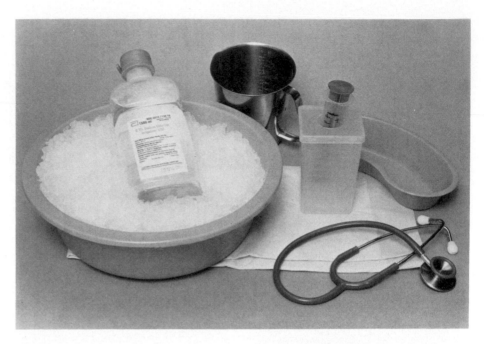

2 Assemble the following equipment: the prescribed amount of irrigant, usually 1000–1500 mL of normal saline, which should be kept cold on ice; a measured container for evaluating the amount of aspirate; irrigation set, preferably with a 50-mL piston syringe; a bed-saver pad; emesis basin; and a stethoscope. You should also have blood pressure–monitoring equipment, a rectal or axillary thermometer, and blankets at the bedside. *Note: You may pour the irrigant into a metal container for faster chilling, but do not pour the solution directly over ice because you would dilute the irrigant and make it difficult to keep accurate intake and output records.*

3 Place the client in a semi-Fowler's or Fowler's position. If this position is contraindicated because of hypovolemia or other conditions, lower the head of the bed, but place the client in a side-lying position to prevent aspiration. Drape the client with a bed-saver pad and confirm correct stomach placement of the nasogastric tube by aspirating gastric contents with the 50-mL syringe. Rather than reinstill the aspirate, inject it into a measured container for later disposal.

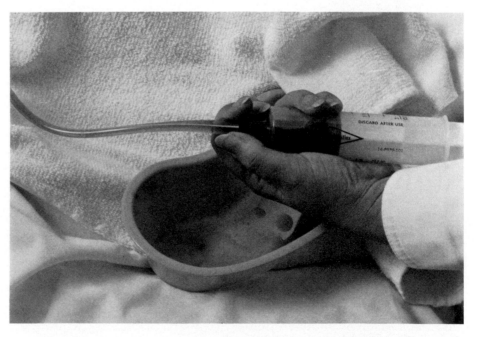

(Continued on p. 246)

Implementing

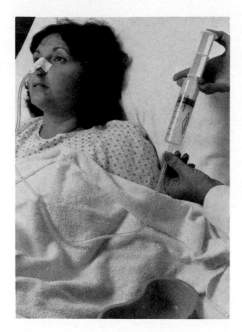

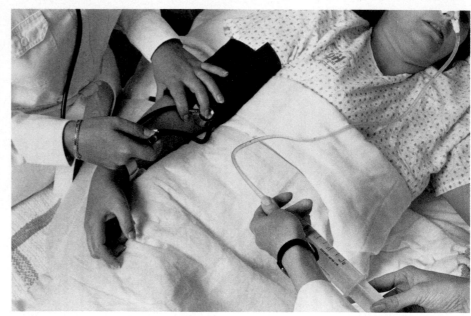

4 Draw up approximately 50 mL of the iced solution into the syringe and instill it into the tube using gentle pressure. Do not use force. Wait 30 seconds to allow the icy solution to stimulate vasoconstriction.

6 Have a co-worker monitor vital signs as you perform the lavage. If a decrease in blood pressure occurs, lower the head of the bed. Cover the client with blankets if her temperature drops

because of the icy lavage. After an hour (or the prescribed amount of time) if the aspirate has not become clear or pink-tinged, the physician should be notified for medical intervention.

Evaluating

7 Accurately record the amounts of both the irrigant and return to evaluate the quantity of blood loss. Continue to monitor the variations in blood pressure and pulse rates as an assessment for hypovolemia and potential shock. Provide materials for oral and nasal hygiene; document the procedure describing the type and amount of irrigant, the amount and character of the return, and your assessment of the client's condition and tolerance of the procedure.

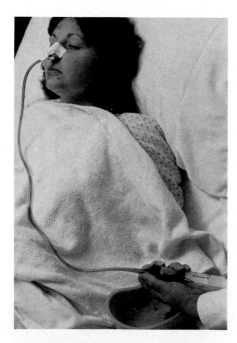

5 Aspirate and inject the return into the measured container. Continue to instill and aspirate until the returns are clear or pink-tinged.

ASPIRATING STOMACH CONTENTS FOR GASTRIC ANALYSIS

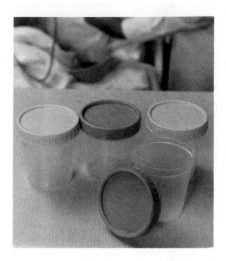

If possible, explain the procedure to the client at least a day ahead of time because he or she must fast for at least 8 hours before the test. A gastric analysis evaluates the amount of acid produced by the parietal cells when the stomach is in a state of rest. Therefore fluids, smoking, and anticholinergics are also contraindicated because they will affect the gastric contents. At the prescribed time, insert a nasogastric tube (see steps, pp. 231–236) and aspirate the residual stomach contents with a 50-mL syringe. Usually, you will discard the first aspirate unless the physician wishes to test the residual. After waiting the prescribed amount of time, aspirate all the stomach contents again and place them in a specimen container that has been properly labeled, dated, and numbered. Send the container to the laboratory. You will probably do this three or four more times at 15-minute intervals. Depending on the type of test ordered, you may be required to repeat the procedure after administering subcutaneous histamine to the client. Histamine not only stimulates acid secretion, it rapidly dilates capillaries as well, resulting in a potential drop in blood pressure, increased pulse rate, and headache. Assess the client's pulse and blood pressure immediately after the histamine administration.

GIVING GASTROSTOMY TUBE FEEDINGS

Assessing and Planning

1 If tube feedings have been ordered for your client who has a gastrostomy tube, determine whether the client has a history of food allergies or medically related alterations in nutrition. If the client has already received a tube feeding, inspect and palpate the abdomen to assess for gastric distention. If the abdomen is distended, the previous feeding may not have been adequately absorbed. Monitor the client for indications of intolerance to the previous feeding: alterations in bowel elimination, flatulence, and nausea. Assess the client's understanding of the procedure and intervene accordingly.

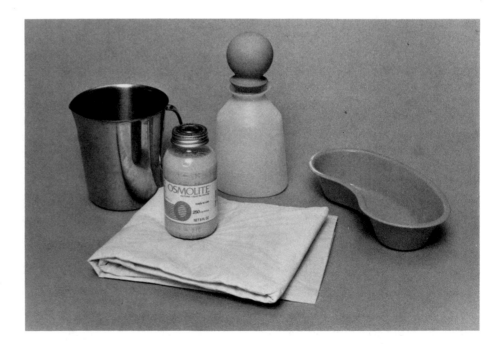

Assemble the following materials and equipment for an intermittent feeding: irrigation set with a 50-mL bulb or piston syringe; 30–50 mL of water; a measured container; emesis basin; a bed-saver pad; and the prescribed solution for tube feeding, which should be warmed to room temperature to minimize the potential for cramping and vasoconstriction. *Note: To administer feedings via continuous drip, follow procedure, pp. 243–244.*

(Continued on p. 248)

Managing Intestinal Tubes

Nursing Guidelines for Managing Intestinal Tubes

Single-Lumen Tubes

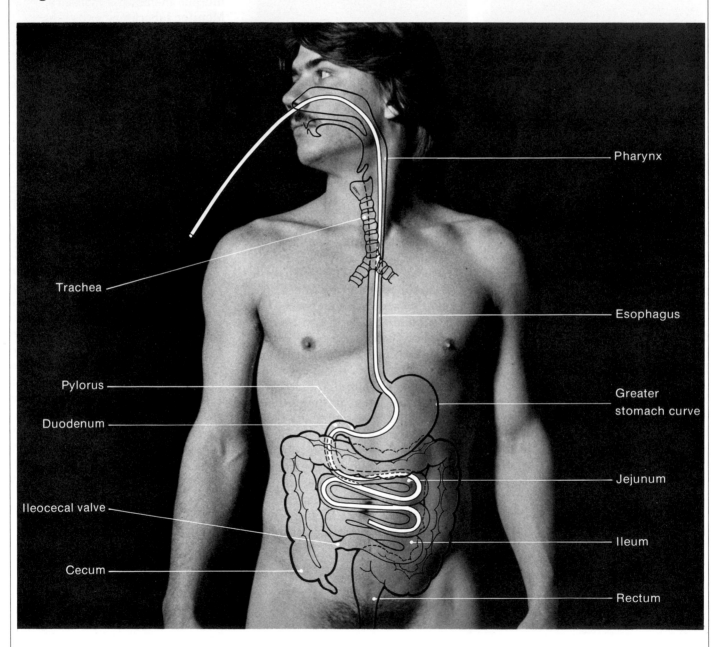

Description	91–300 cm (36 in.–10 ft); made of silicone, rubber, or polyurethane. Most are mercury-weighted at the distal end and have centimeter markings at 25, 50, and 75.
Sizes	Decompression tubes usually 16–18F Feeders usually 8–16F
Uses	Gavage, decompression, medication instillation, splinting of the small bowel after anastomosis
Nursing Considerations	■ The tubes are usually inserted by the physician. ■ The insertion of the tube into the stomach is similar to that of the nasogastric tube. ■ For decompression, connect the tube to intermittent suction. ■ Ensure intestinal placement by checking pH of aspirate: a reading greater than 7 indicates intestinal contents; one less than 7 indicates gastric contents. ■ Tube feedings are usually begun with water, advanced to half-strength of the formula, and finally to full strength, according to client tolerance. ■ Reposition the client frequently when the tube is in position to facilitate drainage. ■ Use infusion pumps to deliver feedings if continuous feedings are prescribed. ■ Provide oral and nasal hygiene at least three to four times daily.

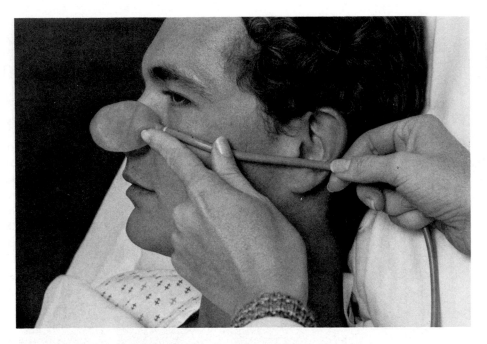

6 The tube is measured from the nostril to the ear.

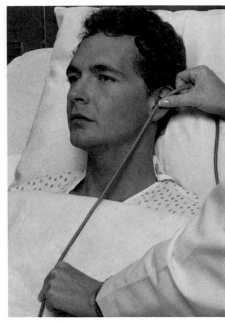

7 It is then measured from the ear to the tip of the xiphoid process. The total NEX measurement is then marked on the tube with indelible ink or remembered if the measurement equals the centimeter markings on the tube.

Implementing

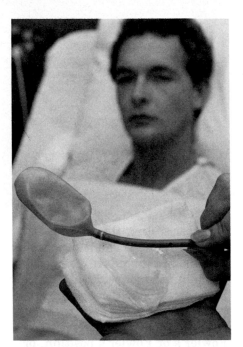

8 Generously lubricate the first 15 cm (6 in.) of the tube with water-soluble lubricant for ease of insertion.

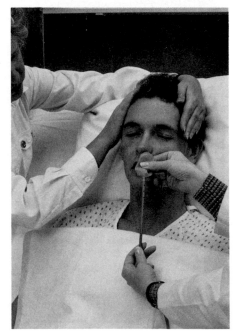

9 As the physician begins to insert the tube, help the client hold his head in an erect or slightly flexed position.

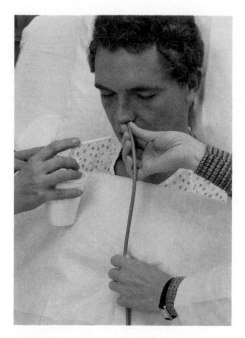 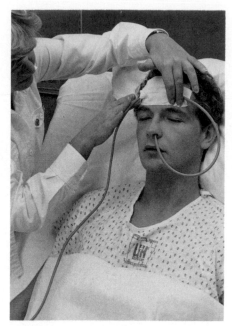 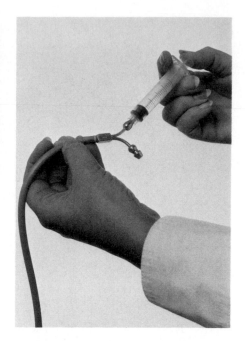

10 After the tube has been inserted 15 cm (6 in.), instruct the client to flex his head forward. This will lessen the chance of activating the gag reflex and prevent the insertion of the tube into the trachea. He should then take sips of water (or dry swallow if fluids are contraindicated). The physician will advance the tube 5–10 cm (2–4 in.) with each swallow. When the predesignated mark is at the level of the client's nostril, confirm correct stomach placement (see procedure, p. 235).

11 After confirming stomach placement, prepare a gauze sling for the tubing by folding a gauze pad in half and inserting the tubing into the fold. Tape the sling to the client's forehead. This will keep the tube stabilized as it advances into the intestine. Do not tape the tube to the client's nose because doing so could hamper the tube's advancement and the tension on the tube could injure the client's nose.

12 For double-lumen tubes the physician will then inject 3–10 mL of mercury, air, water, or saline (depending on the type of tube) into the balloon port. Any one of these substances will act as a bolus for easier advancement past the pylorus. The syringe is then often taped to the balloon port to prevent accidental instillation or aspiration. Tape can instead be placed over the balloon port.

(Continued on p. 260)

Evaluating

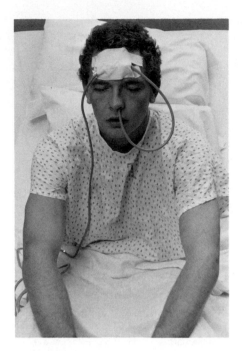

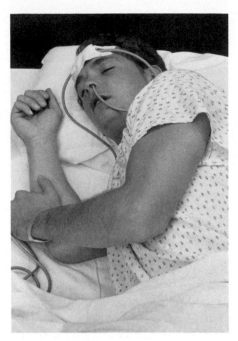

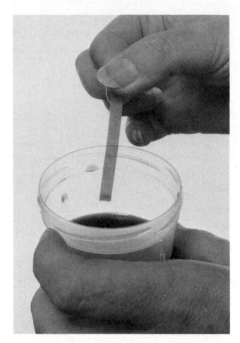

13 If the client is able, instruct him to lean forward with his arms extended to help advance the tube through the pylorus to the duodenum.

14 If you have been asked to insert the tube a prescribed distance, lubricate the tubing with water-soluble lubricant and gradually advance the tube 5–10 cm (2–4 in.) every 2 hours. Do not force the tube if you meet resistance. A peristaltic wave could be preventing its advancement. Wait a few minutes and try again. With every tube advancement, instruct the client to change positions to facilitate the tube's movement. The client should alternate side-lying positions with a supine position. Provide oral and nasal hygiene at regular intervals. When an X-ray film has confirmed the tube's proper position, attach the excess tubing to the client's gown. Then attach the open lumen to intermittent suction, or as prescribed by the physician. Document the procedure.

15 Prior to tube feedings or instillations, or as a means of assessing for correct intestinal position, aspirate intestinal contents through the open lumen to confirm alkalinity. A pH greater than 7 (or a test strip that turns blue) indicates intestinal placement; a pH less than 7 indicates gastric placement.

If the tube is connected to suction, assess the character and amount of drainage and change the suction container (or empty it) according to agency protocol. Reposition the client frequently to facilitate drainage. Monitor and record the client's intake and output and assess for the presence of peristalsis by auscultating the abdomen for bowel sounds. Continue to provide materials for oral and nasal hygiene.

REMOVING AN INTESTINAL TUBE

Assessing and Planning

1 Prior to removing the intestinal tube, assess the client's abdomen by auscultating for bowel sounds and inspecting and palpating for distention. If you do not hear bowel sounds or if the abdomen is quite distended, check with the physician to make sure the tube should be removed. Assess the client's knowledge of the procedure and explain why the tube will be removed. Familiarize yourself with the steps for the removal of a nasogastric tube, p. 238. Because the client may become nauseated during the procedure, you should check to see if an antiemetic has been ordered. *Note: If the tube has passed through the ileocecal valve, the physician may allow it to pass through the rectum rather than removing it through the nose.*

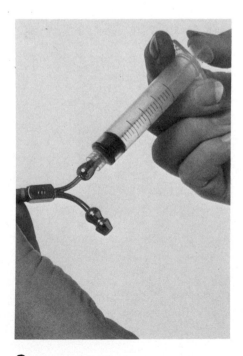

2 If you are removing a Miller–Abbott tube, attach a syringe to the balloon part (as shown) and aspirate the mercury or ballon-inflating substance.

Implementing

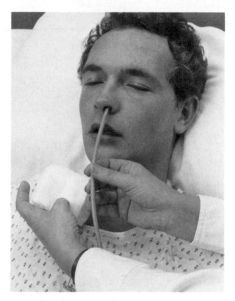

3 Protect the client's gown with a bed-saver pad. Assist him into a semi-Fowler's or Fowler's position to help prevent aspiration of the drainage. If the tube is connected to suction, turn off the suction machine and detach the tube from the client's nose. Pinch or clamp the tubing as you withdraw 5–10 cm (2–4 in.) every 5–10 minutes. Ask the client to exhale as you withdraw the tube because doing so will relax the pharynx. Blot the tube with a gauze pad or paper towel as you withdraw it, to remove gastric and intestinal drainage.

5 If you have removed a Cantor tube, aspirate the mercury from the bag at the distal end of the tube. Dispose of the mercury or return it to the central supply area, according to agency protocol.

Evaluating

6 To evaluate his tolerance to the tube's removal, continue to assess the client for indications of distention, nausea, vomiting, or ileus.

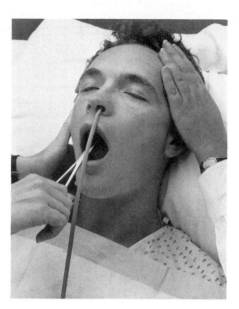

4 If the intestinal tube is disposable, you may wish to grasp the balloon with a hemostat when it reaches the client's oropharynx and snip it off with scissors, removing the balloon through the client's mouth to avoid passing it through the nose. If the tube is not disposable, gently pull it through the client's nose. Remove the tube from the client's bedside, and provide materials for oral and nasal hygiene. Document the procedure.

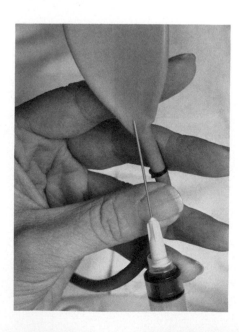

Managing Stoma Care

Nursing Guidelines for Managing Ostomies

Ascending Colostomy

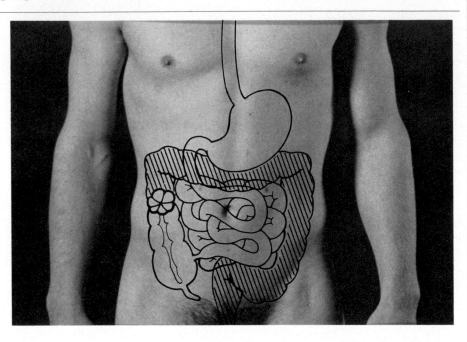

Surgical Indications

Perforating sigmoid diverticulitis, Hirschsprung's disease, obstructed colon, trauma (for example, gunshot or stab wounds), rectovaginal fistula, and inoperable tumors in the colon.

Nursing Considerations

- This is the least common colostomy.
- The surgery is performed on clients of all ages.
- The stoma location is on the right upper or middle quadrant of the abdomen, and it usually protrudes.
- This ostomy is managed as if it were an ileostomy.
- The client will have watery or semisolid stools that flow almost continually.
- The effluent contains digestive enzymes that are damaging to the skin.
- Peristomal skin assessment, skin care, and a properly fitting appliance are essential for preventing skin breakdown.
- Full-time use of an appliance (usually a drainable pouch) with a skin barrier is necessary.
- Irrigation is contraindicated.
- Odor control is usually not a major problem.

Transverse Colostomies

Surgical Indications   Same as ascending colostomies. These ostomies are usually
                             temporary.

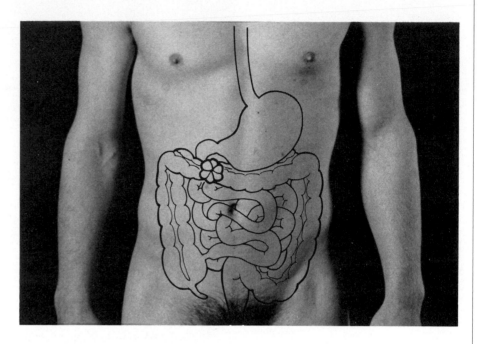

Nursing Considerations for   ■ The surgery is performed on clients of all ages.
the Single-Barrel Colostomy   ■ The stoma location is usually high on the abdomen, at waist level
                                     and near the midline. It usually protrudes.
                                   ■ The stools are usually semisolid, although formed stools are possible.
                                   ■ A drainable pouch is recommended.
                                   ■ The enzymatic, watery stools can lead to peristomal skin excoriation.
                                   ■ The rectum is not removed, so the client may feel the urge to defecate.
                                   ■ Although this ostomy is not controllable, it is more predictable than
                                     an ascending colostomy as to when it will function.

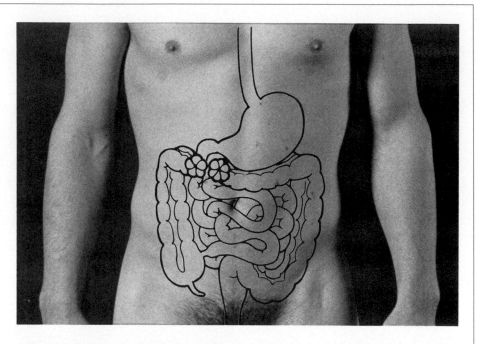

Nursing Considerations for the Double-Barrel Colostomy

- This is often a temporary intervention for resting the colon, with a possible anastomosis at a later date.
- The client has two stomas: the proximal stoma is active and discharges feces; the distal stoma is inactive and discharges mucus. The inactive stoma may be eventually covered with a gauze pad to absorb mucus.
- Postoperatively, the client may use a loop ostomy appliance or an open-end drain with a skin barrier.
- The client may experience occasional rectal drainage of stool or mucus.

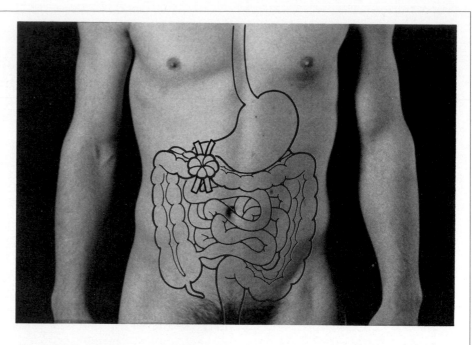

Nursing Considerations for the Loop Colostomy

■ An intact segment of the colon is looped through the abdomen rather than severed.
■ The loop is held exterior to the body and stabilized with a plastic bridge or glass rod for 7–10 days postoperatively.
■ Fecal material is released through an incision on the anterior section of the loop.
■ This type of fecal diversion is usually performed in emergency situations; therefore the client is often ill-prepared both physiologically and psychologically.

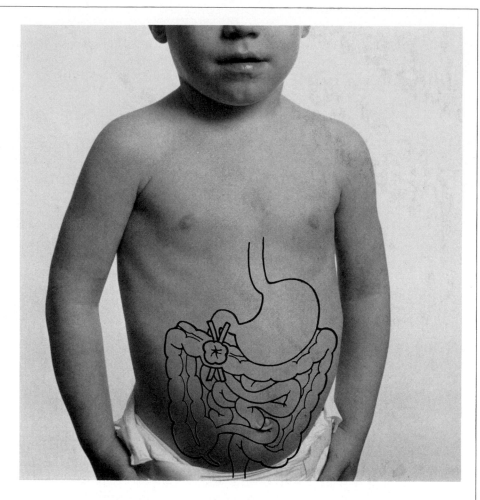

Nursing Considerations for the Pediatric Colostomate

- For the child, a pediatric postoperative pouch and skin barrier are used during the first 3–5 postoperative days. Thereafter pediatric drainable pouches are frequently used.
- The use of skin barriers and close observation of peristomal skin is crucial because of the watery, enzymatic feces.
- For the infant, a diaper alone might be used until discharge from the hospital. Follow agency protocol.
- Closely monitor the infant and child for weight loss and indications of dehydration.

Descending or Sigmoid Colostomy

Surgical Indications

Cancer of the sigmoid colon or rectum, chronic diverticulitis, congenital anomaly, or trauma.

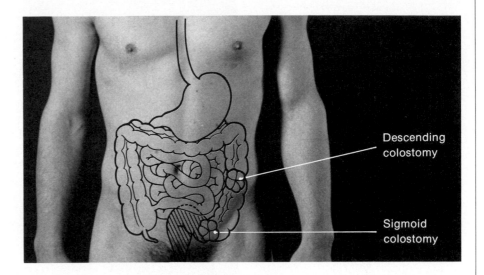

Descending colostomy

Sigmoid colostomy

Nursing Considerations

- This is the most commonly occurring fecal diversion.
- The surgery may be performed on clients of all ages, but most clients are 40 years of age or older.
- The stoma is located in the left lower quadrant, and it might be either flush or protruded.
- After recovery, the regulated client wears a closed pouch, stoma cap, or stoma dressing.
- After the initial postoperative period, the stools become formed.
- This is the easiest ostomy to control.
- Elimination may be regulated by irrigation and diet.
- Teach the client how to manage elimination by increasing intake of foods high in bulk and decreasing intake of foods known to give the individual loose stools, flatus, and odor. Increase the intake of fluids as well.
- Encourage the intake of parsley, yogurt, and cranberry juice as odor preventatives.

Ileostomy

Surgical Indications

Ulcerative colitis (80%), Crohn's disease, cancer, trauma, familial polyposis.

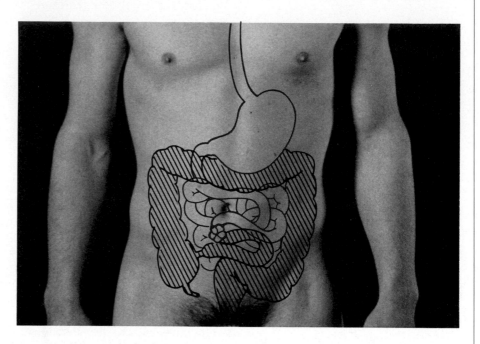

Nursing Considerations

- This procedure is performed most frequently on young adults including teenagers, with 40 years as the average age.
- The stoma is located in the right lower quadrant, and it usually protrudes.
- The pouch must fit properly to prevent skin breakdown potentially caused by the enzymatic effluent.
- Change the pouch immediately if leakage occurs at the peristomal area or if the client complains of itching or burning around the stoma.
- Because of a potential fluid volume deficit from colon loss, encourage a fluid intake of 2–3 L/day.
- Because of electrolyte loss, increase the client's intake of sodium and potassium through foods, fluids, and supplements.
- Instruct the client to decrease roughage in the diet, which can cause a blockage, and to thoroughly chew the food.
- Change the appliance when the ileostomy is more quiescent, for example, in the morning before eating or 2–4 hours after meals.
- The maximum wearing time for the pouch is 7 days, although some clients change their pouches as frequently as every 3 days and others change them every 5 days.

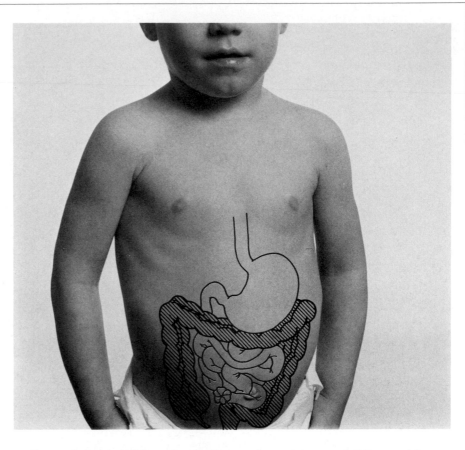

Nursing Considerations for the Pediatric Ileostomate

- Care of these children is similar to that given to children with pediatric transverse loops.
- The fecal output is very caustic, and therefore the use of skin barriers and close observation of the peristomal skin is essential.

Continent Ileostomy (Kock Pouch)

Surgical Indications

Ulcerative colitis and familial polyposis. It is often contraindicated for clients with Crohn's disease.

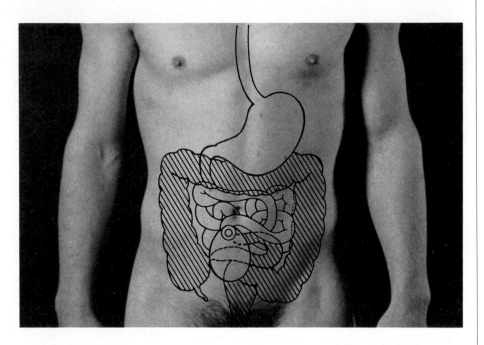

Nursing Considerations

- The age group involved is the same as that for the ileostomy.
- The stoma is located on the right lower quadrant, and it is flush with the skin.
- The intraabdominal pouch (reservoir) is created from the looped ileum. It collects feces, making external collection pouches unnecessary.
- A gastrostomy tube is often sutured into the stomach during surgery for decompression.
- A 28F catheter is inserted into the reservoir and sutured to the client's skin during surgery; it remains in place for 14–21 days to provide pouch decompression. It is irrigated with normal saline every 4–6 hours, or as prescribed.
- At 14–21 days postoperatively, the reservoir is intubated and drained every 3–4 hours with a lubricated silastic catheter. This is decreased to every 6 hours by week 8 or 9.
- The stoma is covered with a bandage or a gauze pad between intubations to absorb leaks or mucus.
- Instruct the client to avoid gas-forming foods, decrease roughage, and chew the food thoroughly to prevent clogging the silastic catheter.
- The adjustment to the body change is usually less traumatic for these clients than for those with conventional ileostomies.
- The reservoir gradually increases in size and may attain a capacity of 500 mL.

PATCH TESTING YOUR CLIENT'S SKIN

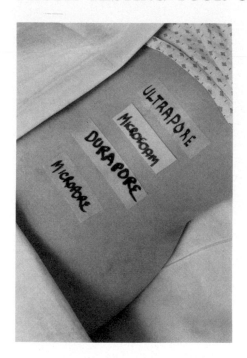

At least 24 hours prior to ostomy surgery, perform skin patch testing to assess for allergies your client may potentially have to tape that will be used to adhere the ostomy appliance to the abdominal skin. Test the abdomen on the nonoperative side, rather than testing the inner arm. The inner arm is not as sensitive as the abdomen and the test results may not be as accurate.

Test at least four different types of tape that are used by your agency. This will provide you with more options should the client prove to be allergic to more than one type. The photo depicts the testing of foam, silk, and two types of paper tape on the client's abdomen. If you are patch testing skin on a client with abdominal hair, clip the hair with scissors as close to the follicle as possible before applying the tape. Unless the client complains of itching and burning before the 24-hour period has elapsed, remove the tape at the scheduled time, using a tape solvent if necessary. Thoroughly cleanse the area with water and a gentle soap or skin cleanser; assess for redness, swelling, and other indicators of an allergic reaction. Document the test's results in the chart. If your client does have an allergic reaction to any of the tapes, note the type(s) on the front of the chart, stating "Allergic to _____ Tape." This will alert both the surgical team before their application of the postoperative pouch and the nursing staff during followup care.

APPLYING A POSTOPERATIVE POUCH

A postoperative pouch is typically worn during the early part of the client's hospital stay. It is usually clear to provide optimal observation of fecal drainage, and the pouch openings can readily be adapted to fit most stoma sizes and sites.

Assessing and Planning

1 To apply a postoperative pouch, assemble the following materials: the postoperative pouch, a pectin wafer skin barrier, straight scissors, curved scissors (optional), a binder clip or a rubber band, skin cleanser (optional), stomal measurement guide, 4 × 4 gauze pads, and 2.5-cm hypoallergenic tape if you plan to "picture frame" the appliance to enhance the seal (see procedure, p. 284). In addition, keep a supply of bed-saver pads at the client's bedside.

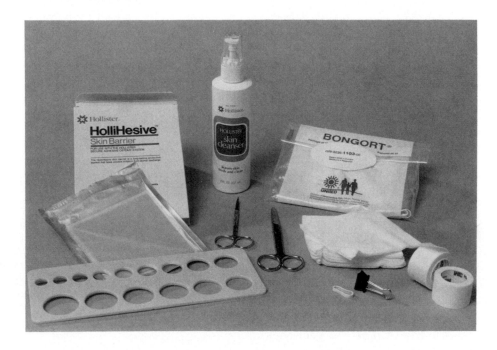

(Continued on p. 272)

2 Explain the procedure to the client, and lower the head of the bed to decrease the angle at the peristomal area. Assess the client's reaction to her stoma and let her know that you have as much time as she needs for answering her questions and assisting her with future pouch applications. If she is psychologically ready, encourage her to inspect and touch her stoma so that she can begin to develop a realistic appraisal of her altered appearance and body function. It is essential that you project a positive reaction to the client's ostomy.

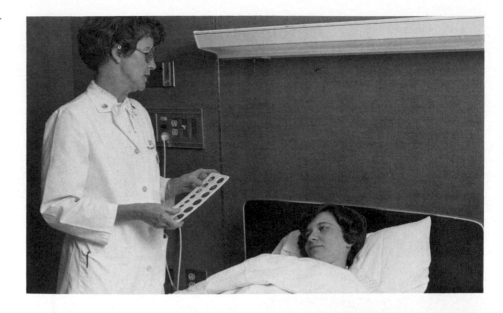

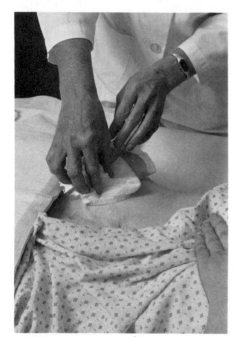

3 To protect the client's gown and bed from fecal drainage, place a bed-saver pad under the pouch. Then, moisten a 4 × 4 gauze pad or cloth with warm water and lift up the uppermost inside corner of the skin barrier. Position the moistened gauze pad at the loosened corner and gently depress the skin as you peel back the adhesive material. This method will facilitate the removal of the appliance as quickly and painlessly as possible.

4 After removing the appliance, assess the color of the stoma. It should be a healthy red, similar in color to the mucosal lining of the inner cheek. Report immediately a darker, purplish cast or a very pale stoma, which would suggest impaired blood circulation to the area. Also assess for impaired peristomal skin integrity potentially caused by leakage of fecal effluent, an allergic reaction to the tape or skin barrier, or infected hair follicles (folliculitis). Plan skin care and/or appliance changes accordingly. Cleanse the peristomal area with warm water and either a skin cleanser or a nonoily soap such as Ivory. Be sure to avoid using soaps that contain creams or lanolin because the residue left on the skin could prevent the appliance from adhering properly. Rinse and dry the skin thoroughly.

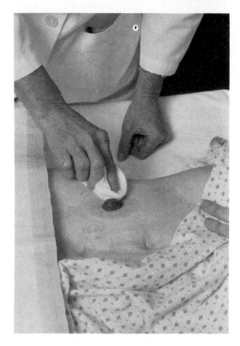

5 A pectin wafer skin barrier protects the client's peristomal skin from contact with the effluent and pouch adhesive. If you are using a pectin wafer with squared edges, curve the edges (as shown) to prevent them from jabbing your client's skin. Set the skin barrier aside.

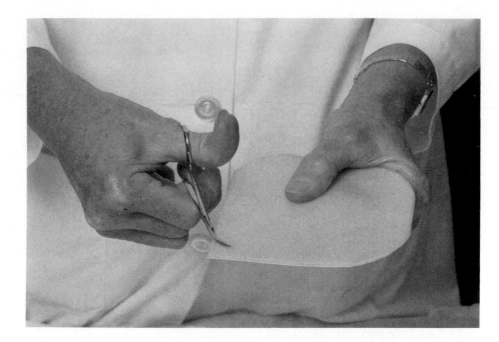

Implementing

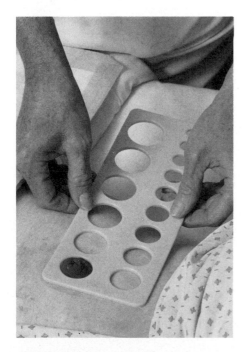

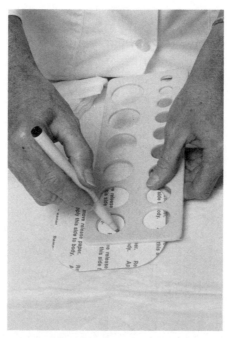

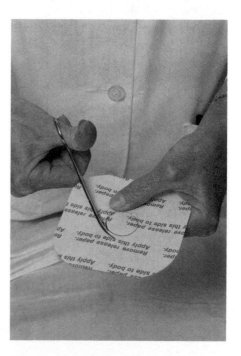

6 Measure the stoma with a stomal measuring guide. You will need to measure the stoma frequently during the postoperative period because the stoma will continue to shrink in size, with the majority of the shrinkage occurring during the first 2–3 months.

7 Trace the exact measurement of the stoma on the back and in the center of the skin barrier.

8 Cut out the circle from the skin barrier.

(Continued on p. 274)

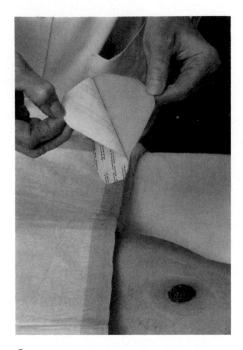

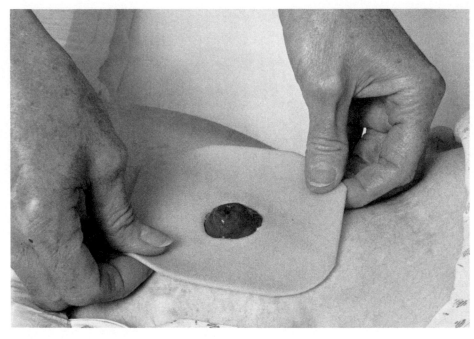

9 Remove the adhesive backing from the back of the skin barrier.

10 Place the skin barrier directly over the stoma, and gently press around its surface to adhere it to the client's skin.

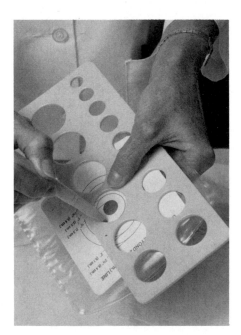

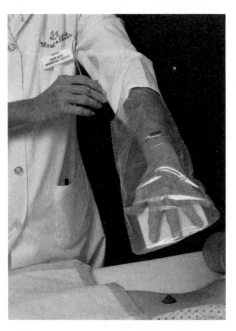

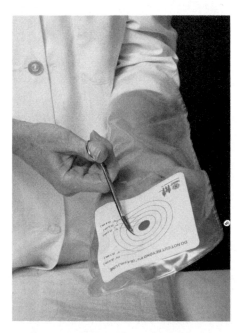

11 Add $\frac{1}{8}$–$\frac{1}{4}$ in. to the stomal measurement, and trace that circle on the back of the postoperative pouch. Making this circle slightly larger than the circle you cut out of the skin barrier will help to ensure an adequate seal, thereby protecting the peristomal skin.

12 Fan your fingers inside the pouch to separate the front from the back.

13 Keep your hand inside the pouch while you cut out the circle you traced. This will prevent you from cutting through the pouch. *Note: A shortcut taken by many nurses is folding the pouch vertically to cut out the circle. Avoid doing this because the crease created by the fold can form a conduit for fecal drainage.*

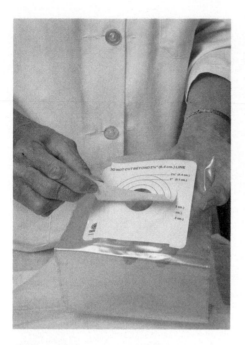

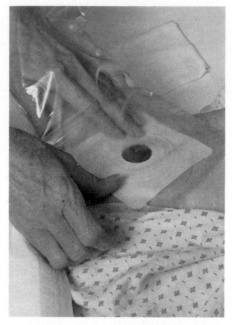

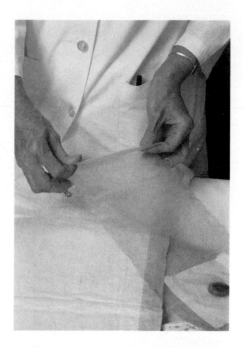

14 Remove the protective paper backing from the back of the pouch.

15 Place your hand inside the pouch again and position the opening of the pouch directly over the stoma. Gently press your fingertips around the attached surfaces of the appliance (as shown). Note that the pouch angles toward the side of the bed. This facilitates emptying the pouch into a basin or bed pan during the early postoperative period. It should be angled in this manner only during the period in which the client is on bed rest.

16 To close the appliance, fold the bottom of the pouch up into two or three 1-in. folds.

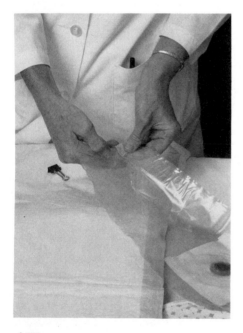

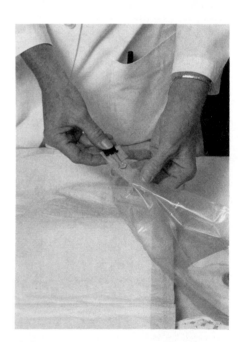

17 Fold the pouch crosswise into three or four equal "curtain folds."

18 Secure the folds with a binder clip or rubber band. Record the procedure, noting your evaluation of the stoma and the peristomal skin, and the amount and character of the effluent. Also evaluate and record the client's reaction to the stoma and note her readiness to participate in her own care.

(Continued on p. 276)

Evaluating

19 Continue to monitor the client for alterations in fluid and electrolyte balance, impairment of stomal and peristomal skin, nutritional deficits, and daily changes in body weight. In addition, it is especially important in the early postoperative period to be alert to indications of paralytic ileus or peritonitis. Inspect and palpate the abdomen for the presence of distention or rigidity, and auscultate the abdomen to ensure there are bowel sounds. Although an absence of fecal output is one indicator of ileus, an ileostomy usually does not function until the first 12–24 hours; a lack of fecal output during the first 24–36 hours is often normal for a colostomy. Keep accurate daily records of the amount, color, and consistency of fecal output and compare the output to the client's intake.

When the pouch becomes one-third full, detach the rubber band or binder clip and empty the pouch into a basin or bedpan. If the pouch is allowed to become full of effluent, its seal with the skin can break, resulting in leakage of effluent onto the client's abdomen.

APPLYING A DRAINABLE POUCH

A drainable pouch is appropriate for the client whose ostomy is unregulated—for example, the client with an ileostomy or an ascending or transverse colostomy. The application of this pouch can be demonstrated to the client after the initial postoperative stomal shrinkage has occurred, usually a few days prior to discharge. This will provide the necessary time for the client to become comfortable with performing the procedure independently.

Assessing and Planning

Note: The procedure for pouch application and the materials used will vary from agency to agency. Follow your own agency's protocol, using the following guidelines.

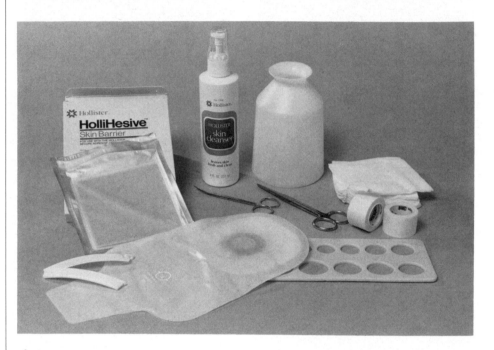

1 Before applying a drainable pouch, determine the client's most recent stomal measurement, and gather together the following materials: a premeasured drainable pouch with or without a karaya seal, a pectin wafer skin barrier, skin cleanser (optional, you may use a gentle, nonoily soap instead), tap water, 4 × 4 gauze pads or a clean washcloth, straight scissors, curved scissors (optional), pouch clamp, 2.5-cm of hypoallergenic tape if you will "picture frame" the pouch for added security (see procedure, p. 284), and the stoma measurement guide. *Note: If your client is obese or has a stoma that is flush with the peristomal area, preventing good adherence of the pouch, it is advisable to use an ostomy belt (not shown with this equipment).*

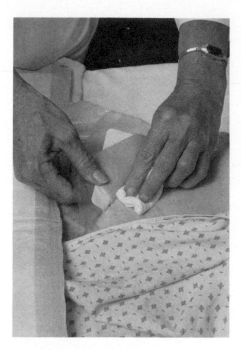

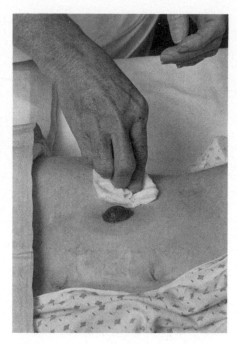

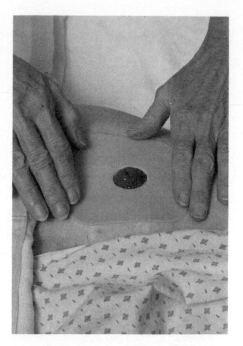

2 Drape the client with a bed-saver pad and remove the used pouch following the steps, p. 272.

3 Cleanse the peristomal area with warm water and either skin cleanser or soap such as Ivory. Rinse and dry the area thoroughly because skin barriers will not adhere to the skin unless it is totally dry and free of soap film. Assess the color of the stoma and evaluate the integrity of the peristomal skin. If the client's skin is irritated from leaking fecal material or a reaction to the pouch adhesive, either apply a skin barrier paste, sprinkle the site with a powdered skin barrier, or apply a skin care product such as Op-Site to the area. *Note: If the client's stoma continues to drain during the pouch change, instruct the client to place a gauze pad around the stoma to absorb fecal material, preventing its contact with the skin.*

4 Depending on agency policy, you will either apply a pouch with an attached karaya seal directly to the skin, a pouch without a karaya seal over a pectin wafer skin barrier, or apply both the karaya seal and the pectin wafer for added skin protection. Many enterostomal therapists recommend the use of both because the pectin wafer protects the peristomal skin from the highly enzymatic effluent, while the karaya seal protects the stoma from irritation or abrasions. To adhere the skin barrier to the peristomal skin, follow the steps, pp. 273–274.

(Continued on p. 278)

Implementing

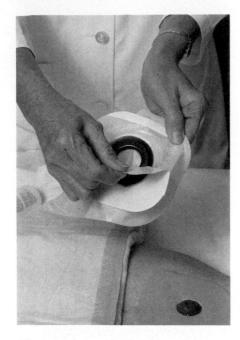

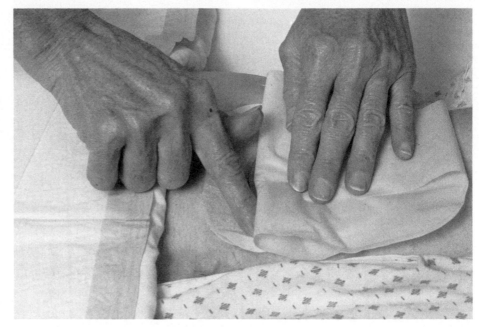

5 Remove the protective paper backing from the back of the pouch, retaining the protective white tabs that are on both sides. These tabs will enable you to hold the pouch without touching the adhesive.

6 Center the pouch opening directly over the stoma. To adhere the distal section of the pouch to the skin barrier, fold the tail of the pouch toward the client's head.

7 Fold over the proximal end of the pouch and adhere the proximal section to the skin barrier.

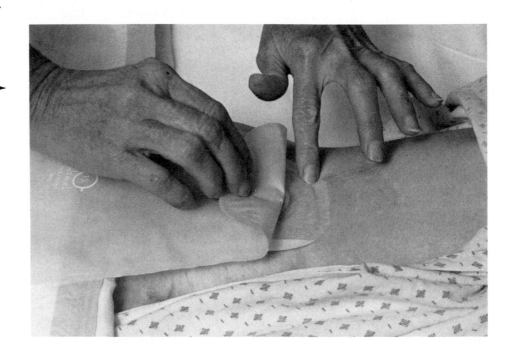

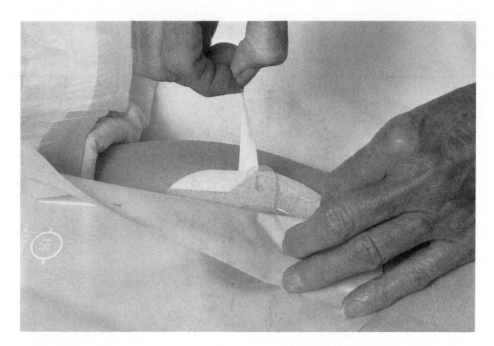

8 Remove the protective tabs and adhere the lateral sections of the pouch to the skin barrier.

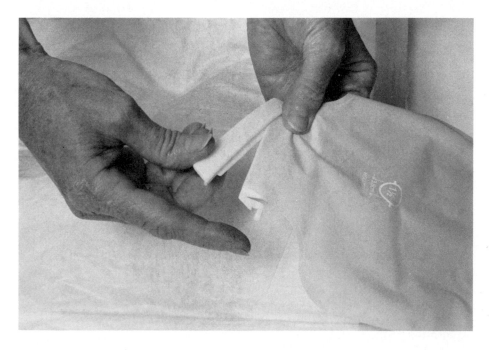

9 Secure the end of the pouch with the pouch clamp (for detail, see p. 286). This type of pouch clamp is easily lost during pouch changes. Remember to remove it prior to discarding the disposable pouch. Be certain that the pouch is emptied when it becomes one-third full. If it is allowed to contain larger amounts of fecal drainage, the increasing weight could break the seal of the pouch. Allow the effluent to drain into a bedpan or basin. Rinse the pouch through the distal (draining) end, using paper cups full of water to cleanse the inner surface of the pouch.

(Continued on p. 280)

Evaluating

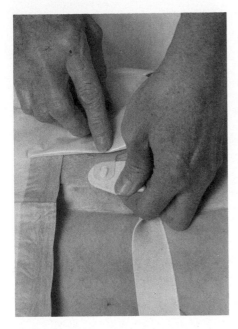

10 If the client requires an ostomy belt, position it around her waist and connect it to the flanges of the face plate (as shown).

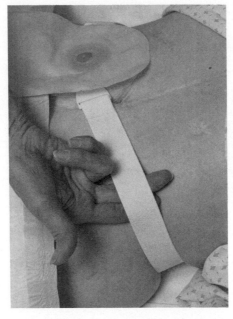

11 Ensure that two fingers can comfortably fit between the belt and the client's skin. Document the procedure, noting the stomal measurement, the appearance of the peristomal skin, and the amount and character of the fecal output. In addition, note and record your client's reaction to the stoma and her readiness to participate in her own care.

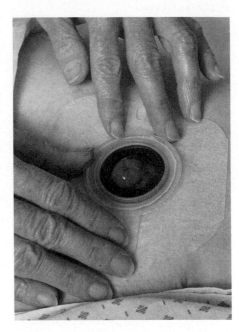

12 The top portion of a disposable pouch has been cut away to show you a correct fit. Notice how the karaya ring fits snugly around the stoma.

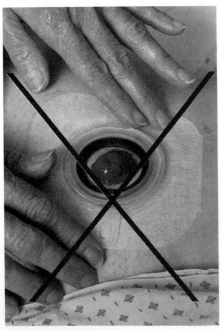

13 The top portion of a disposable pouch that no longer fits because of typical stomal shrinkage occurring during the postoperative period has been cut away. Because the exposed peristomal skin can readily become excoriated after contact with caustic fecal effluent, it is essential that the appliance be changed as soon as stomal shrinkage occurs and the skin is exposed. Similarly, if your client has an irregularly shaped stoma, you should use karaya paste to fill in the exposed area, or cut a pectin wafer skin barrier to fit the stoma.

14 Continue to monitor the client for potential alterations in fluid and electrolyte balance, alterations in the integrity of the stoma and peristomal skin, nutritional deficits, and changes in body weight.

APPLYING A REUSABLE POUCH

Two weeks after the client's surgery, the stoma has usually healed, and approximately 50% of the shrinkage will have occurred. At that time, the client may be fitted with a reusable pouch if it is appropriate for the client's needs, life style, or stomal character. The faceplate, which is an integral part of this appliance, is often indicated for clients with large abdomens or poor muscle tone, or for those whose stomas are flush with their abdomens.

Assessing and Planning

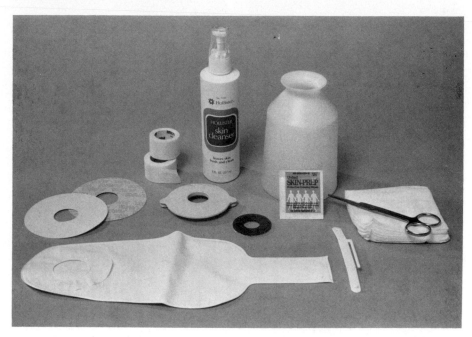

1 If a reusable pouch is indicated for your client, you will probably demonstrate the application procedure a few days prior to her discharge. Usually, the properly sized materials will already have been ordered, based on the most recent stomal measurement. Those materials include the reusable pouch, karaya ring, faceplate, and double-faced adhesive disc. Because the karaya ring is expansive and should hug the stoma, order one that is ⅛ in. smaller than the client's stoma. The openings of the faceplate and double-faced adhesive disc, however, should be ⅛ in. larger than the stoma to ensure an adequate seal. *Note: A pectin wafer skin barrier can be used instead of the karaya ring if a longer wearing time is desired. The karaya ring can wash out after 3 days, while the pectin wafer can be worn for at least 5 days.* You will also need the following materials for applying a reusable pouch: skin protector wipes; skin cleanser or a mild, nonoily soap; a container of water for cleansing the skin; 2.5-cm tape cut into either four or eight 7.5-cm (3-in.) strips for "picture-framing" the appliance; scissors; a pouch clamp; 4 × 4 gauze pads or a wash cloth for cleansing the peristomal skin; and a bead-o-ring or lock ring for securing the pouch to the faceplate (not shown).

(Continued on p. 282)

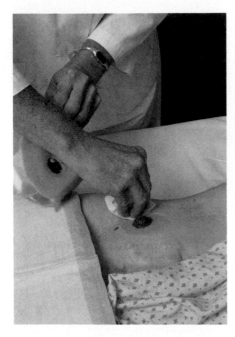

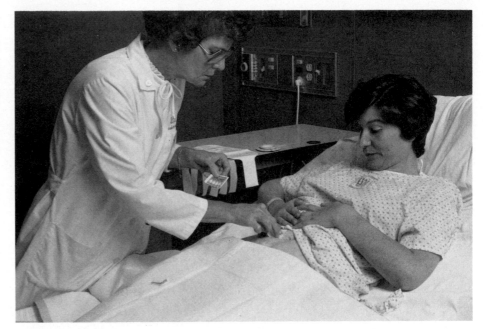

2 Position the client so that she can both observe and participate in the procedure. It may also be appropriate to involve a significant other or family member in the teaching segment of this procedure. Drape the client with a bed-saver pad, remove the used appliance, and clean, dry, and inspect the stoma and peristomal area (see p. 272).

3 Swab the peristomal area with a skin barrier wipe or liquid skin barrier to protect the skin from irritation that can be caused by the tape or pouch adhesive. The skin will appear shiny after 30 seconds, which is the time it

takes for the skin barrier to dry. *Note: If you use a skin barrier spray rather than a wipe or liquid, hold an inverted medicine cup over the stoma or ask the client to cover the stoma with a rolled gauze pad.*

4 If your client has continuous drainage from the stoma, she should hold a gauze pad over it to protect the peristomal skin. Demonstrate removing one of the protective paper strips from the double-faced adhesive disc. Apply the sticky side of the disc to the back of the faceplate (below). Set the faceplate aside.

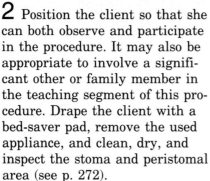

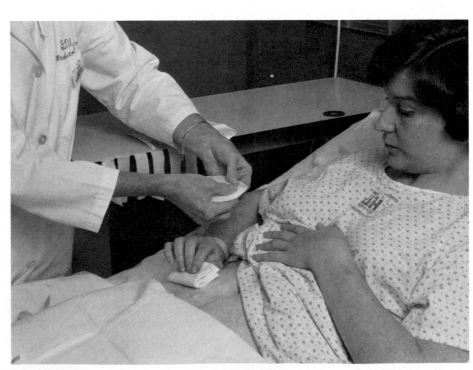

Implementing

5 Remove the strip of protective paper from the back of the karaya ring and gently stretch the ring around the stoma. Adhere it to the peristomal skin by pressing around the karaya ring in a circular fashion.

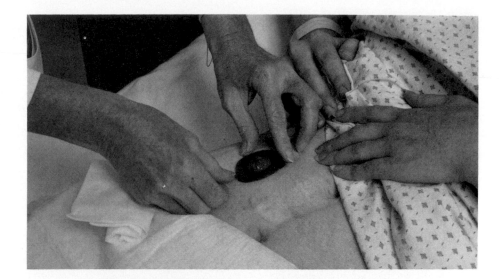

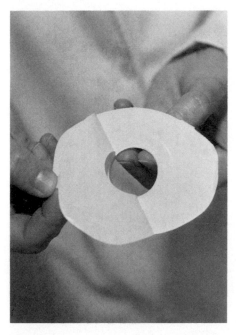

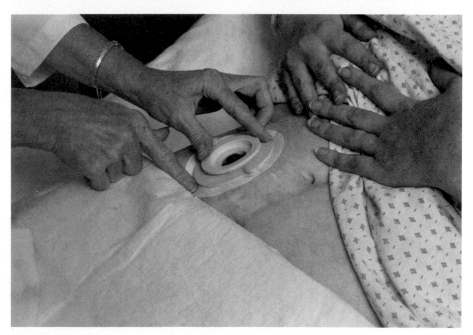

6 Remove the remaining protective paper strip from the double-faced adhesive disk on the faceplate (above). Center the faceplate over the karaya ring and press the sticky surface to your client's skin. Hold the faceplate against the client's skin for a few moments to enhance the seal. Then gently press your fingertips around the periphery of the adhesive (as shown).

(Continued on p. 284)

7 Tape the faceplate to the client's abdomen, making a square with four of the tape strips. This is called "picture framing." It enhances the seal and helps to evenly distribute the weight of a full pouch.

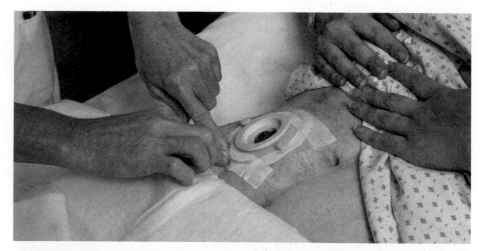

8 If desired, four tape strips may be applied along the diagonals of the pouch to further enhance the seal.

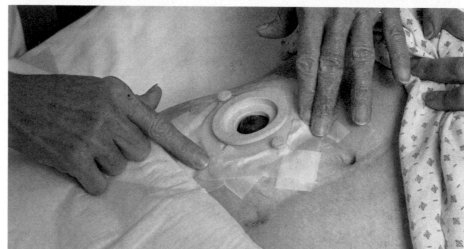

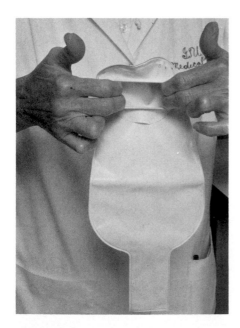

9 Gently stretch the opening on the back of the pouch to facilitate its attachment to the faceplate.

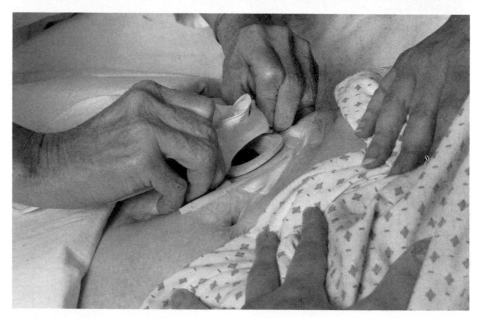

10 Position the pouch opening over the base of the faceplate, and ease it over the entire flange.

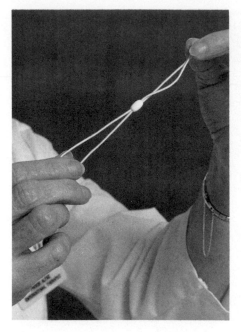

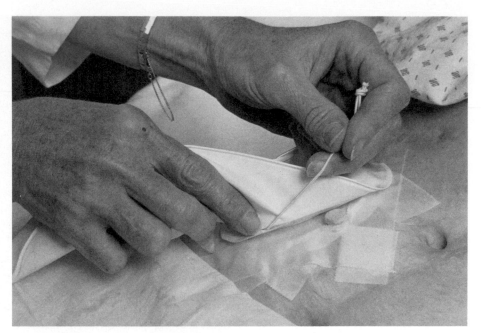

11 Show the client the bead-o-ring (or lock ring, if that is what you are using), and explain that it is placed between the pouch and flange of the faceplate to ensure a tight fit.

12 Place the bead-o-ring under the tail of the pouch and position it between the pouch and the faceplate flange (as shown).

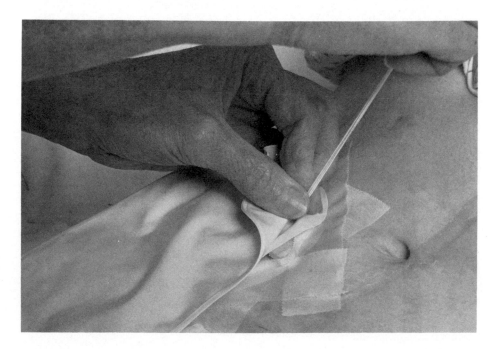

13 Hold the bead between your thumb and index finger as you tighten the elastic string. This will produce a tension that will help secure the pouch to the faceplate.

(Continued on p. 286)

14 Place the end of the pouch over the pouch clamp and roll the tail three times.

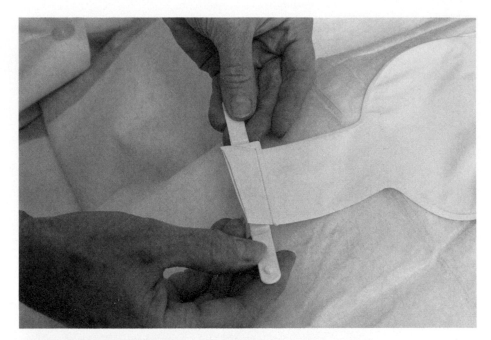

15 Snap the clamp shut, making sure the snap is in the back of the pouch. Closing it in the back will prevent the rolled pouch tail from protruding through the client's clothing. Attach an ostomy belt if one is indicated (see procedure, p. 280). Record the procedure, noting your client's response to her stoma and, if she assisted in the procedure, to her performance.

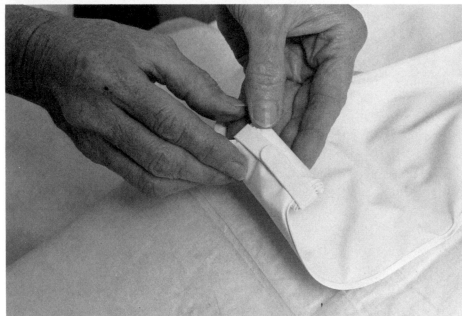

Evaluating

16 Continue to monitor and document the amounts of fecal elimination, the stomal and peristomal skin integrity, nutritional status, and any indications of a fluid volume deficit.

DILATING A STOMA

Stoma dilation is performed to stretch and relax the stomal sphincter and to assess the direction of the proximal colon prior to a colostomy irrigation. Check for a physician's order prior to dilating a client's stoma, because the procedure is not done for all colostomates.

Assessing and Planning

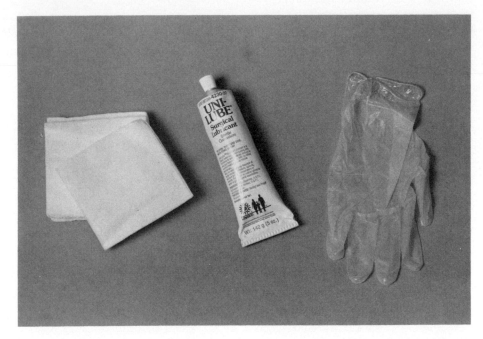

1 Assemble the following materials: gauze pads, water-soluble lubricant, and a disposable glove.

Be sure that you also have bed-saver pads on hand. Then ask the client to remove her appliance.

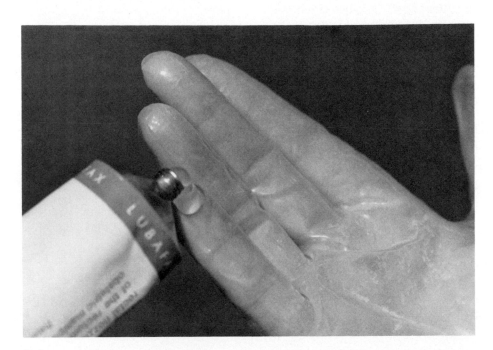

2 Instruct the client to put on the disposable glove and generously lubricate the small and index fingers of her gloved hand with the water-soluble lubricant.

(Continued on p. 288)

Implementing

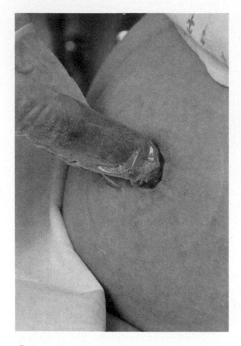

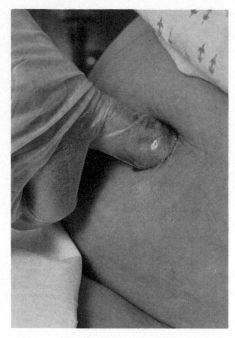

3 Drape the client's lap with a bed-saver pad and position a gauze pad under the stoma to collect drainage. Instruct the client to introduce her small finger gently into the stoma and to maintain the position for 1 minute to relax the sphincter.

4 She may then insert her index finger, gently rotating the finger to midknuckle or 5 cm (2 in.) to assess the direction of the proximal colon. This assessment will enable her to correctly position the tip of the irrigation cone.

Evaluating

5 Because the stoma comprises a vast number of capillaries, there may be slight bleeding from this procedure; however, copious bleeding is abnormal and should be reported immediately. Document the procedure and your client's performance.

IRRIGATING A COLOSTOMY

Colostomy irrigations are performed to evacuate the bowel of stored fecal content, allowing clients control over their fecal elimination. They are most appropriate for clients with ostomies of the descending or sigmoid colon. Check for a physician's order prior to performing this procedure. Irrigations are not performed for all colostomates; and they are contraindicated for infants, clients with diarrhea, or for those receiving radiation therapy.

Assessing

1 To ensure that your client does not have an obstruction or paralytic ileus, assess the client's abdomen before initiating the procedure by palpating for distention and auscultating to determine the presence of bowel sounds.

Planning

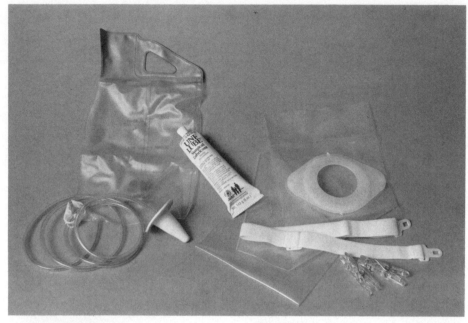

2 Assemble the following equipment: an irrigation bag with tubing and a cone, irrigation sleeve and belt, water-soluble lubricant, and plastic spring clips. You will also need an IV pole or a bathroom hook and the prescribed amount of irrigant, which is usually warm tap water. Unless otherwise ordered, the amount of the first postoperative irrigation is 500 mL, and it is gradually increased by 250 mL up to 1000 mL until the effective amount is determined by a complete and comfortable evacuation.

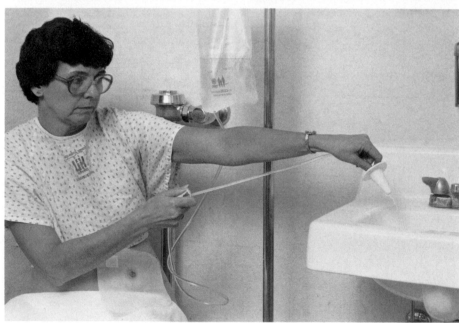

3 Although the procedure can be performed in bed, if the client is ambulatory set up the equipment in the bathroom. Ideally, at this stage in the client's recovery, she should perform as much self-care as possible, with your assistance. This photo shows 750 mL of warm tap water hung on an IV pole. The bottom of the irrigation bag should be positioned at shoulder level to ensure an effective rate of flow. Instruct the client to open the clamp on the irrigation tubing, and allow the irrigant to flow through the tubing and irrigation cone to remove the air from the irrigation set (as shown). She should then remove her used appliance and perform stomal dilation (if prescribed) to relax the sphincter and to assess the direction of the proximal colon (see steps in preceding procedure).

(Continued on p. 290)

Implementing

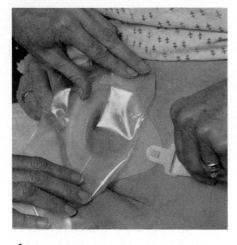

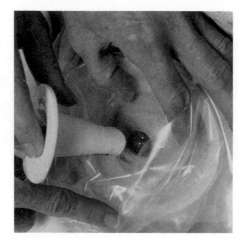

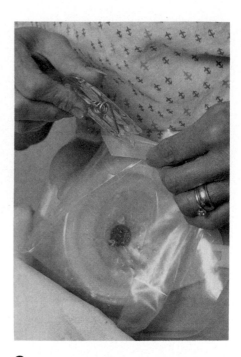

4 Assist the client with applying the irrigation sleeve and belt, and instruct her to place the tail of the sleeve between her legs so that the irrigation return can drain directly into the toilet. If the client is in bed, the tail of the sleeve can be placed into a bedpan.

6 Assist the client with placing the cone into the proximal end of the irrigation sleeve and gently centering the tip of the cone into the stoma until it fits snugly, facing the direction of the proximal colon.

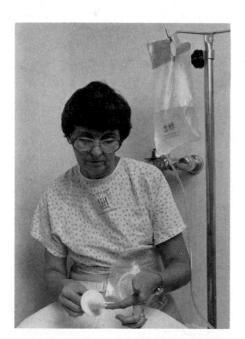

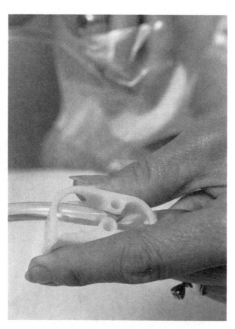

5 Squeeze some water-soluble lubricant onto a paper towel and have the client generously lubricate the tip of the irrigation cone. An irrigation cone is preferred to a straight catheter as a means of delivering the irrigant, because the latter has a greater potential for perforating the bowel.

7 Control the speed of the irrigational flow by adjusting the regulator. Instruct the client to stop the flow if she begins cramping. Once the cramps have subsided, she can slowly restart the flow. However, if the cramps continue, the irrigation should be discontinued.

8 When the irrigant has finished draining, instruct the client to fold the top end of the irrigation sleeve twice and to secure it with a plastic spring clip. This will protect her from the forceful rush of the return. It will usually take around 45 minutes for a complete evacuation, with the initial return occurring within the first 15–20 minutes. During the final 15–20 minutes, the client should be encouraged to ambulate to facilitate evacuation. If there is no return, instruct the client to massage her abdomen or drink warm fluids to stimulate peristalsis. *Note: If you are keeping output records, you will need to measure the return. To do this, either fold up the tail of the irrigation sleeve and secure it with the other spring clip or allow the return to flow directly into a bedpan. Subtract the amount of irrigant from the return.*

DRAINING A CONTINENT ILEOSTOMY (KOCK POUCH)

Assessing

1 To assess the need for draining the internal pouch, inspect the client's abdomen and gently palpate the abdomen exterior to the pouch to determine the amount of fecal content. Assess the client's knowledge of the procedure and explain why it is performed.

Planning

2 Assemble the following equipment: an irrigation set with a 50-mL syringe; 30–40 mL of warm water; a #28 silastic or teflon-coated catheter; water-soluble lubricant; and a stoma cap (as shown) or a bandage, depending on your client's need for drainage absorption. If the client is ambulatory, perform the procedure in the bathroom.

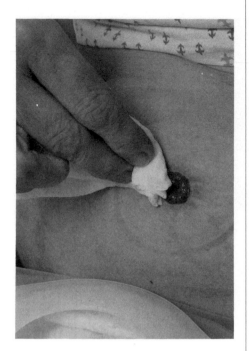

9 When a complete evacuation has been achieved, the client should remove the irrigation equipment and clean the peristomal skin with water and cleanser or a gentle soap. The stoma may be lightly patted with a soft cloth. When the peristomal skin has been rinsed and dried, the client may then apply a drainable pouch or the appliance appropriate for her needs.

Evaluating

10 Inspect and palpate the client's abdomen to assess for gastric distention, which can be indicative of an incomplete evacuation. Assess the stoma and peristomal skin for color and integrity. Document the procedure, noting the amount of irrigant and the character and amount of the return. If client teaching took place, document the client's performance.

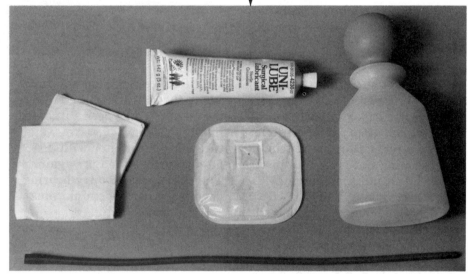

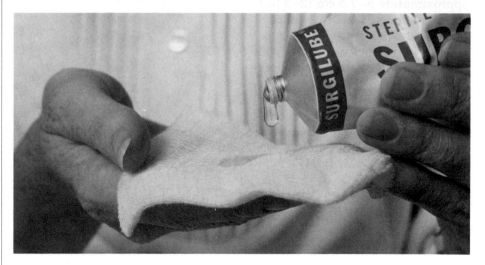

3 Squeeze some water-soluble lubricant onto a gauze pad or paper towel and instruct the client to lubricate 7.5 cm (3 in.) of the catheter's tip.

(Continued on p. 292)

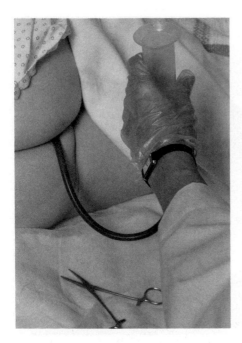

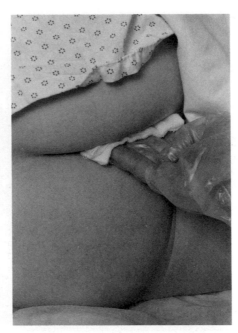

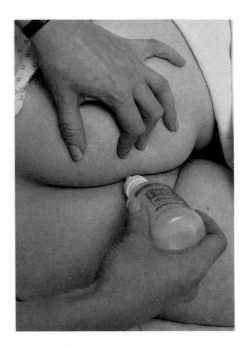

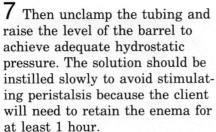

7 Then unclamp the tubing and raise the level of the barrel to achieve adequate hydrostatic pressure. The solution should be instilled slowly to avoid stimulating peristalsis because the client will need to retain the enema for at least 1 hour.

8 When the solution has been instilled, gently remove the tube and press firmly on the client's anus for a few moments, using a gauze pad or toilet paper (or the client may wish to do this herself). Advise the client to lie flat for 30 minutes to help prevent the stimulation of peristalsis. Before leaving the room, be sure a call light and bedpan are within reach in case she is unable to retain the solution. When the prescribed retention time has elapsed, assist the client into the bathroom or onto a bedpan as indicated. *Note: If the client is unable to retain an enema solution, a Foley catheter can be inserted, following the steps for inserting a rectal tube in the next procedure. After insertion past the external and internal sphincters, inflate the balloon with the designated amount of air. Then pull the balloon gently against the anal sphincter to seal the rectum.*

9 If a Fleets enema has been prescribed, separate the client's buttocks and gently insert the prelubricated tip into the anus. Then raise the base of the container to avoid instilling air into the rectum and squeeze the container to instill the solution.

Evaluating

10 If the procedure necessitates your observation of the return, do so at this time. If an oil-based retention enema was instilled, determine whether a cleansing enema needs to be instilled next. Document the procedure.

INSERTING A RECTAL TUBE

Assessing and Planning

1 A rectal tube can be inserted to relieve gastric distention when the distention is caused by flatus. However, you should first auscultate the client's abdomen for bowel sounds. An absence of bowel sounds in a rigid abdomen can mean that an obstruction or paralytic ileus, rather than flatus, is causing the distention; either condition necessitates immediate medical intervention.

2 Assemble the following materials: a rectal tube or a catheter, 22–24F for adults or 12–18F for children; water-soluble lubricant; hypoallergenic tape; bed-saver pad; and a disposable glove. You will also need a flatus bag, or receptacle to collect potential fecal discharge, such as a stool specimen container. Or wrap the draining end of the tube or catheter with gauze and tape. Explain the procedure to the client and provide privacy.

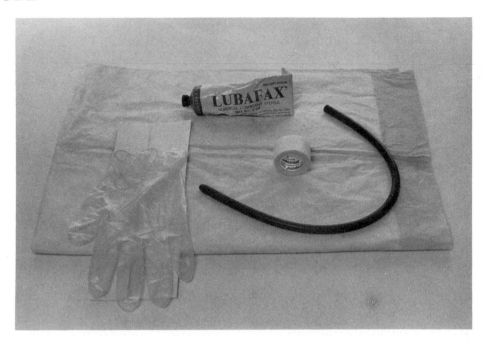

Implementing

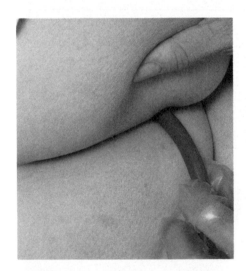

3 Assist the client into a Sim's position, and place a bed-saver pad under the buttocks. Lubricate the tip of the tube with water-soluble lubricant, and insert the tube into the rectum 7.5–10 cm (3–4 in.), past both the external and internal sphincters. (For a child, insert the tube 2.5–7.5 cm [1–3 in.].)

Evaluating

5 Continue to assess the client for distention and intervene accordingly.

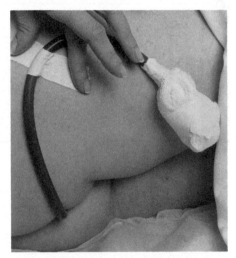

4 If relief from distention is not immediate, tape the tube to the thigh so that the client can have mobility without dislodging the tube. *Caution: To minimize the potential for rectal irritation or a loss in sphincter tone, do not leave the tube indwelling for longer than 20–30 minutes.* At the appropriate time, remove the tube and clean or discard it, depending on agency policy. Wash your hands, and document the procedure.

Percussing

Percussion will help you determine whether underlying structures are solid or filled with air or fluid. Percussion of the thorax is performed by placing a middle finger over an intercostal space and sharply striking that finger with the opposite middle finger to elicit sounds. Hollow sounds, referred to as resonance, will mostly be heard over the greater portions of the healthy lung. Hyperresonance, which is booming and low in pitch, may normally be heard in children with thin chest walls. It will also be found in clients with hyperinflated lungs or where there is an increase in pleural air, for example in clients with emphysema or a pneumothorax. Dullness will be elicited over dense lung areas in clients with pneumonia or atelectasis, but it is normally heard over the heart and liver. When percussing, you can follow the same pattern used for auscultating (see p. 312). The assessment should progress down one side of the chest, going from right to left (or vice versa) so that each side is checked against the symmetrical area on the opposite side, and repeated on the posterior (or anterior) chest.

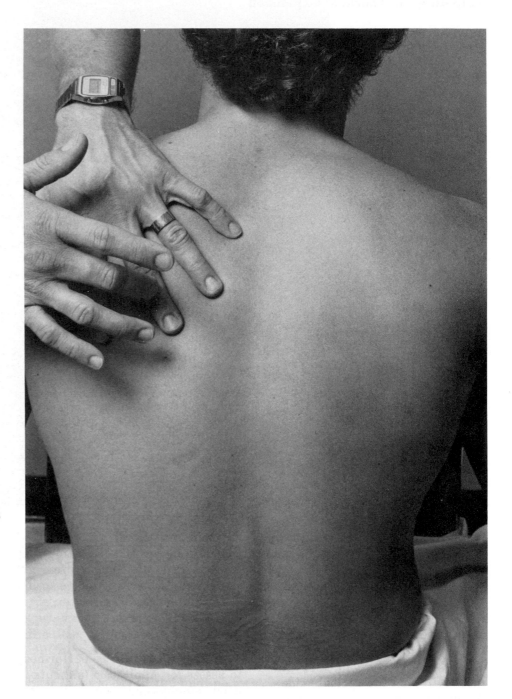

Auscultating

Warm the diaphragm of the
stethoscope between your hands
before placing it on the client's
skin. Instruct the client to
breathe through his mouth, more
slowly and deeply than usual.
Listen to at least one full breath
in each position, comparing one
side of the chest to the symmetrical area on the opposite side of
the chest. (See next page for auscultation patterns.)

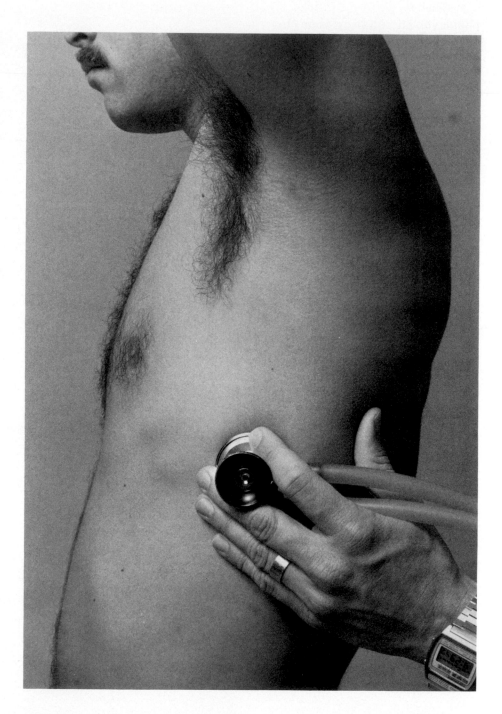

Follow the pattern in these photos for auscultating your client's chest. Listen for normal breath sounds, which include vesicular, bronchial, and bronchovesicular sounds; note their intensity, decrease in intensity, or absence from one auscultation site when compared to its symmetrical opposite. Vesicular sounds are soft and swishing and are considered normal when heard over the peripheral lung, but they are abnormal when heard over the large airways. A decrease in their sound over a segment of the peripheral lung might be found with emphysema, or in the presence of pleural fluid, or with a pneumothorax. Bronchial sounds are louder and coarser, of longer duration, and can be heard over the trachea and bronchi during inhalation and exhalation. They should not be heard over the normal peripheral lung, but they may be elicited over lungs of clients with some type of consolidation, such as a lung tumor or atelectasis. Bronchovesicular sounds are moderate in both pitch and intensity and are heard at the sternal borders of the major bronchi. Assume there is an abnormality if they are heard over the peripheral lung, which can occur with consolidation.

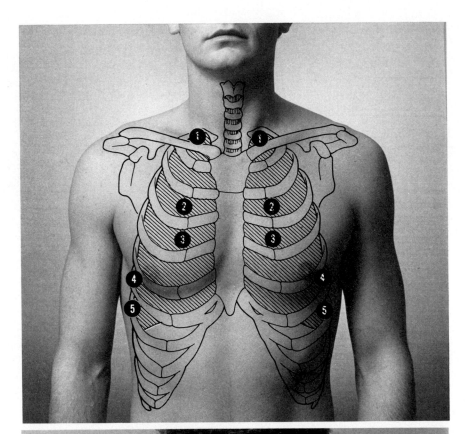

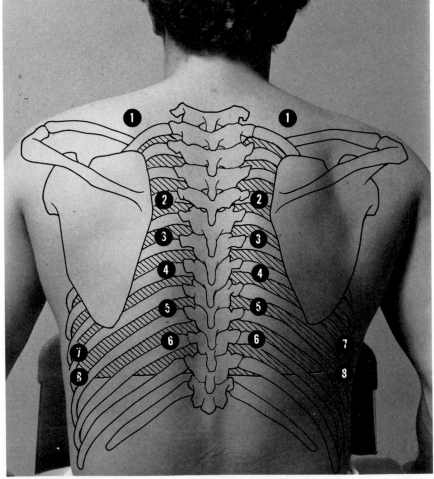

Table 6–1. Adventitious Sounds*

Acoustic characteristics	Time-expanded waveform	ATS recommended term†	ACCP report‡	A current British usage	Other terms(s)	Some common clinical associations
Discontinuous, interrupted, explosive sounds—loud, duration of about 10 msec. Low in pitch initial deflection width§ averaging 1.5 msec.		Coarse crackle	Rale	Crackle	Bubbling rales Coarse crepitations	Pulmonary edema Resolving pneumonia
Discontinuous, interrupted, explosive sounds—less loud than above and of shorter duration. They average less than 5 msec in duration and are lower in pitch. Initial deflection width§ averages about 0.7 msec.		Fine crackle	Rale	Crackle	Fine crepitations	Interstitial fibrosis
Continuous sounds—longer than 250 msec, high-pitched, dominant frequency of 400 Hz or more; a hissing sound.		Wheeze	Sibilant rhonchus	High-pitched wheeze	Sibilant rale Musical rale	Airway narrowing
Continuous sounds—longer than 250 msec, low-pitched, dominant frequency about 200 Hz or less; a snoring sound.		Rhonchus	Sonorous rhonchus	Low-pitched wheeze		Sputum production

*Used with permission from American Thoracic Society.
†From 1977, American Thoracic Society (ATS) ad Hoc Committee on pulmonary nomenclature.
‡From 1974 ATS/American College of Chest Physicians (ACCP) committee on pulmonary nomenclature.
§Time in msec from the onset of the crackle until the first deflection returns to the baseline.

Review Table 6-1 to help you identify adventitious (added or abnormal) breath sounds. Regardless of the terminology used in your agency to describe adventitious sounds, it is important that you determine whether the added sounds you hear are continuous or discontinuous, low or high in pitch, fine or coarse, and whether they are heard during inhalation or exhalation. Coarse crackles (rales), associated with resolving pneumonia or pulmonary edema, are often heard during inhalation and may be eliminated by coughing when they are caused by secretions in the airway. Fine crackles, found in interstitial lung disease or heart failure, are heard late during inspiration, usually over lung bases, and are rarely cleared by coughing. Wheezes (sibilant rhonchi) are musical and high in pitch and are most often associated with bronchial asthma or COPD. They are best heard over the larynx during exhalation; however, wheezes of different pitches and sounds might at times be heard simultaneously over all lung fields.

Rhonchi occur with increased sputum production and are usually heard during exhalation as air passes through passages narrowed by mucosal swelling or secretions. They are usually cleared or lessened by coughing.

A pleural friction rub sounds like two pieces of sand paper rubbing together, and it is caused by the loss of normal pleural lubrication. It is typically heard over the anterolateral chest, and it can be caused, for example, by pleurisy.

Maintaining Patent Airways

Nursing Guidelines to Artificial Airways

Oropharyngeal Tube

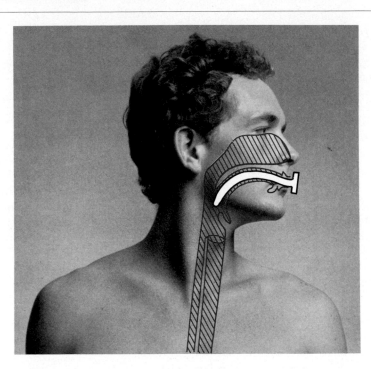

Description	S-shaped, plastic device that fits over the tongue and extends into the posterior pharynx. Available in infant, child, and adult sizes.
Uses	For clients requiring an assisted airway immediately postanesthesia, or for those who are semiconscious and in danger of obstructing their own airways with a displaced tongue. It can also be used when suctioning is required on a short-term basis, or as a bite blocker when used with an endotracheal tube.
Nursing Considerations	■ To facilitate insertion and to keep the client's tongue from falling back into the pharynx, the client should be supine with a hyperextended neck unless it is contraindicated by head and neck injuries.
	■ After insertion, keep the client's head turned to the side to prevent aspiration from vomitus and secretions.
	■ Remove the airway every 4 hours and provide oral hygiene.
	■ The airway should not be discontinued until the client is conscious, can swallow on his own, and his gag and cough reflexes have returned.
	■ This airway is contraindicated in the conscious client because it stimulates the gag reflex.

Nasopharyngeal Tube

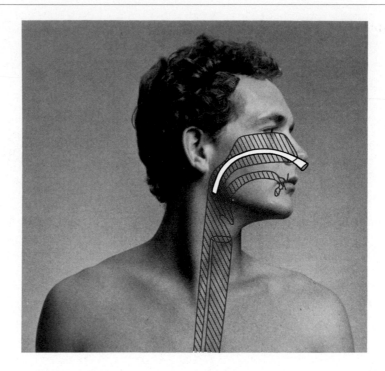

Description

Rubber or latex tube (also called trumpet) that extends from the naris to the hypopharynx. Large variation in sizes accommodates the infant to the adult.

Uses

For clients requiring short-term airway management when the oral route is contraindicated, or for those with a sensitive gag reflex. Also inserted to protect the nasal mucosa during nasopharyngeal or nasotracheal suctioning.

Nursing Considerations

- Prior to insertion, lubricate the tube with water-soluble lubricant, or topical anesthetic, if ordered.
- For optimal fit, the diameter of the tube should be only slightly smaller than the diameter of the naris.
- To prevent pressure areas, rotate the tube to the alternate naris at least every 8 hours.
- Provide nasal hygiene to both nares.
- Nasotracheal suctioning should be done only when necessary because it can stimulate the vagus nerve and may potentially lead to bradycardia and cardiac arrest.

Endotracheal Tube

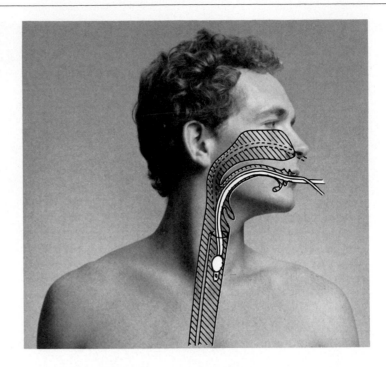

Description

Polyvinyl chloride curved tube that extends from the mouth or nose to just above the bifurcation of the trachea (carina). Inner and outer diameters of the tube are measured in millimeters, the length in centimeters. Sized to accommodate the newborn to the adult, with cuffed tubes available in adolescent and adult sizes.

Uses

Most commonly for clients receiving general anesthesia or in short-term emergency situations to provide a patent airway, facilitate suctioning, or provide a means for mechanical ventilation.

Nursing Considerations

- Turn the client to the side to prevent aspiration from vomitus and secretions.
- Keep the airway taped securely in place. Accidental extubation can be life threatening.
- To monitor tube slippage, mark the tube at the nose or mouth with indelible ink.
- Provide frequent oral and nasal hygiene.
- Oral tubes should be repositioned to the opposite side of the mouth every 8 hours to prevent pressure areas in the mouth. With nasal tubes, the nares should be evaluated frequently for breakdown.
- To prevent unconscious clients from biting down on oral tubes, an oropharyngeal airway or a bite block can be inserted to keep the jaws apart.
- Provide means for communication; keep the call light within the client's reach.
- Frequently monitor cuff pressure to prevent tracheal necrosis. It should not be greater than 20 mm Hg.
- Continuous humidification or aerosol therapy via a T-piece is necessary to prevent drying of membranes and respiratory complications.
- Review Nursing Considerations for the tracheostomy tube. The nursing care plan is basically the same.

Tracheostomy Tube

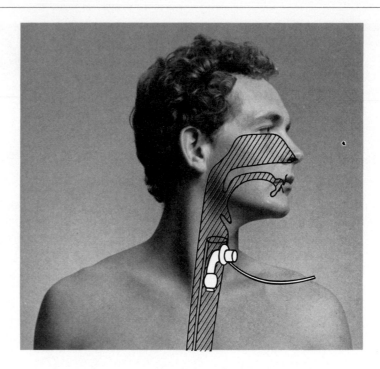

Description

Plastic, metal, or foam tube that extends from an incision in the anterior neck directly into the trachea. Available in infant to adult sizes, but smaller sizes generally come without cuffs. Single-cannula tubes indicated for short-term use; tubes with both inner and outer cannulas are most often used in long-term care. Can attach to mechanical ventilator with an adaptor.

Nursing Considerations

- To assess need for suctioning and patency of airway, frequently auscultate lung fields and trachea for breath sounds.
- To minimize the potential for infection and for client comfort, change the dressing around the tracheostomy as soon as blood and secretions collect.
- Hyperinflate the client's lungs with high concentrations of oxygen before, during, and after suctioning to minimize hypoxemia.
- Encourage turning, coughing, deep breathing, and range of motion exercises to help mobilize secretions.
- Continuous humidification or aerosol therapy via T-piece or tracheostomy collar is necessary to prevent drying of membranes and respiratory complications.
- If heated humidity is delivered, monitor the temperature frequently to prevent injury to the trachea. Keep it within 34–36 C.
- Inflate cuffed tracheostomy tubes during eating, intermittent positive pressure breathing (IPPB), and mechanical ventilation.
- Provide a means for communication and keep the call light within reach.
- Secure the tube carefully to prevent accidental dislodgement.

Tracheostomy Button

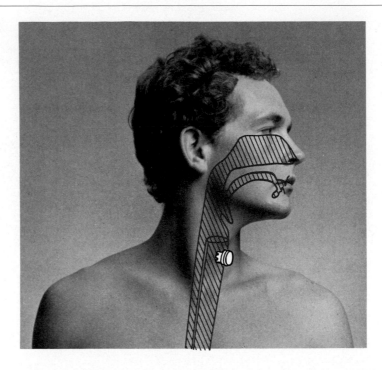

Description	Short tube that extends from tracheal stoma to just inside the tracheal wall. Most come with adaptors, for use with IPPB and manual resuscitator, and plugs for closing the button.
Uses	Maintains stoma for emergency airway management after the tracheostomy tube has been removed. It also can be used to wean client from ventilatory support.

Nursing Considerations

- The button allows the client to cough and breath more easily than does a tracheostomy tube.
- Remove closure plug for suctioning and/or ventilating.
- Insert IPPB adaptor plug for ventilating.
- The client can speak when the button is plugged.
- To prevent skin irritation, keep stomal area clean with hydrogen peroxide. Dry thoroughly after rinsing with sterile water.
- Clean the cannula often, according to agency protocol, by immersing in hydrogen peroxide solution and rinsing with sterile water.

INSERTING ARTIFICIAL AIRWAYS

Inserting an Oropharyngeal Airway

Assessing and Planning

1 Choose the correct airway size. Generally, they are available in infant, child, and adult sizes. Wash your hands and explain the procedure to the client, even though he is semiconscious. Position him so that his neck is hyperextended unless this position is contraindicated by a head or neck injury. You can also roll a large towel or small pillow and place it under the client's shoulders to further increase the angle of the head tilt. Positioning him in this manner will open his airway and help keep the tongue away from the pharynx.

2 To open his mouth, employ the crossed-finger technique (as shown). In this position, your fingers will pop out of his mouth should he have a seizure or clamp down with his teeth. *Note: If you use a tongue blade instead, depress the tongue and place the airway directly over the tongue and into the back of the mouth.* Before inserting the artificial airway, make sure the client's airway is clear of obstructions.

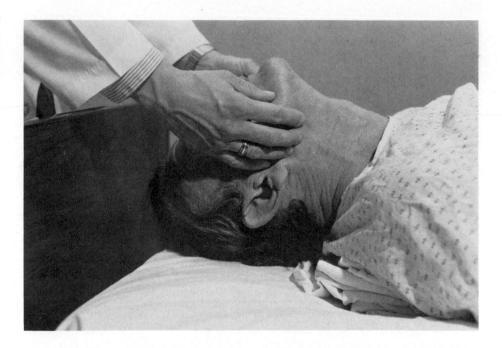

Implementing

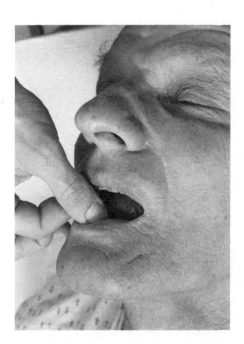

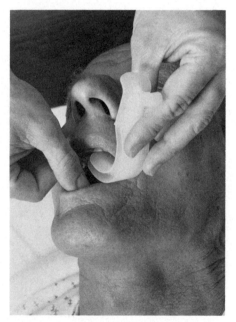

3 With your other hand, position the airway so that it is upside down, with the tip pointing upward toward the roof of the mouth. Insert it into the back of the mouth. Positioning it in this manner will depress the tongue and prevent tongue displacement into the posterior pharynx.

(Continued on p. 320)

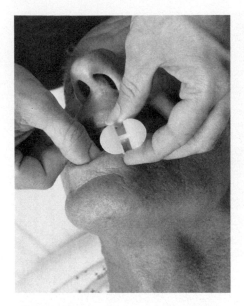

4 Turn the airway 90° so that it is positioned sideways.

Evaluating

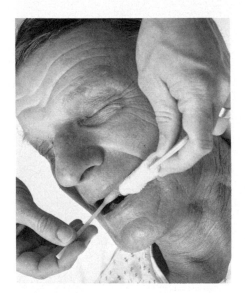

7 At least every 4 hours, remove the airway by gently pulling it downward and outward following the natural curve of the mouth. Use a gauze-covered tongue depressor to keep the client's mouth open while assessing the oral cavity and providing hygiene. The photo illustrates swabbing the mouth with a lemon-glycerine solution.

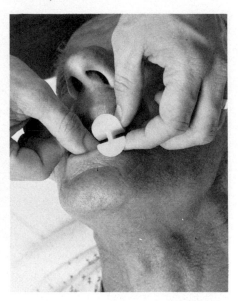

5 Turn the airway another 90° so that its curve fits over the tongue.

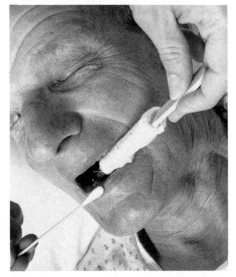

8 Moisturize the client's lips to prevent cracking and breakdown from the pressure of the airway's flange. The photograph illustrates the use of a cotton-tipped applicator saturated with a water-soluble lubricant. Following mouth care, reinsert the airway following the steps outlined above. Before discontinuing the airway, ensure that the client is at least semiconscious, can swallow on his own, and that gag and cough reflexes have returned.

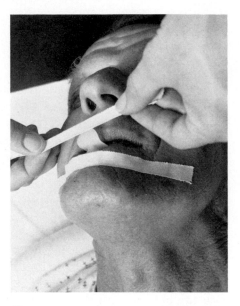

6 Apply a skin preparation and tape the airway in place with two strips of hypoallergenic tape that are 1.25-cm (½-in.) wide. *Caution: Be sure the airway is not obstructed by the tape and that you have allowed ample access for suctioning.* Turn the client to his side to prevent aspiration from vomitus and secretions. Wash your hands and document the procedure.

Inserting a Nasopharyngeal Airway

Assessing and Planning

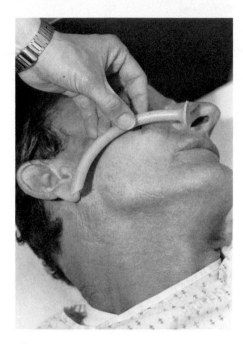

1 Explain the procedure to your client. Place him in semi-Fowler's to high-Fowler's position to enhance his respirations unless this position is contraindicated. Select an airway that extends from the earlobe to the naris. For optimal fit, the outer diameter of the airway should be only slightly smaller than that of the naris.

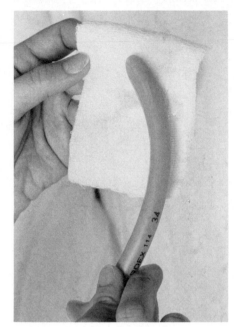

2 If you have an order for an anesthetic jelly, lubricate the entire length of the airway with the topical anesthetic. Otherwise, lubricate the airway with a water soluble lubricant to facilitate its insertion.

Implementing

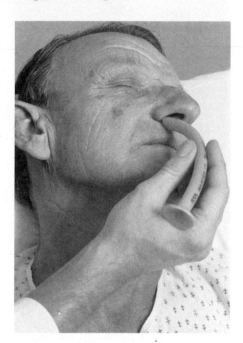

3 Select the naris that looks more patent; gently insert the airway while pushing up the tip of the nose so that the tube follows the curve of the nasopharynx. If the naris you selected proves to be obstructed, intubate the other.

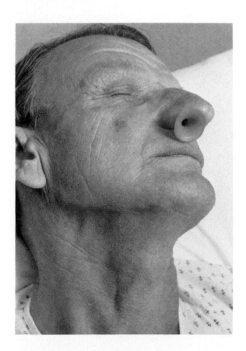

4 When the flange of the airway reaches the naris, the distal end of the airway should be correctly positioned in the hypopharynx.

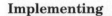

5 To prevent its expulsion, tape the airway in place by looping 1.25 cm (½ in.) of hypoallergenic tape over the area of the airway that is distal to the flange and adhering the rest of the tape to the skin above the client's upper lip. Use a skin preparation first if your client has sensitive skin. Wash your hands and document the procedure.

(Continued on p. 322)

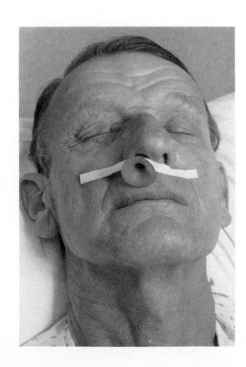

Evaluating

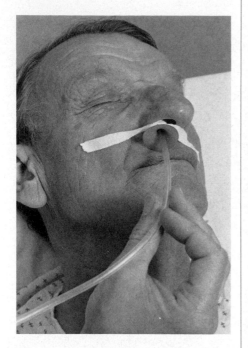

6 Prior to its removal, suction down the airway to remove the secretions. Be sure to rotate the airway to the other naris at least every 8 hours. Assess the naris for breakdown and provide materials for cleansing the naris and moisturizing the nasal mucosa.

MANAGING ROUTINE TRACHEOSTOMY CARE

Suctioning the Client with a Tracheostomy

Assessing and Planning

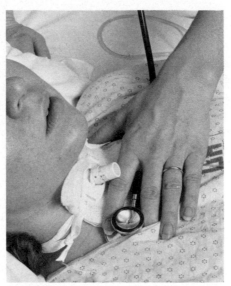

1 Evaluate the client's need for suctioning by bilaterally auscultating the lung fields to identify and locate secretions. If suctioning is needed, explain the procedure to the client and place her in Fowler's position unless it is contraindicated. Remember that suctioning is always done as needed rather than as a standard order; therefore frequent client assessment is crucial.

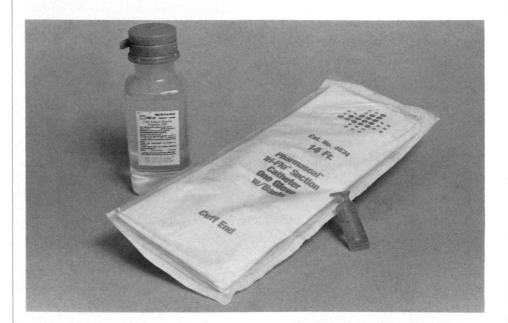

2 Assemble the following materials: sterile solution (usually normal saline), a small vial of normal saline for lavage if your client's secretions are thick (optional), and a sterile suction kit (or a sterile glove, sterile basin, and a sterile catheter). The use of two gloves (one sterile and one clean to protect the nurse's other hand) is recommended by some experts because of the potential for infection from the herpetic virus found in the oral secretions of some clients. *Note: To minimize the potential for hypoxia, make sure the outer diameter of the suction catheter is no greater than half of the inner diameter of the tracheostomy tube.*

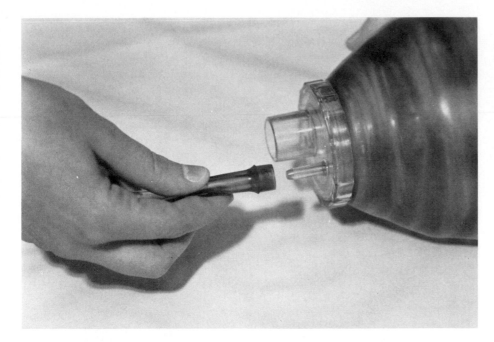

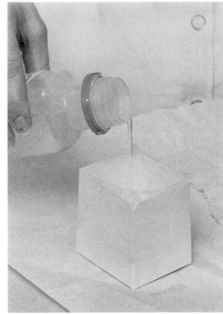

3 In addition, you will need both a suction apparatus and a manual resuscitator such as an Ambu or Laerdal. Attach the resuscitator to source oxygen (as shown). Some agencies also recommend the use of an oxygen reservoir that attaches to the large bore outlet pictured above. The reservoir allows the delivery of higher oxygen concentrations. When hyperinflating the client (using the "sigh maneuver") you will need to adjust the oxygen flowmeter to deliver 12–15 L/min, which will provide the necessary oxygen concentrations.

4 Wash your hands and loosen the cap on the sterile solution bottle. Open the sterile suction kit on a clean surface using the internal wrapping as a sterile field, and fill the sterile basin with the sterile solution.

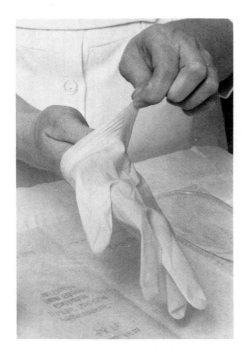

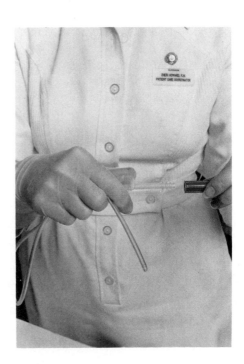

5 Put a sterile glove on your dominant hand.

6 Attach the suction catheter to the suction tubing, holding the sterile catheter in your gloved hand and the suction tubing in your ungloved hand. *Note: The same catheter can be used during the entire procedure provided it does not become contaminated, and it is not used to suction the oropharynx or nasopharynx before suctioning or resuctioning the trachea. If either of these situations occurs, replace the contaminated catheter with a sterile one to prevent contaminating the respiratory tract.*

(Continued on p. 324)

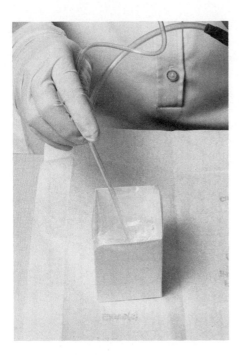

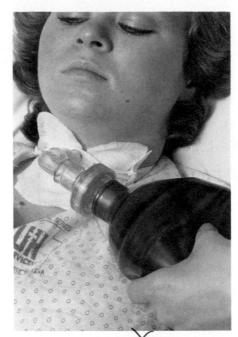

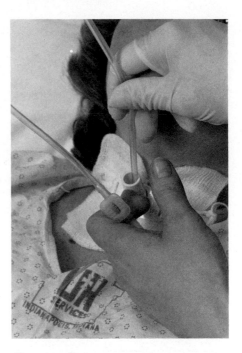

7 Set the suction regulator dial at 120 mm Hg. Submerge the tip of the catheter into the sterile solution and briefly place your ungloved hand over the suction port to produce suction. This not only tests the efficiency of the suction apparatus, but it also lubricates the catheter to facilitate its insertion into the trachea. In addition, it lubricates the inside of the catheter, which helps to prevent tenacious secretions from sticking to the tubing.

8 Using your nondominant hand, oxygenate your client with three to five deep lung inflations to help compensate for the oxygen you will remove during the suctioning process. To do this, turn the oxygen on, position the tracheostomy adaptor of the resuscitator directly over the tracheostomy tube, and compress the bag to deliver the oxygen. Ideally, a second person should "sigh" the client. Because the second person can place both hands firmly around the resuscitation bag, there is less potential for trauma from manipulation of the bag. In addition, the second person can provide greater volume with two hands than that which can be provided with one hand. *Caution: Clients with copious secretions should not be hyperinflated with a resuscitator because their secretions could be expelled deeply into the airway. Keep these clients on their regular oxygen delivery devices and increase the liter flow for a few minutes just prior to suctioning.*

9 Remove the oxygen device. With your dominant gloved hand, gently insert the catheter into the tracheostomy, keeping your nondominant thumb off the suction port. Insert the catheter as far as it will go, but do not use force. When you reach the carina or bronchial wall, withdraw the catheter 1–2 cm to prevent damaging the area.

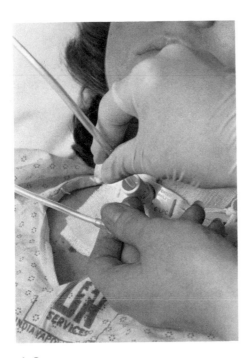

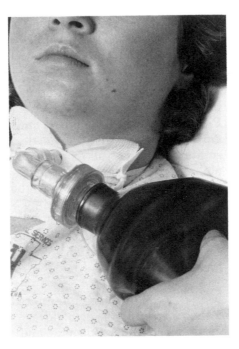

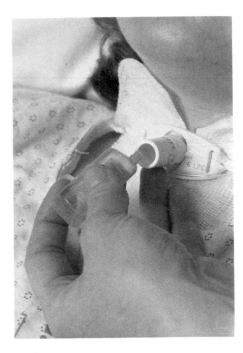

10 Place your nondominant thumb over the suction port to produce suction. Rotate the catheter between your dominant thumb and forefinger, gradually withdrawing the catheter as you apply intermittent suction by moving your nondominant thumb up and down on the suction port. This should prevent the catheter from adhering to the mucosa and damaging the bronchial wall. To minimize hypoxemia, do not suction for longer than 10–15 seconds during each suction attempt. Some experts suggest having the client turn the head to the right while you attempt to suction the left tracheobronchial tree, and the head to the left while you attempt to suction the right tracheobronchial tree. Although this technique is recommended, its efficacy has not been proven.

11 To prevent suction-induced hypoxemia, reoxygenate the client after every suction attempt, following the technique outlined in step 8.

12 If the secretions are tenacious, flush the catheter in the sterile solution and lavage the trachea with at least 3–5 mL of normal saline. This will help liquify the secretions and facilitate their aspiration. Then suction again.

(Continued on p. 326)

Converting a Nonrebreathing Mask to a Partial Rebreathing Mask

Assembling a Venturi Delivery System

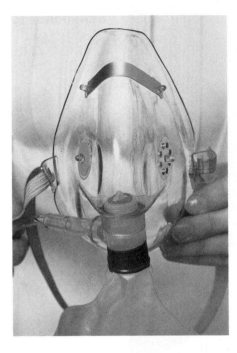

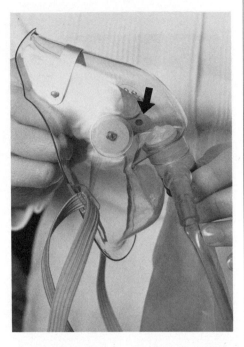

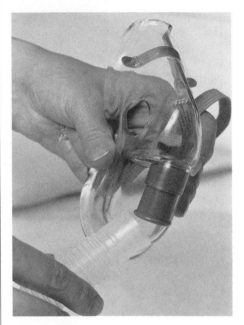

The difference between a nonrebreathing mask and a partial rebreathing mask is that the former has two rubber disks. One disk occludes one of the exhalation ports, and the other occludes the port between the mask and the reservoir bag. These disks allow for the exhalation of gas while also minimizing the inhalation of room air. When it is no longer necessary for the client to receive the higher concentration of oxygen that is provided by the nonrebreathing mask, the physician might prescribe a partial rebreathing mask. You can easily convert the client's existing mask to a partial rebreather.

1 Begin by removing the rubber disk at the port between the mask and the reservoir bag.

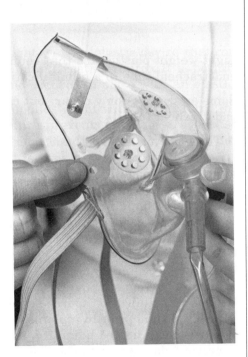

2 Remove the rubber disk at the exhalation port. Save the disks in the event your client might again need the higher oxygen concentrations that require reconversion to a nonrebreathing mask.

1 A venturi mask comes prepackaged with a 15–20-cm (6–8-in.) wide-bore tube, a humidification adaptor, and a variety of jets or adaptors that are usually color coded to coincide with the prescribed concentration of oxygen. To assemble a venturi mask, attach the wide-bore tubing to the mask's adaptor.

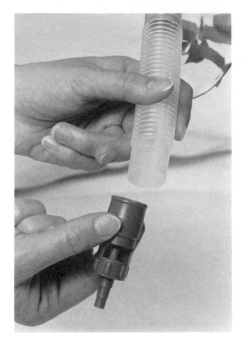

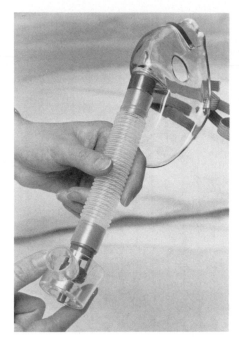

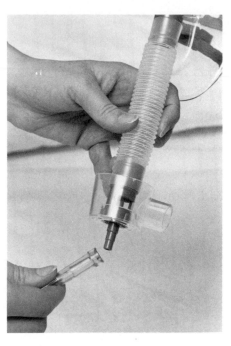

2 The lower hand in the photograph holds the jet adaptor. The size of the jet's opening determines the delivered percentage of oxygen. Slide the jet into the open end of the wide-bore tubing. Keep the remaining jets at your client's bedside in case the physician prescribes a different oxygen concentration at a later time. Most manufacturers imprint the adaptors with concentration and recommended liter flow, for example, 24% (4–6 L/min).

3 Attach the humidity adaptor to the jet, regardless of whether or not humidity has been prescribed. The adaptor will prevent the jet adaptor's air entrainment ports from becoming occluded by blankets or the client's body.

4 Attach the oxygen tubing to the jet's nipple, and the other end of the tubing to the oxygen flowmeter. Adjust the flowmeter to the level prescribed on the nipple.

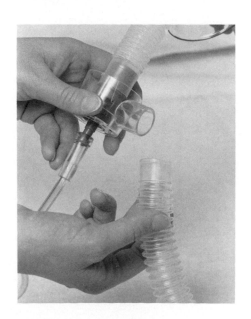

5 If humidification has been prescribed, attach one end of the wide-bore tubing to the humidity adaptor, and the other end to the humidifier or nebulizer.

6 Apply the venturi mask to your client. The client in this photograph is wearing a venturi mask that is attached to humidity. The system can also attach to a T-piece for a client with a tracheostomy.

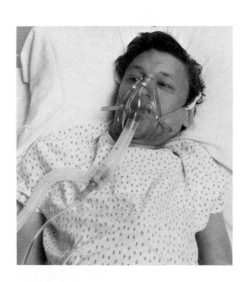

Setting Up an Oxygen System with Humidification

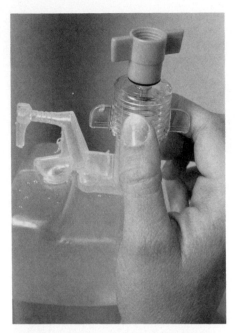

1 Follow these steps to deliver humidified oxygen to your client. A disposable humidifier is used here, but the principles are basically the same if you are using a reusable humidifier. Attach the adaptor to the humidifier. The adaptor is usually packaged with the disposable humidifier.

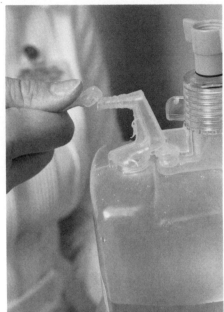

2 Snap off the seal from the outlet port of the humidifier.

3 Connect the humidifier to the flowmeter via the adaptor.

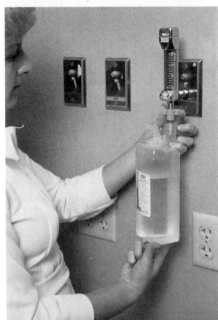

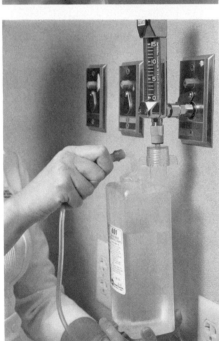

4 Connect small-bore oxygen tubing to the outlet port of the humidifier bottle.

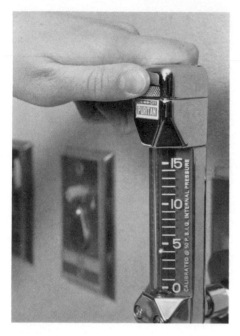

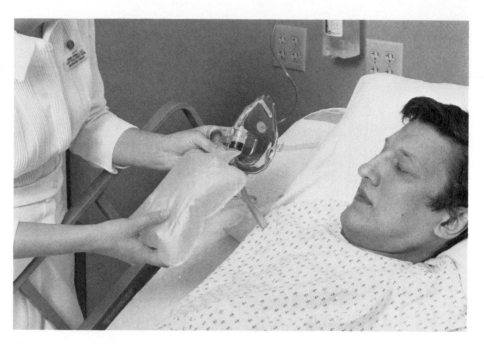

5 Adjust the flowmeter to the prescribed number of liters of oxygen per minute.

6 You are now ready to attach the distal end of the oxygen tubing to one of the following: simple oxygen mask, nasal cannula, par- tial rebreathing mask, or to a nonrebreathing mask as shown here.

Delivering Heated Humidity

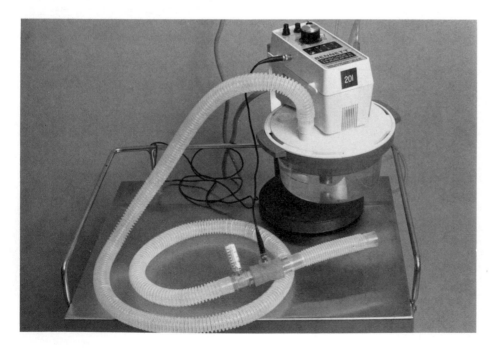

1 A heated servo-controlled cascade humidifier can be used to deliver either warmed oxygen or humidity. In this photo, wide-bore tubing is attached to deliver the humidity. In addition, the reservoir is filled with sterile water. If oxygen has also been prescribed for your client, you will need to attach one end of the small-bore oxygen tubing to the oxygen flowmeter and the other end to the oxygen port of the system. Remember to adjust the flowmeter to achieve the prescribed FiO_2.

(Continued on p. 348)

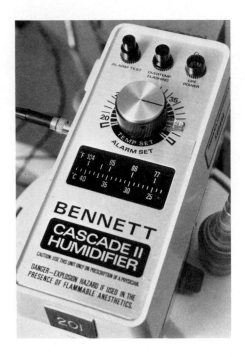

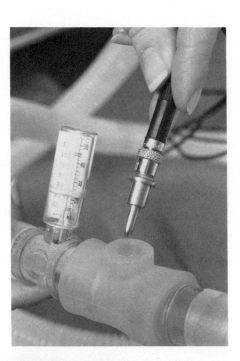

2 Set the temperature control dial to the prescribed temperature (usually as close to body temperature as possible). The unit pictured shows the connection of the temperature probe on the left side.

3 The other end of the probe → attaches to a rubber adaptor, as close to the client's airway as is feasible. The unit will automatically heat and turn off, as needed, to maintain the preset temperature. If the heat surpasses that which you have set on the temperature-control dial, or in the event of an equipment malfunction, an alarm will sound.

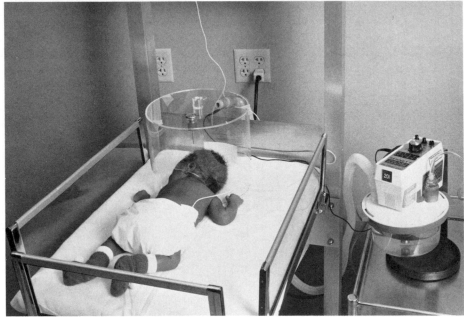

4 You can now attach the free end of the wide-bore tubing to an oxygen hood.

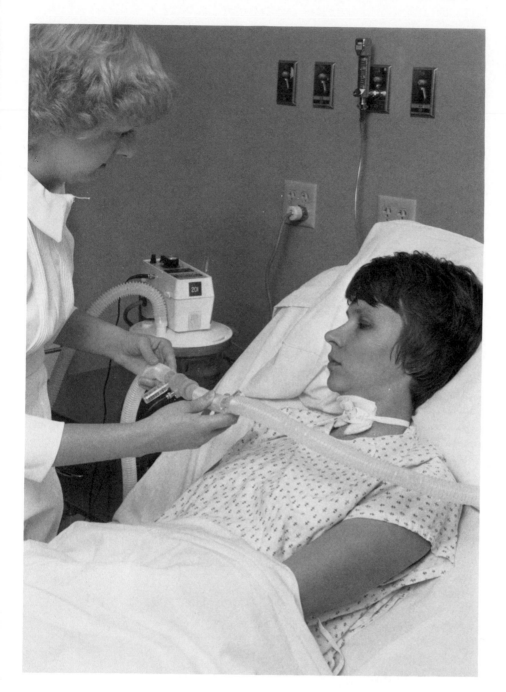

5 Or attach the tubing to a tracheostomy collar or to a T-piece (as shown).

Assembling a Nebulizer

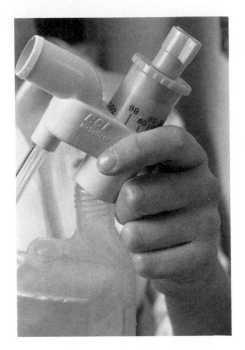

1 A common method for the delivery of aerosol therapy is the use of a pneumatic (jet) nebulizer as outlined in these steps. The first step is to attach a venturi adaptor to the nebulizer bottle.

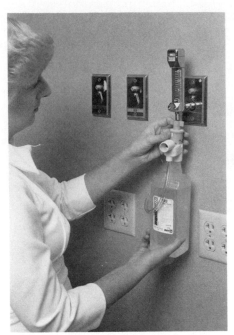

2 Attach the assembled nebulizer to the flowmeter.

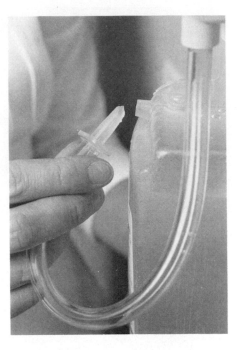

3 This venturi adaptor has a small tube that collects condensate. Connect it to the small outlet on the front of the nebulizer, after first snapping off the outlet's seal.

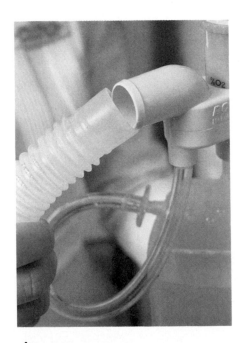

4 Attach wide-bore tubing to the outlet of the venturi adaptor.

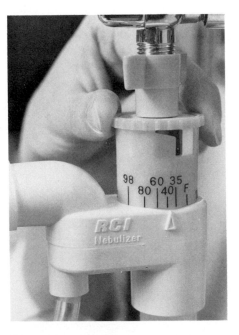

5 If you will also be delivering oxygen, adjust the venturi dial to the prescribed FiO_2. If oxygen has not been prescribed, set the dial to "F" (for Full).

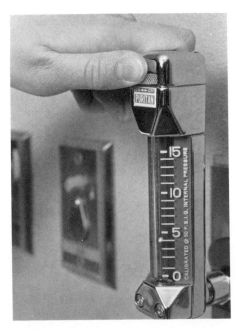

6 Adjust the flowmeter until a visible mist is produced at the distal end of the tubing. The flowmeter is usually turned to its maximum level to ensure adequate gas flow to the client.

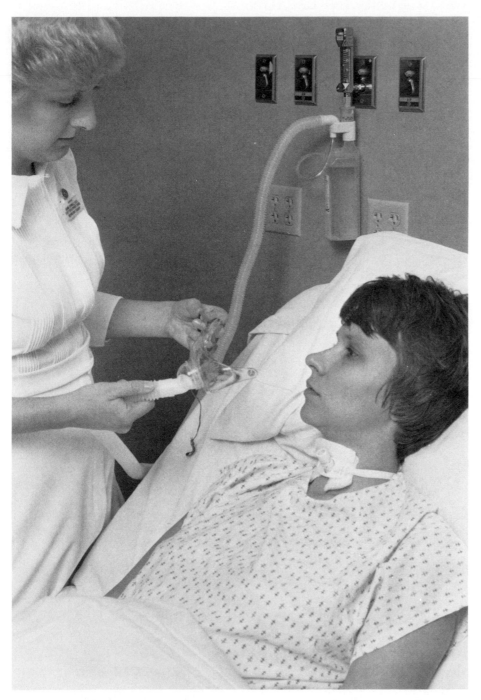

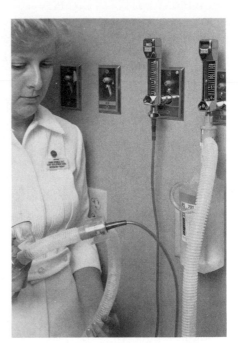

8 The tubing can also be connected to the high humidity adaptor of a venturi mask. Check to make sure the client is receiving adequate gas flow from the nebulizer. Mist should be visible from the delivery device during inspiration and exhalation. If mist is not visible, increase the liter flow by adjusting the flowmeter.

7 Connect the distal end of the tubing to either an aerosol mask, T-piece, or tracheostomy collar (as shown).

EMPLOYING TECHNIQUES FOR LUNG INFLATION

Instructing Clients in Deep Breathing Exercises

Teaching Apical Expansion Exercises: Clients who will benefit from this exercise are those who might be restricting their upper chest movement because of splinting from pain—for example, clients who have had a lobectomy, mastectomy, or gross pleural effusion. Position your fingers below the clavicles and apply moderate pressure. Instruct the client to inhale while pushing his chest upward and forward, expanding against your finger pressure. Encourage him to retain the expansion for a few moments and then exhale quietly and passively. Once you have taught him the technique, he can perform the exercise on his own by positioning his fingers over the same area. When done correctly and frequently, apical expansion will help reexpand remaining lung tissue, eliminate secretions, and minimize flattening of the upper chest wall.

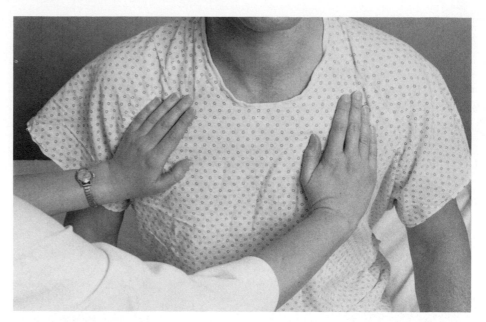

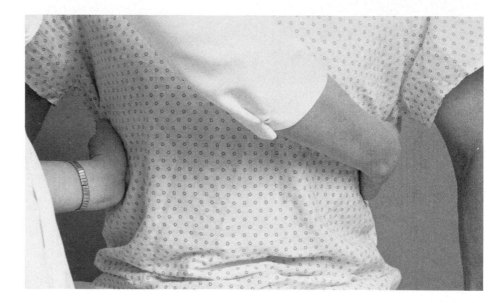

Teaching Basal Expansion Exercises: Lower thoracic exercises are frequently indicated for clients recovering from chest surgery, for whom pain on the affected side inhibits bilateral chest movement. Position your hands on the midaxillary lines in the area of the eighth ribs, and apply moderate pressure as the client inhales. Instruct the client to attempt to move your hands outward as he expands his lower ribs. He should retain his maximum inhalation for 1 or 2 seconds to help promote aeration of his alveoli, and then exhale in a relaxed, passive manner. Clients with COPD, especially, should be closely observed for both a slow, relaxed exhalation and a relaxed upper chest. Encourage clients to perform the exercise on their own by using the palms of their hands. When practiced frequently and correctly, this technique will both promote and maintain lower chest wall mobility.

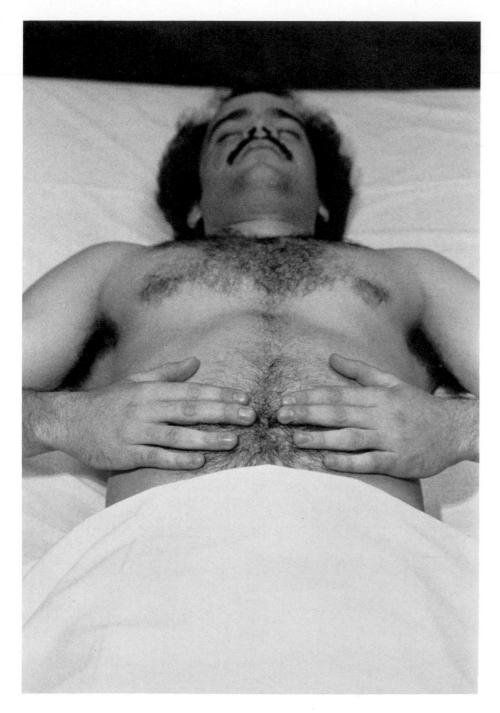

Teaching Diaphragmatic Breathing: Your clients will breathe more efficiently and obtain better lung function when correctly using their abdominal muscles and diaphragms.

To instruct the client in diaphragmatic breathing, have him assume a supine position and flex his knees to relax the abdominal wall. He should then place his hands over his abdomen and breathe in deeply and slowly through his nose as he pushes his abdomen outward. If he does this correctly, his hands will rise during the inspiration. The exhalation should be quiet and passive, with the lower ribs and abdomen sinking downward as the abdomen relaxes. Once the client has been taught diaphragmatic breathing while supine, he may then assume other positions for practicing this technique. Emphasize the need for frequent and regular practice until breathing in this manner becomes automatic and no longer requires a conscious effort. *Note: Clients with COPD should be taught to inhale through the nose and exhale slowly through pursed (puckered) lips. This will help to minimize small airway collapse.*

Assisting with Coughing

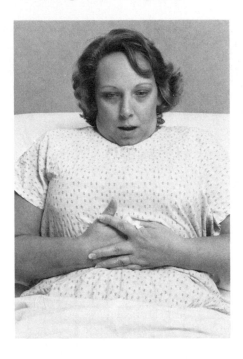

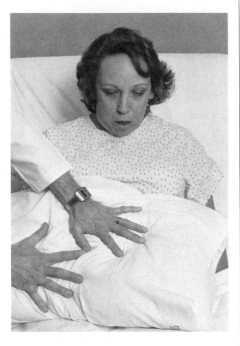

Teaching clients an effective, controlled cough is essential in the management of bronchial secretions, and it should be taught to all clients *before* surgery. Instruct the client to sit with her upper body flexed slightly forward. If this position is contraindicated, she can assume a lateral position, with flexed knees and hips. Either position will promote a forceful cough, while also minimizing strain in the lower back. First, instruct the client to take two or three deep breaths with passive exhalation. She should then take a deep breath, hold it briefly, and cough forcefully.

An alternative method is the "double cough" technique, which is especially recommended for clients with COPD in whom one very forceful cough could cause small airway collapse. The client is instructed to cough from the midinspiratory point rather than from the point of deep inspiration. The client exhales in a rapid succession of two or more abrupt, sharp coughs. The first cough loosens secretions and the following cough(s) facilitates the movement of the secretions toward the upper airway.

To minimize pain, a postoperative client will require splinting over her incisional area during the coughing process. A pillow can be pressed over the affected area, or you can show the client how to splint her own incision by pressing the arm and hand of the unaffected side against the site.

Using Incentive Spirometers

Assessing

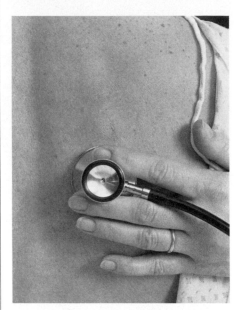

1 Auscultate the client's lung fields to establish a baseline for postexercise comparison. Explain the procedure in detail. Many clients incorrectly *exhale* rather than inhale during the exercise. Incentive spirometry is a goal-oriented and measurable breathing exercise, which helps clients increase their inspiratory volume while also inflating their alveoli.

Planning and Implementation

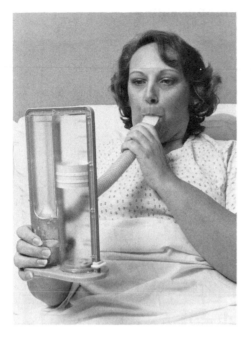

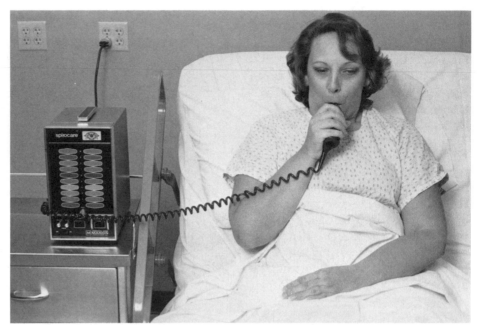

2 Many disposable flow-incentive spirometers have pointers that you can slide to the prescribed inspiratory volume level. Check the operating instructions on the unit used by your agency. Instruct the client to hold the unit upright because tilting it will make the exercise less challenging. She should complete a normal exhalation and then seal her lips tightly around the mouthpiece while inhaling slowly and deeply. Encourage the client to sustain the inspiration long enough to elevate the disk for at least 3 seconds.

3 If your client is using a reusable volume-incentive spirometer, set the prescribed volume by adjusting the volume-control gauge. Position the unit on the bedside table and instruct the client to follow the same steps just outlined. In many volume-incentive spirometers, the area of the prescribed volume will light up when the client achieves the appropriate preset level.

When the client has achieved the appropriate level, instruct her to sustain the inspiration until the device alerts her that she can exhale. With the unit in this photo, the clown on the top will illuminate until the client has sustained the inspiration for the appropriate length of time. Be sure to position the unit so that the side that illuminates is clearly visible to the client. Upon completion of the treatment, remove the mouthpiece, clean it, and store it in the bedside table for the next treatment.

Evaluating

4 Auscultate the client's lung fields for postexercise breath sounds and compare them to your earlier assessment. Document the procedure and the client's response.

SETTING UP A PLEUR-EVAC SYSTEM

1 Familiarize yourself with the nursing guidelines to the Pleur-evac system, pp. 367–369, so that once the chest tube has been inserted you are prepared to manage both the client and the system. In addition to the Pleur-evac, you will need either sterile water or sterile saline and a 50-mL syringe.

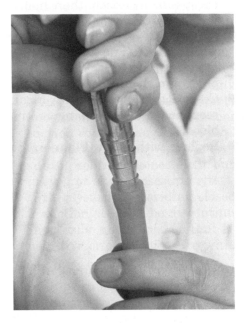

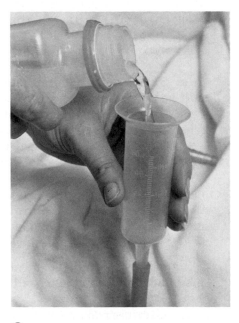

2 Remove the connector from the short rubber tubing of the water seal chamber.

3 Remove the bulb from an asepto syringe or plunger from a 50-mL piston syringe. Attach the barrel of the syringe to the rubber tubing. Pour sterile solution to the 2-cm line of the chamber. Remove the barrel and reattach the connector to the tubing.

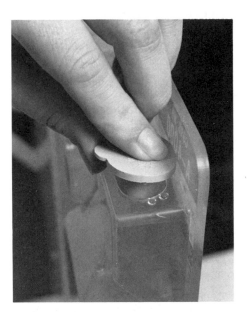

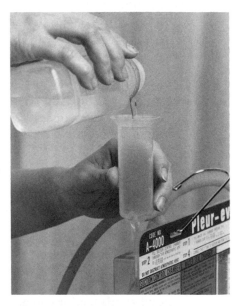

4 If suction has been ordered, remove the diaphragm from the suction control chamber.

5 Connect the syringe barrel directly to the vent of the suction chamber, and pour sterile solution to the prescribed level, which is usually 20–25 cm. Reattach the diaphragm.

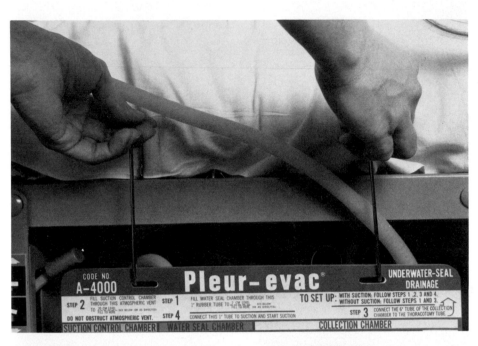

6 Attach the Pleur-evac to the bed frame or onto a bedside holder. *Caution: At all times keep the Pleur-evac lower than the client's chest to prevent a backflow of fluid into the client's chest cavity.*

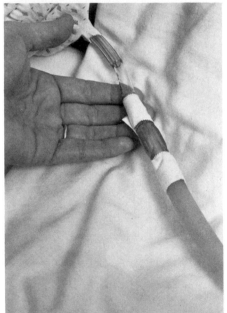

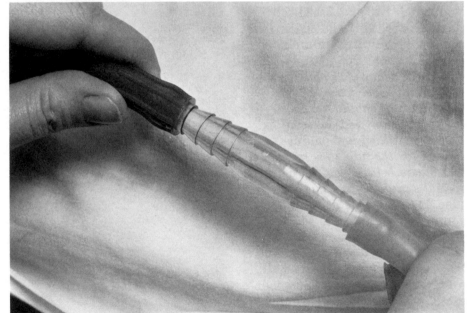

7 When the physician has inserted the chest tube, connect the longer of the two rubber tubes to the chest tube. Then tape the connector sites to ensure that the connection is air tight. To ensure that drainage is visible, the tape should not completely cover the connector.

8 If the physician has ordered suction rather than gravity drainage, attach the short rubber tube to suction via the tube connector. Turn the suction control knob slowly until gentle bubbling ap-

pears in the suction control chamber. If suction has not been ordered, keep the short rubber tube unclamped to maintain negative or equal pressure in the system.

(Continued on p. 372)

OBTAINING A CHEST DRAINAGE SPECIMEN

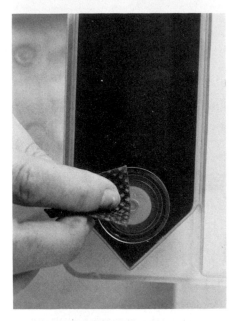

1 Most disposable drainage systems have a self-sealing diaphragm on the back of the drainage collection chamber. To obtain a specimen, wipe the diaphragm with a povidone–iodine swab, allowing it to dry completely.

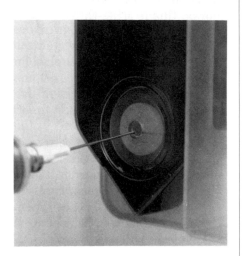

2 Insert a sterile 18- or 20-gauge needle, which is attached to a syringe large enough to contain the desired amount of the specimen. When you have aspirated the specimen, attach the needle protector, label the syringe, and send it directly to the lab with a requisition form.

ASSISTING WITH THE REMOVAL OF A CHEST TUBE

Assessing

1 Assess your client's respiratory status by auscultating the lung fields for the presence of normal breath sounds and palpating to ensure improved bilateral chest expansion. Determine the need for a pain medication. If one has been ordered, administer it 30 minutes prior to the removal of the chest tube. In many instances, the chest tube will have been clamped for a period of time (1–2 days prior to removal) to evaluate the client's tolerance.

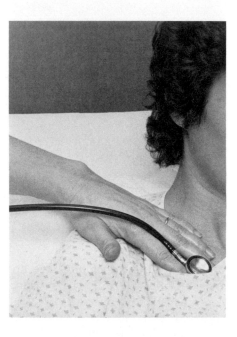

Planning

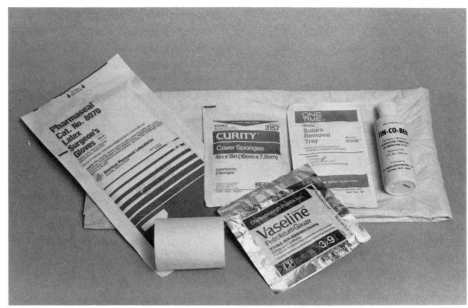

2 You will need to assemble a suture-removal kit, sterile 4 × 4 gauze pads, 3-in. tape, a petrolatum gauze pad, and tincture of benzoin for tape adherence. An impervious drape should be placed under the client's chest to protect the bed from drainage.

3 Explain the procedure to your client. Instruct her in the Valsalva maneuver so that she can hold her breath and bear down as the physician removes the tube. This will increase intrathoracic pressure, thereby lessening the potential for air to enter the pleural space.

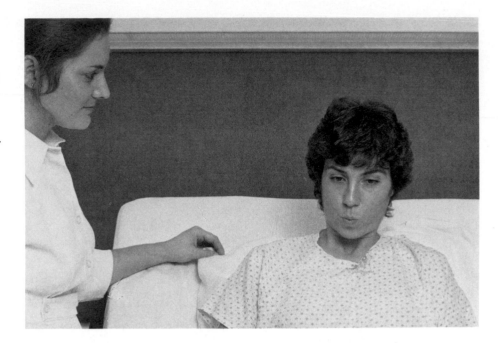

Implementing

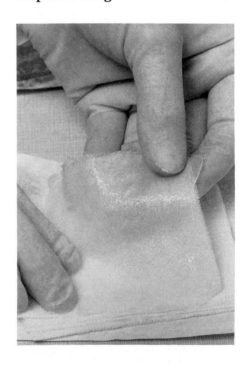

4 Prior to the chest tube removal, prepare the sterile dressing using aseptic technique. After opening the packages, put on sterile gloves and place the petrolatum gauze pad on top of the sterile 4 × 4. The physician will then apply the dressing to the insertion site immediately after removing the chest tube. This will minimize the potential for air to enter the chest wall.

5 Tape the dressing in place. To seal the site from inrushing air, cover the entire dressing with wide strips of air-occlusive tape.

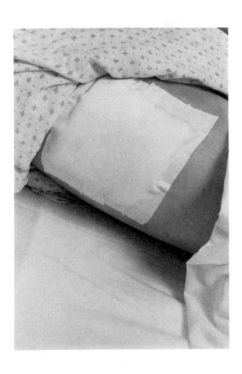

Evaluating

6 Continue to monitor your client's respiratory status. Observe for indications of a pneumothorax and/or for the condition that necessitated the chest tube's insertion. Assess the dressing for copious drainage, and document the procedure and your assessments.

References

Albanese, A., and Toplitz, A. April 1982. A hassle-free guide to suctioning a tracheostomy. *RN* 45:24–29.

American Heart Association. 1980. Standards and guidelines for cardiopulmonary resuscitation (CPR) and emergency cardiac care (ECC). *JAMA* 244:453–509.

Billings, D. M., and Stokes, L. G. 1982. *Medical-surgical nursing.* St. Louis: C.V. Mosby.

Bricker, P. Nov. 1980. Chest tubes. *RN* 43:21–26.

Brown, I. May 1982. Trach care? Take care—infection's on the prowl. *Nursing '82* 12:44–49.

Brunner, L. S., and Suddarth, D. S. 1982. *The Lippincott manual of nursing practice,* 3rd ed. Philadelphia: J.B. Lippincott.

Burton, G., et al. 1977. *Respiratory care, a guide to clinical practice.* Philadelphia: J.B. Lippincott.

Centers for Disease Control. 1981–1984. *Guidelines for the prevention and control of nosocomial infections.* Atlanta, Ga.: U.S. Department of Health and Human Services.

Cystic Fibrosis Foundation. 1980. *Segmental bronchial drainage.* Rockville, Md.: Cystic Fibrosis Foundation.

Ericson, R. May 1981. Chest tubes: they're really not that complicated. *Nursing '81* 11:34–43.

Gaskell, D. V., and Webber, B. A. 1980. *The Brompton hospital guide to chest physiotherapy,* 4th ed. Oxford, England: Blackwell Scientific Publications.

Harper, R. 1981. *A guide to respiratory care: physiology and clinical applications.* Philadelphia: J.B. Lippincott.

Hirsch, J. and Hannock, L. 1981. *Mosby's manual of clinical nursing procedures.* St. Louis: C.V. Mosby.

Holloway, N. N. 1984. *Nursing the critically ill adult,* 2nd ed. Menlo Park, Calif.: Addison-Wesley Publishing.

King, R. C. Aug. 1982. Examining the thorax and respiratory system. *RN* 45:55–63.

Louden, R. G. Fall 1982. Auscultation of the lung. *Clini Notes Res Dis* 21:3–7.

McPherson, S. 1981. *Respiratory therapy equipment,* 2nd ed. St. Louis: C.V. Mosby.

Nursing Photobook. 1981. Providing respiratory care. Horsham, Pa.: Intermed Communications.

Reports of the ATS AdHoc Committee on Pulmonary Nomenclature. 1977. Updated nomenclature for membership reaction. *Amer Thor Soc News* 3:5.

Saxton, D., et al. 1983. *The Addison-Wesley manual of nursing practice.* Menlo Park, Calif.: Addison-Wesley Publishing.

Shapiro, B. A., et al. 1979. *Clinical application of respiratory care,* 2nd ed. Chicago: Yearbook Medical Publishers.

Smith, S. F., and Duell, D. 1982. *Nursing skills and evaluation.* Los Altos, Calif.: National Nursing Review.

Sorenson, K. C., and Luckmann, J. 1979. *Basic nursing: a psychophysiologic approach.* Philadelphia: W.B. Saunders.

Spearman, C., et al. 1982. *Egan's fundamentals of respiratory therapy,* 4th ed. St. Louis: C.V. Mosby.

Spence, A. P. 1982. *Basic human anatomy.* Menlo Park, Calif.: Benjamin/Cummings Publishing.

Thompson, J., and Bowers, A. 1980. *Clinical manual of health assessment.* St. Louis: C.V. Mosby.

Visich, M. A. Nov. 1981. A guide to assessing breath and heart sounds. *Nursing '81* 11:64–72.

Wade, J. F. 1982. *Comprehensive respiratory care,* 3rd ed. St. Louis: C.V. Mosby.

Chapter 7

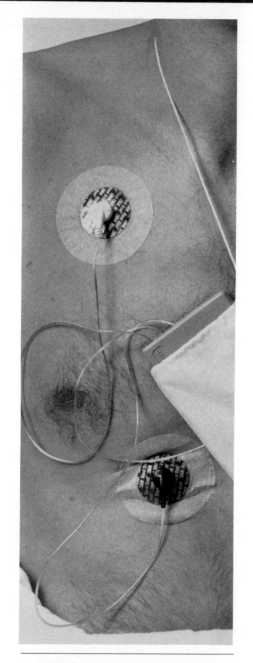

Managing
Cardiovascular
Procedures

CHAPTER OUTLINE

Assessing the Cardiovascular System

THE CARDIOVASCULAR SYSTEM

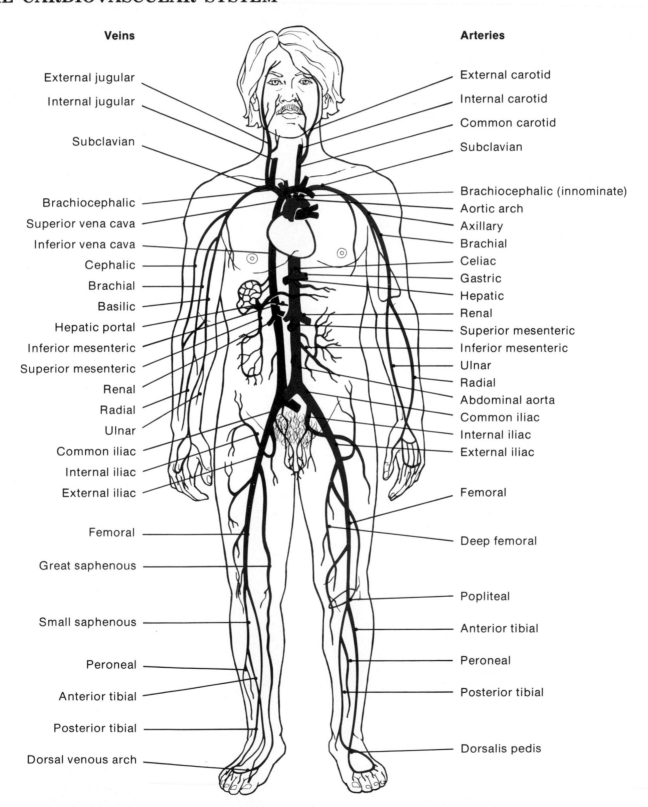

Veins

External jugular
Internal jugular

Subclavian

Brachiocephalic
Superior vena cava
Inferior vena cava
Cephalic
Brachial
Basilic
Hepatic portal
Inferior mesenteric
Superior mesenteric
Renal
Radial
Ulnar
Common iliac
Internal iliac
External iliac

Femoral

Great saphenous

Small saphenous

Peroneal

Anterior tibial

Posterior tibial

Dorsal venous arch

Arteries

External carotid
Internal carotid
Common carotid
Subclavian

Brachiocephalic (innominate)
Aortic arch
Axillary
Brachial
Celiac
Gastric
Hepatic
Renal
Superior mesenteric
Inferior mesenteric
Ulnar
Radial
Abdominal aorta
Common iliac
Internal iliac
External iliac

Femoral

Deep femoral

Popliteal

Anterior tibial

Peroneal

Posterior tibial

Dorsalis pedis

NURSING ASSESSMENT GUIDELINE

To assess your client's cardio-vascular system, you need to inteview him or her for subjective data, take vital signs, examine the cardiac area, and monitor pulses. A comprehensive nursing care plan includes a complete evaluation for the following subjective data:

Personal factors: age, sex, race, nationality, occupation, marital status

History or family history of: cardiac or coronary artery disease (especially prior to the age of 60), diabetes mellitus, gout, hypertension, cerebrovascular accident (CVA), congenital heart defects, rheumatic heart disease, angina, congestive heart failure

Risk factors: smoking, type-A personality, major life change units, excessive stress, obesity, lack of exercise

Dietary habits: intake in approximate amounts of calories, cholesterol, sodium, fluids, "fast foods," alcohol; food allergies

Medications: for example, nitroglycerin, diuretics, cardiotonics (such as digoxin), quinidine, antiarrhythmics, beta blockers, antihypertensives, calcium antagonists; over-the-counter; drug allergies

Pain: location, intensity, duration, character, precipitating factors, methods of alleviation

Cyanosis: precipitating factors, sites

Peripheral vascular alterations: coldness, numbness, discolorations, blanching, edema, sites

Limitations of activities: exercise intolerance, dyspnea on exertion, precipitating factors

Sleep patterns: need for pillows, nocturia, night sweats

Diaphoresis

Syncope, dizziness

Palpitations

Nausea, vomiting

Edema, digital clubbing

Headaches

EXAMINING THE CARDIAC AREA

Explain the procedure to your client and examine him in a warm, quiet, and private environment. Assist the client into a supine position, with his head slightly elevated. Ask him to uncover his chest, but provide a robe or blanket for warmth and privacy. For optimal inspection and to facilitate palpation of the cardiac area, approach the client on his right side.

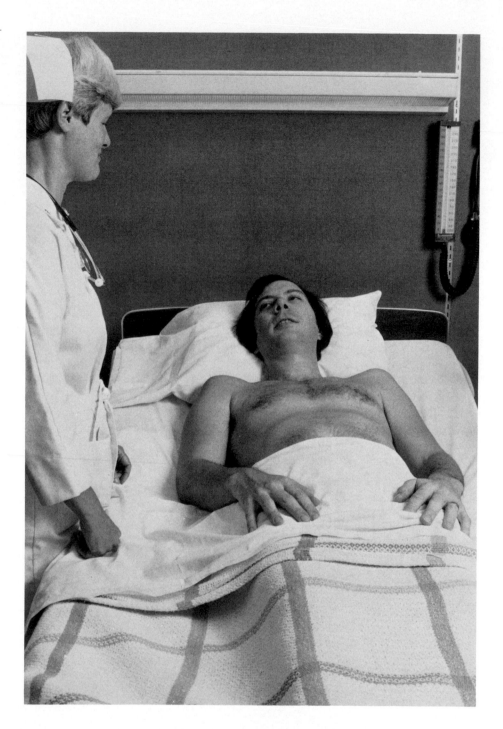

To assist you with your examination and documentation of sites, familiarize yourself with these anatomic landmarks.

Inspecting and Palpating

Identify these areas for cardiac palpation on your client's chest. Begin by inspecting the apical area for the point of maximal impulse (PMI) at the fifth intercostal space, near the left midclavicular line. Normally, it is seen in the male client as a pulsation covering an area no greater than 2 cm. If the PMI is not observable, for example, in clients with barrel chests, obese males, and in females, you may need to palpate for it. A pulsation that covers a larger area may indicate left ventricular hypertrophy or an aneurysm.

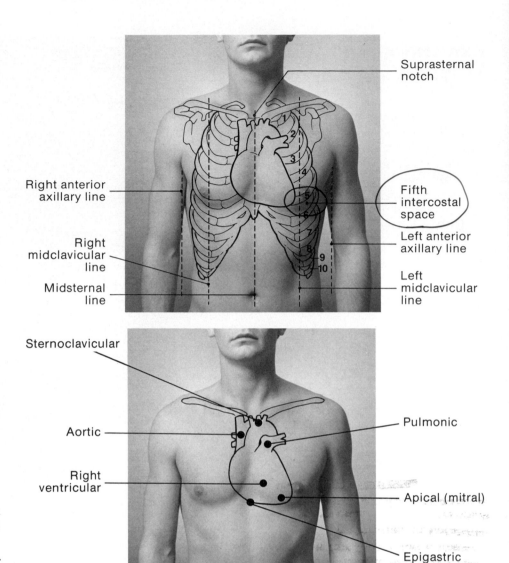

Suprasternal notch

Right anterior axillary line

Right midclavicular line

Midsternal line

Fifth intercostal space

Left anterior axillary line

Left midclavicular line

Sternoclavicular

Aortic

Right ventricular

Pulmonic

Apical (mitral)

Epigastric

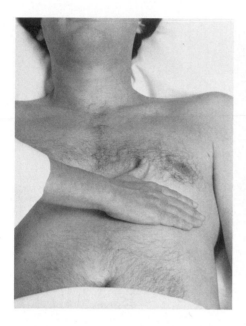
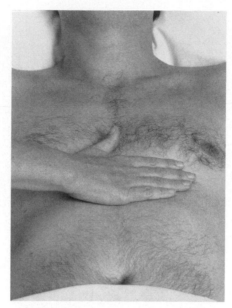

Palpate the apical area to assess duration and strength of the beat. An abnormally strong and sustained pulsation is often found in clients with left ventricular hypertrophy. However, anemia, fever, or hyperthyroidism can produce moderately strong pulsations. Also, palpate for thrills by using the palmar surface of your hand (as shown). Thrills give the sensation of water running through a hose. They are most often indicative of ventricular or atrial septal defects. *Note: If you are able to palpate a thrill, you will probably also detect a murmur over the same area during auscultation.*

Palpate these areas using the palmar surface of your hand and the fat pads of your fingers: right ventricular, aortic, pulmonic, sternoclavicular, and epigastric (as shown). Note the presence or absence of pulsations. In addition to the apical area, they normally may be felt over the aortic and right ventricular areas; you might detect a light pulsation at the sternoclavicular area. Bounding pulsations at the epigastric or sternoclavicular areas, however, could be indicative of an aortic aneurysm.

Auscultating

Familiarize yourself with these areas for cardiac auscultation. Remember that a valve's sound is better heard in the direction of its blood flow rather than directly over the valve itself. Use this guideline as you develop your own pattern for cardiac auscultation.

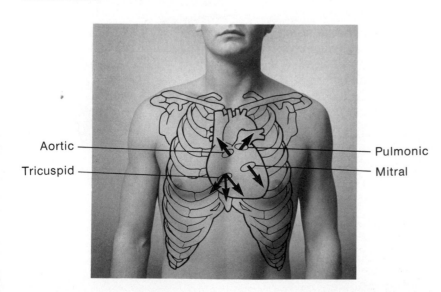

Aortic —
Tricuspid —
— Pulmonic
— Mitral

(Continued on p. 386)

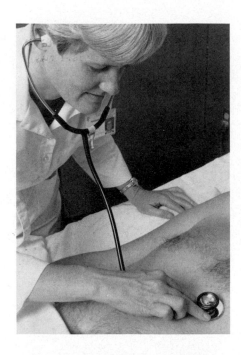
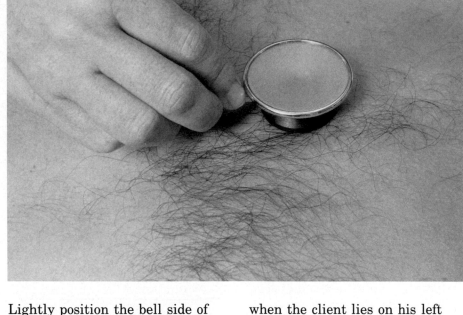

Use the diaphragm of the stethoscope to auscultate normal heart sounds, S_1 and S_2. S_1 ("lub") is best heard over mitral and tricuspid areas, and S_2 ("dub") is best heard over aortic and pulmonic areas. Both sounds are more easily heard when the client is supine. If the heart sounds are distant, for example, in clients who are obese or who have large thoraxes, ask the client to turn slightly toward his left side so the heart is closer to the chest wall.

Lightly position the bell side of the stethoscope against the client's chest to detect adventitious heart sounds such as murmurs and gallops. Follow the guideline, p. 385, for auscultating normal heart sounds. Murmurs may be heard during systole (between S_1 and S_2) at the pulmonic and mitral area, or during diastole (between S_2 and S_1) over most of the cardiac area, but the latter are more often pathologic and are found in heart disease or congenital defects. Murmurs may be palpated as thrills over the same area. Note the timing, location, intensity, and pitch of murmurs when recording your findings. S_3 (ventricular gallop) is a dull and low-pitched sound, "lub-dub-dee" (S_1-S_2-S_3), and it is best heard over the apical and right ventricular areas during exhalation

when the client lies on his left side. In this position gravity enhances ventricular filling and thereby exaggerates the sound. Because a ventricular gallop is one of the first clinical signs of congestive heart failure, early detection can avert advancing cardiac failure. Normally it may be heard in children and in young adults. S_4 (atrial gallop) has a higher pitch, and if present, it is elicited in the mitral area (apex). It sounds like "dee-lub-dub" (S_4-S_1-S_2). Clients with congestive heart failure might have both S_3 and S_4 as well as an increased heart rate. A pericardial friction rub might be heard in postmyocardial infarction clients when they lean forward and exhale deeply. It sounds like two pieces of sand paper rubbing against each other.

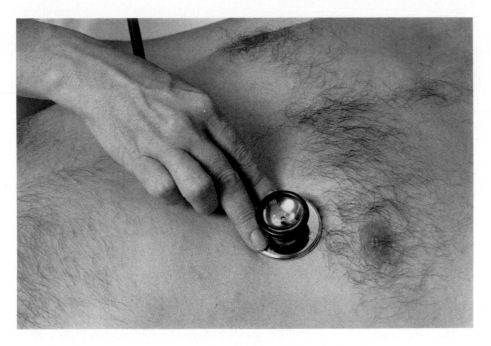

Auscultate the chest for the apical pulse (as shown) for 1 minute to determine the rate and rhythm of the heart. Irregular rhythms, bradycardia (less than 60 beats per minute) in nonathletes, or tachycardia (greater than 100 beats per minute) are considered abnormal in adults. Palpate the brachial or radial pulse as you auscultate the apical pulse to assess for a potential pulse deficit in the peripheral artery. A peripheral pulse deficit occurs when the cardiac systole is not strong enough to produce a palpable arterial pulse. It can occur with atrial fibrillation. If a pulse deficit is found, ask an associate to count peripheral pulsations while you auscultate the apical pulse. Document both pulse rates.

PALPATING ARTERIAL PULSES

Review these anatomic landmarks to assist you in locating the arterial pulse points. For infants, pulses can range between 80–180 beats per minute. At 4 years old, children can have pulses ranging from 80–120, and at age 10, 70–110. From 14 years on, pulses can range from 50–100, with women averaging a slightly faster pulse than men.

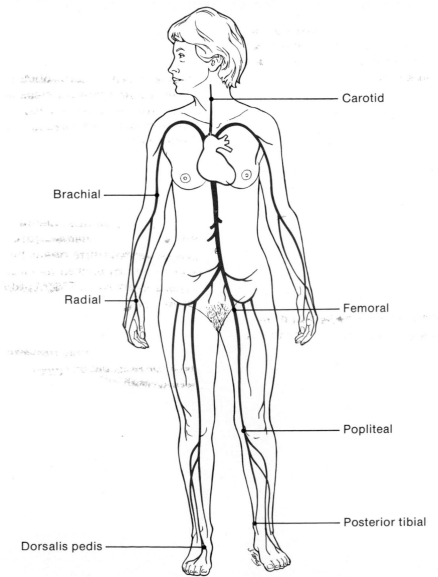

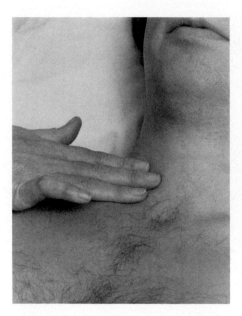 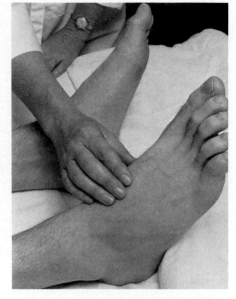

Begin your assessment of the arterial pulses by palpating the carotid artery to evaluate rate, rhythm, and amplitude of the pulse. Use a light touch to avoid arterial occlusion and the precipitation of bradycardia by carotid sinus massage. Palpate *only* one artery at a time to ensure adequate cerebral blood flow. The artery should feel soft and pliant to the touch, but clients with atherosclerosis may have cordlike arteries. Palpate the opposite artery and compare the two pulses. An abrupt cessation of one pulse with accompanying chest or back pain suggests an aortic aneurysm.

Palpate the peripheral pulses for rate, rhythm, and amplitude; compare each pulse to its corresponding pulse on the opposite side. Begin by palpating the brachial arteries, and then palpate the radial arteries. Palpate the femoral and popliteal arteries and complete the assessment with the arteries farthest from the heart: posterior tibial and dorsalis pedis (as shown). The posterior tibial pulse can be palpated behind and slightly inferior to the medial malleolus; the dorsalis pedis pulse is best palpated over the dorsum of the foot, with the foot slightly dorsiflexed.

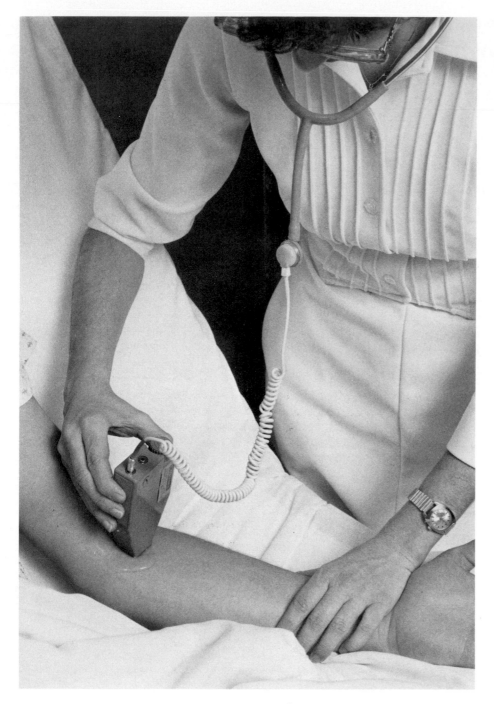

Using a Doppler Ultrasonic Probe:
If you are unable to easily palpate peripheral arterial pulses, a Doppler ultrasonic probe may be used to elicit sounds that will identify the flow of arterial blood. In this photo, the nurse has positioned the probe's transducer over the client's brachial pulse site, which she has lubricated with a conducting gel. The earphones enable her to hear wavelike "whooshing" sounds, which are produced by the reflection of red blood cells as they flow through the artery. The Doppler can also be used to evaluate the patency of veins and arteries for clients with a potential for thrombus or embolus, or for those who have undergone vein grafts. After using the Doppler, record either the presence or the absence of pulsations. Be sure to describe the rate and character of the sound you hear, including its intensity and frequency.

Monitoring the Cardiovascular System

INSPECTING THE JUGULAR VEIN

To inspect the jugular vein, elevate the head of the client's bed to a 45° angle. Assess the highest level of distention and pulsation in the interior jugular vein in centimeters, using the sternal angle (the point at which the clavicles meet) as a reference point. If you find the level to be 3 cm above the sternal angle, the client's central venous pressure is probably elevated. The client in the photo does not have a distended jugular vein.

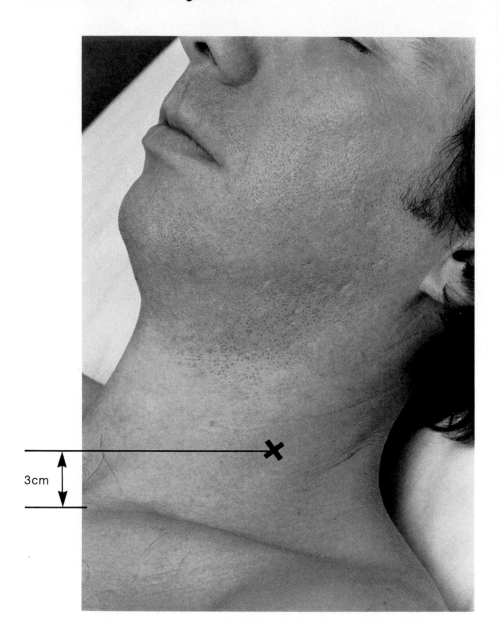

3cm

MEASURING ARTERIAL BLOOD PRESSURE

Assessing and Planning

1 Assess your client's knowledge of the procedure and follow up accordingly, stressing the importance of regular blood pressure monitoring. Determine whether the client has exercised, eaten, drunk, or smoked within the last 30 minutes. These activities, in addition to pain, urinary bladder distention, or merely having the blood pressure measured, can alter the reading. It is also important that you have the correct bladder and cuff size. The bladder from an adult-sized cuff has been removed here to help you envision its width and length. To ensure an accurate reading, the width of the bladder should be 40% of the circumference of the midpoint of the limb on which it is used (or approximately 20% wider than the diameter of the same site). The length of the bladder should be equal to 80% of the limb's midpoint circumference. For the average adult arm, bladder widths of 12–14 cm are recommended, but remember, it is the circumference of the limb, not the client's age, that determines cuff size.

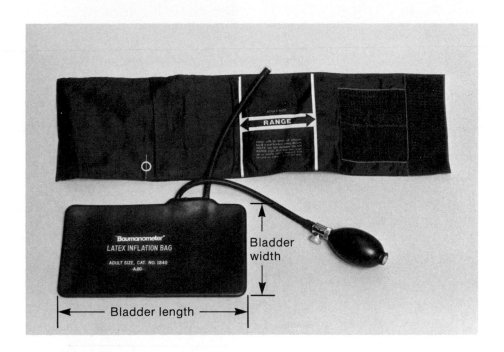

Bladder width

Bladder length

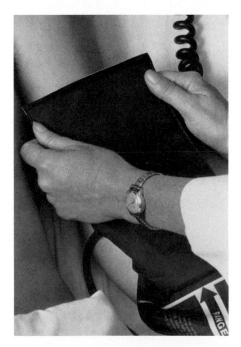

2 For example, in this photo the width of the cuff is being compared to the diameter of the client's upper arm to ensure the cuff's bladder is 20% wider than the arm's diameter. If the bladder is too narrow, the blood pressure reading may be falsely high; if it is too wide, the reading may be falsely low.

(Continued on p. 392)

Implementing

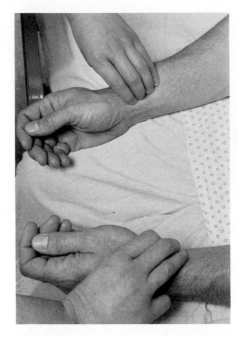 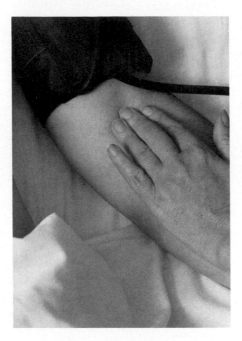 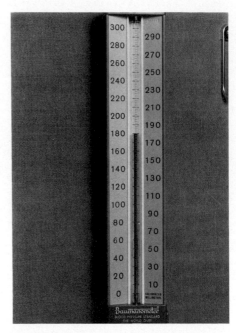

3 If this is an initial screening, you should measure the blood pressure in both arms; if it is a routine assessment, first compare the quality of the pulses in both arms by palpating both radial pulses simultaneously (as shown). Measure the blood pressure in the arm with the stronger pulse if the pulses are unequal; if they are equal, measure the pressure on the right arm if you are right-handed, or on the left arm if you are left-handed. This is recommended for your comfort and convenience, to facilitate the procedure.

4 Support and position the client's arm at his heart level, and place the center of the cuff's bladder over the brachial artery. Wrap the cuff snugly around the upper arm 2.5 cm (1 in.) above the antecubital space to allow room for the diaphragm of the stethoscope. While you palpate the brachial (or radial) artery, inflate the cuff until you feel the pulse disappear.

5 When you feel the pulse disappear, immediately note the reading on the manometer. This is the palpated systolic blood pressure. Read the gauge at eye level to ensure a correct reading. Then rapidly deflate the cuff and wait 30 seconds to allow for a decrease in venous congestion. A failure to do so could cause an alteration in the reading.

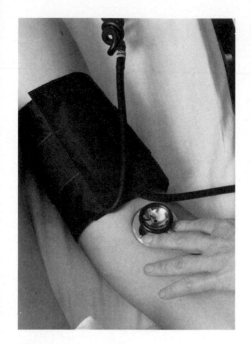

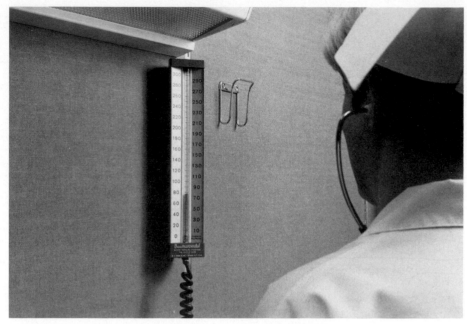

6 Place the stethoscope over the brachial artery and rapidly reinflate the cuff to a point 30 mm Hg above the palpated systolic pressure, which is referred to as the point of maximum inflation. You must inflate to this point to ensure that the first sound (systolic pressure or Korotkoff I) is heard, and that you have inflated above the auscultatory gap that occasionally occurs in hypertensive clients. *Note: To minimize extraneous sounds, the diaphragm of the stethoscope should contact neither the cuff nor any clothing.*

7 Slowly deflate the cuff at a rate of 2–4 mm Hg per heart beat and note the systolic pressure when the first sound is heard (Korotkoff I) for both adults and children. To be sure that the first sound you hear is not an extraneous noise, make sure the initial sound is accompanied by at least one other consecutive beat. The diastolic pressure is recorded for children when the sound muffles (Korotkoff IV), and for both children and adults when the sound disappears and silence begins (Korotkoff V). Thus, for children, three numbers should be recorded: Korotkoff I, Korotkoff IV, and Korotkoff V; for adults, only Korotkoff I and Korotkoff V are recorded, unless sounds are heard all the way down to zero. If this occurs, record three numbers: systolic, muffled sound, and the disappearance (zero); for example, 100/40/0. After completely deflating the cuff, wait 2 minutes for venous congestion to decrease and repeat the procedure in the same arm to verify the reading. *Note: If this is the initial screening, measure the blood pressure three times in both arms, averaging each of the last two readings.*

(Continued on p. 394)

Evaluating

8 Document your client's blood pressure, noting the limb(s) on which the blood pressure was taken, the client's position during the reading, and the cuff size. If you have been the first to detect hypertension or related significant findings, refer the client for further evaluation. For the adult, diastolic pressures of 90 mm Hg and greater are considered hypertensive, and diastolic pressures of 115 mm Hg and greater are considered dangerously elevated. Systolic pressures of 160 mm Hg and greater are significant in the older adult, as are systolic pressures of 150 mm Hg and greater in clients under 35 years of age (The 1980 Report of the Joint National Committee on Detection, Evaluation and Treatment of High Blood Pressure 1981:6). Clients with systolic pressures less than 90 mm Hg and diastolic pressures less than 60 mm Hg may be considered hypotensive if illness or medications are the cause, and you should evaluate and follow up accordingly. However, if it is your client's typical pattern, low pressure readings are considered to be both normal and desirable. Establish your client's baseline blood pressure status early upon admission so that you will have an adequate database from which to evaluate the integrity of each body system.

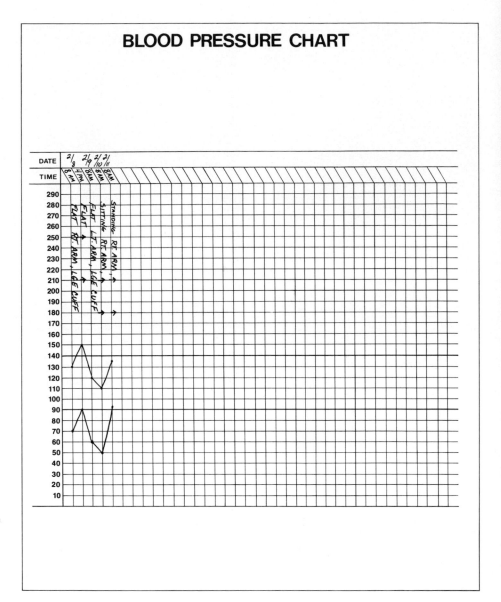

NURSING GUIDELINES FOR IDENTIFYING COMMON TELEMETRY LEAD SITES

If your agency utilizes telemetry monitoring, it will employ either a two-electrode or a three-electrode monitor. Review these common lead sites to assist you with electrode placement. Negative, positive, and ground lead positions will vary, depending on the telemetry unit you will use; however, the electrode placement will be the same, regardless of the telemetry unit. Position the upper electrodes just under the clavicular hollows at the midclavicular line. This will minimize artifact from muscles and arm movement. Lower electrodes are placed at the intercostal spaces, either at the right sternal border, fourth or fifth intercostal space, or at the left midclavicular line, sixth or seventh intercostal space. If necessary, vary the electrode placement slightly to accommodate your client's anatomy. For example, obese clients may require electrode placement over bony surfaces to decrease artifact from adipose tissue.

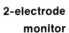

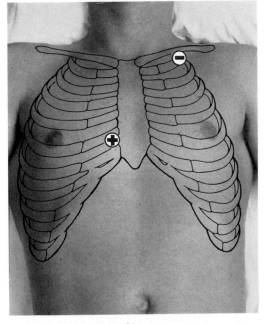

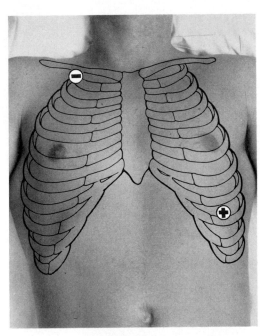

MCL₁

Lead II

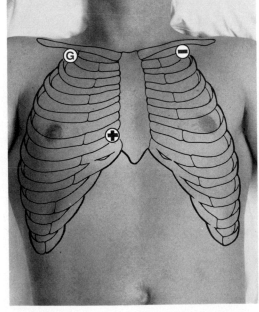

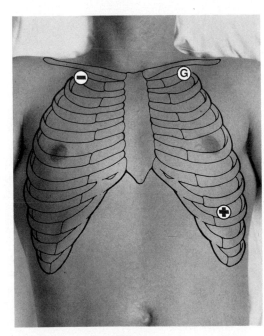

MCL₁

Lead II

APPLYING DISPOSABLE ELECTRODES FOR TELEMETRY MONITORING

Assessing and Planning

1 The procedure for applying disposable electrodes is the same, regardless of the type of cardiac monitoring equipment that is used. In these photos the steps for initiating telemetry monitoring are also included. If the physician prescribes telemetry for your client, study the operational guidelines for the telemetry unit your agency employs. Determine the prescribed lead site position, and familiarize yourself with the guidelines for identifying common telemetry lead sites, p. 395. Assemble the electrodes, 4 × 4 gauze pads, tincture of benzoin, and scissors or a razor (optional). Explain the procedure to your client.

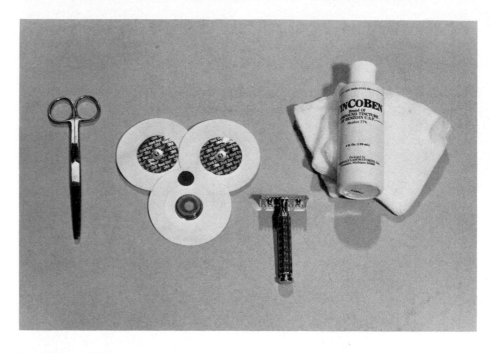

Implementing

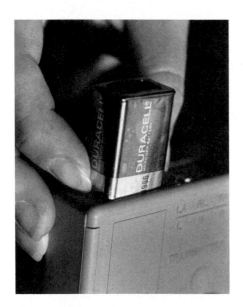

2 Insert the battery into the transmitter. *Note: Many transmitters have a test light on the back that lights up when pressed if the battery is functioning.*

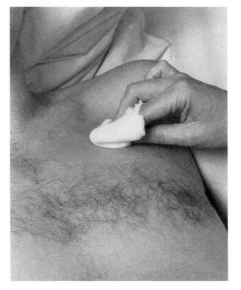

3 If necessary, and with your client's permission, shave or clip his chest hair at the lead sites to allow for better conductivity. Briskly rub the sites with a dry 4 × 4 gauze pad to produce erythema and to remove the skin oils that can interfere with electrical conductivity. A gauze pad saturated with acetone or alcohol can also be used to remove the skin oils.

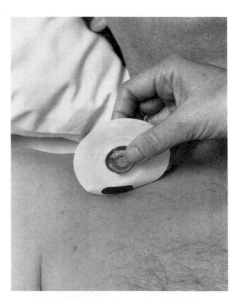

4 *Note: To further enhance electrical conductivity, some disposable electrodes have rough patches for slightly abrading the skin at the lead site. If your client's electrode does not have this feature, you may instead lightly scrape the skin with a tongue blade.*

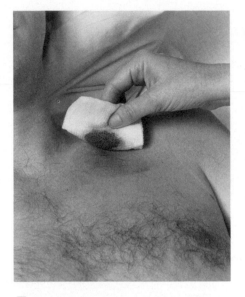

5 If your client is not allergic to tincture of benzoin, apply a small amount to the lead sites with a clean gauze pad. This will facilitate electrode adherence and inhibit skin breakdown. Let it dry thoroughly.

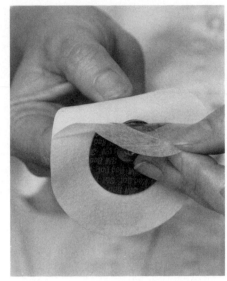

6 Remove the electrode's paper backing, but touch the adhesive surface only minimally.

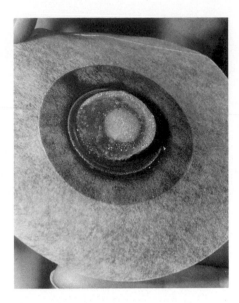

7 Inspect the spongy center of the electrode's adhesive surface. If it is not covered with a moist gel, replace the electrode with a new one.

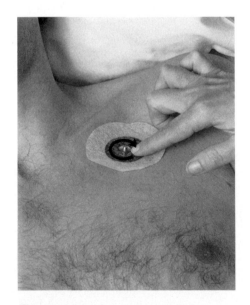

8 Press the center of the electrode down in a circular manner to distribute the conductive gel.

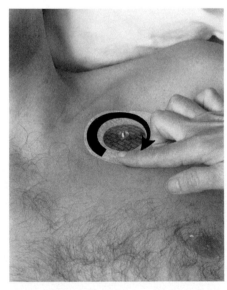

9 Press along the outer perimeter of the electrode to adhere the adhesive backing to your client's skin.

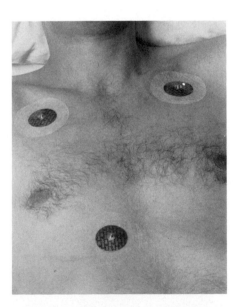

10 Position the remaining electrodes to form the desired pattern. Electrodes should be placed near but not over bony surfaces unless the client is obese. In that case, you may place them over bones to minimize artifact from adipose tissue. And, to minimize artifact from muscles or arm movement, position the upper electrodes just below the clavicular hollows at the midclavicular line.

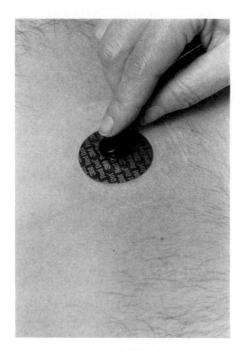

11 You may now attach the specified lead wires to the corresponding electrodes. Apply slight pressure as you snap the lead onto the electrode button. The monitoring system your agency employs will identify the positive, negative, and lead sites. The lead wires will be coded either by color, symbols, or initials.

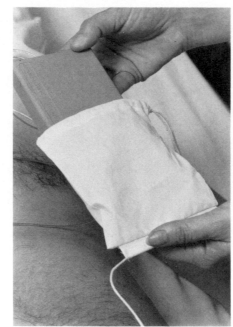

13 Insert the transmitter into a cloth carrying pouch.

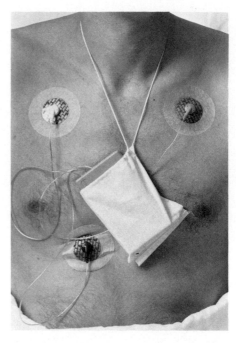

14 Tie the pouch around your client's neck, making sure it is positioned comfortably and does not obstruct the electrodes. You may also place it in a pajama top pocket.

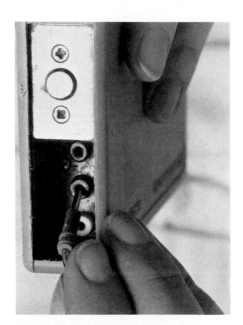

12 Ensure that the lead wires are firmly connected to the telemetry transmitter.

Evaluating

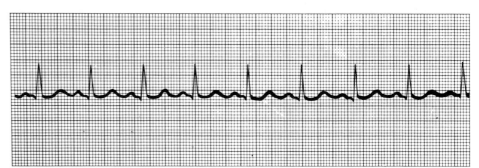

15 At the central console, press the recorder button on the unit reserved for your client. When the waveform has been printed, tear off the printout sheet. Evaluate the waveform and file a 6-second printout in your client's chart as a baseline for future readings. Set the alarm's limits to those ordered by the physician—for example, at a low of 50 and a high of 120.

ASSESSING THE POSTCARDIAC CATHETERIZATION CLIENT

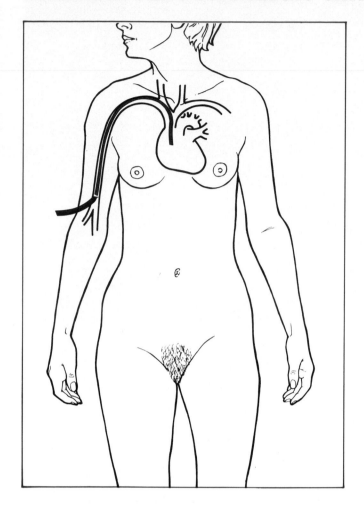

Antecubital site

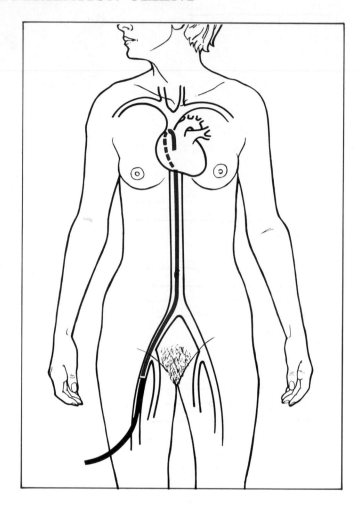

Femoral site

A cardiac catheterization is an invasive procedure performed to assess cardiac anatomy and function. It is frequently performed for clients with chest pain of unknown origin, congenital heart disease, or pulmonary hypertension. It is a valuable diagnostic tool for the preoperative cardiac client, and it is performed postoperatively, as well, to assess the results of cardiac surgery. It is usually performed in conjunction with angiography, during which a contrast medium is injected for envisioning the ventricle, aorta, and coronary arteries.

When the client has been given a local anesthetic, a radiopaque catheter is introduced into the vascular system, usually via the median cubital, basilic, or femoral vein; it is threaded into the great vessels and finally into the right atrium and right ventricle with the aid of fluoroscopy. Catheterization of the left side of the heart may also be performed, usually via retrograde catheterization of the left ventricle or by transseptal catheterization (puncturing the atrial septum). The entire procedure usually lasts 2–4 hours.

When the client has been returned to your care after cardiac catheterization, make her as comfortable as possible; explain that routine assessments will be performed over the next 24 hours so that she does not become unnecessarily alarmed, thinking her condition has deteriorated. The protocol for assessment will vary from agency to agency. The following are general procedures for assessment and its frequency. Be sure to follow the protocol outlined by your agency.

(Continued on p. 400)

1 Measure and record the blood pressure every 15 minutes until it is stable on at least three successive checks. Once it is stable, measure it every 2 hours for the next 12 hours, and every 4 hours thereafter. If the catheterization site was the antecubital area, be sure to measure the blood pressure in the opposite arm. Notify the physician and lower the head of the bed if the client's systolic pressure drops 20 mm Hg lower than that already recorded. Hypotension can be a result of cardiac tamponade, a vagal response, a hematoma at the catheterization site, or hypovolemia. The hypotonic dye used during the catheterization can cause osmotic diuresis, so be sure to monitor the urinary output carefully.

If the client is not being continuously monitored on a cardiac monitor, auscultate the apical pulse with each blood pressure check. Be alert to an irregular pulse rate, which could be indicative of arrhythmias. Remember that an acute myocardial infarction can occur as a complication of cardiac catheterization; therefore, you must monitor the client closely for arrhythmias as well as for diaphoresis, a thready pulse, and complaints of chest pain.

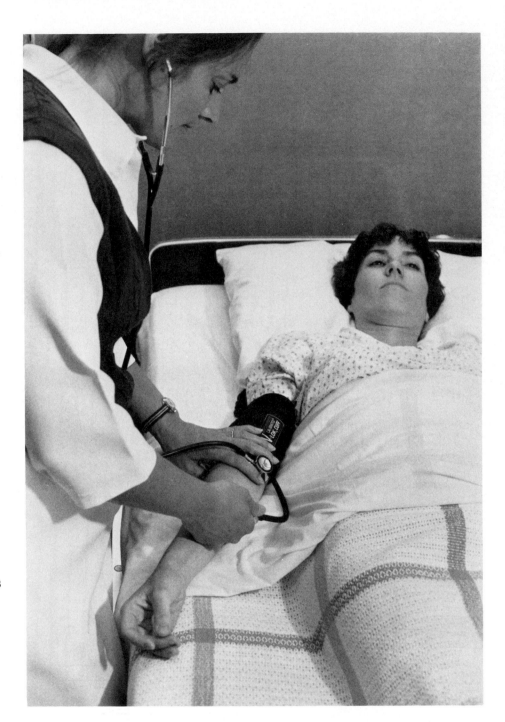

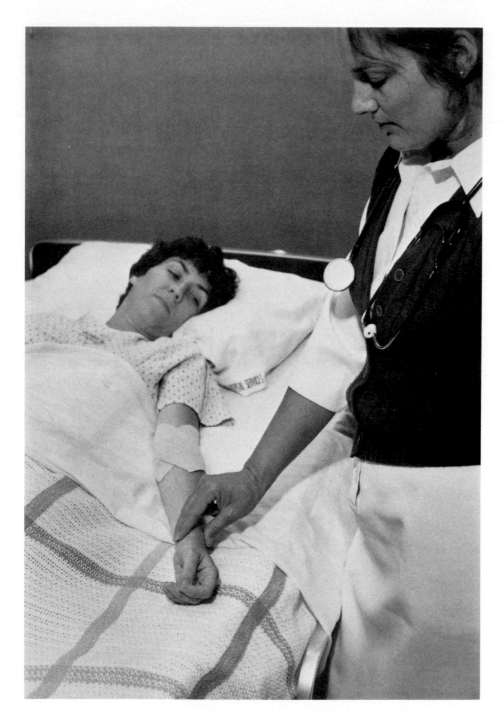

2 Assess the limb distal to the CTS catheterization site to ensure that the color, temperature, sensation, and pulse(s) are adequate. If the catheterization site was in the upper extremities, palpate the radial pulse. Palpate the popliteal, dorsalis pedis, and posterior tibial pulses if the site was in the lower extremities. In addition, the client should be able to easily move her fingers or toes. A faint pulse; pain at the catheterization site; or coolness, numbness, or tingling at the distal extremity can be indicative of an embolus, thrombus, or arterial insufficiency in the involved limb and should be reported to the attending physician immediately. Instruct the client to alert you if any of these conditions occur.

3 Inspect the pressure dressing over the catheterization site for the presence of bleeding. <u>Ask</u> the client <u>about pain or tenderness at the site</u>, <u>which could be indicative of a hematoma formation</u>. If bleeding does occur, elevate the limb and apply pressure to the site. Then recheck the vital signs and notify the physician. The client should also be instructed to <u>apply pressure</u> and to alert you immediately if she detects bleeding at the site.

<u>Keep the limb in extension to prevent bleeding</u>, and encourage the client to <u>keep it immobile</u> during the first day. In many instances, the client will be on bed rest until the next morning. Check the orders for ambulation and follow through accordingly. Carefully document every assessment.

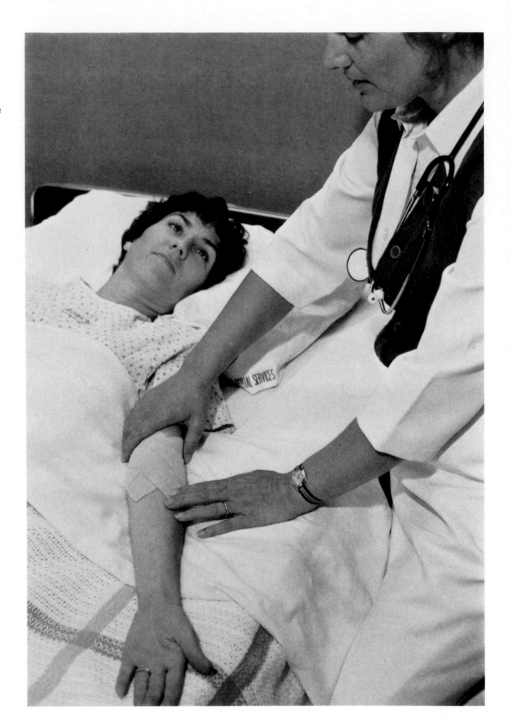

MEASURING CENTRAL VENOUS PRESSURE (CVP)

Assessing and Planning

1 Explain the procedure to your client. Check the intake and output record, measure his pulse and blood pressure, and auscultate his cardiac area for heart sounds. This assessment will provide you with a baseline from which to evaluate his CVP.

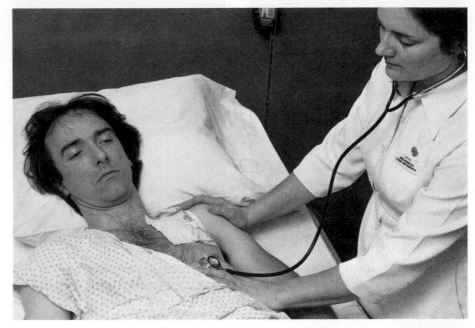

2 To minimize inaccuracies, the client should neither cough nor strain, and he must be in the same position for every reading. If the supine position is not contraindicated (and if previous readings were taken with the client in this position), place him flat in bed and remove his pillow. This will increase intrathoracic venous pressure and minimize the risk of an air embolism during the negative phase of inspiration. Make sure the IV solution is running well, and, to further minimize the potential for an air embolism, ensure that all IV connections are securely attached.

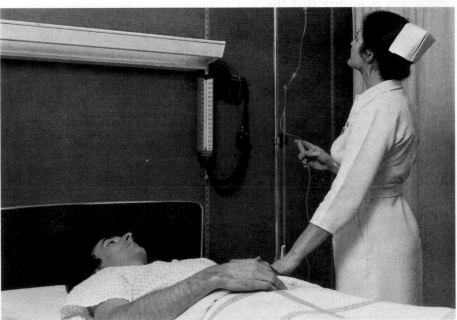

(Continued on p. 404)

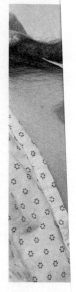

8 Adjust the stopcock so that it is open to the solution, open to the client, and off to the manometer. Adjust the flow rate to the prescribed rate, and return the client to a comfortable position.

Evaluating

9 Compare the client's CVP to his baseline to ensure it is within his norm. Consider also his cardiac assessment, blood pressure, level of consciousness, skin turgor, diagnosis, fluid intake, and hourly urine output. Review the guidelines the physician has ordered for reporting CVP readings and follow up accordingly. Rates near zero may indicate hypovolemic shock, while rates above 15 cm H_2O may indicate hypervolemia or poor cardiac contractility. Both extremes necessitate further assessment and evaluation. Document the procedure, the CVP reading, and the client's position during the procedure.

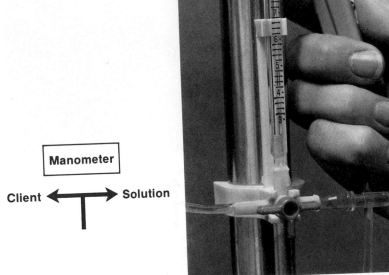

3 Locate
right atriu
intercostal
lary line. I
delible ink
pressure is
this point.

Implemen

5 *Note: If*
nects to an
the pump o
the stopcoc
is off to the
manometer,
tion to allov
the manome
ter fill slowl
or 10–20 cm
pressure rea
will normall
5–15 cm H_2(
at least 10 cı
norm will en
most reading

Caring for Clients with Vascular Disorders

APPLYING ELASTIC (ANTIEMBOLIC) STOCKINGS

Assessing and Planning

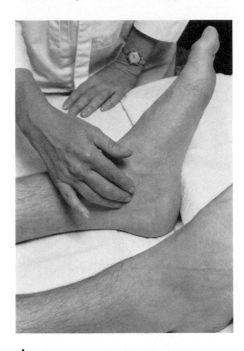

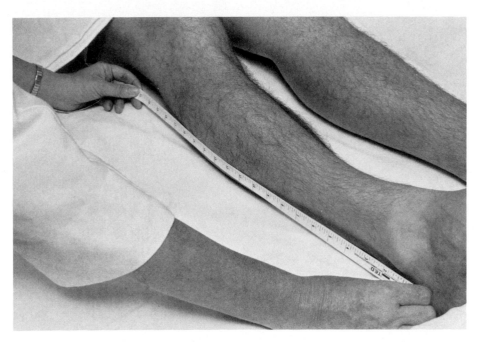

1 The best time for applying elastic stockings is early in the morning before swelling has occurred in your client's legs and feet. Determine the type of stocking the physician has ordered, either thigh-high stockings or below-the-knee stockings. Explain the procedure to your client. Drape his thighs as you remove the top linen. Assess both legs and feet for ulcers or infections, the absence of peripheral pulses below the femoral artery, or unequal pulses. These conditions, in addition to peripheral edema secondary to congestive heart failure, are contraindications for applying these hose. Also, evaluate the color and temperature of both extremities. If you find them cool or cyanotic, alert the physician. *Note: The stockings can be applied easily if talc or corn starch is sprinkled on the legs and feet first to absorb perspiration.*

2 To ensure a correct fit, measure the leg from the Achilles tendon to the popliteal fold (as shown) for the below-the-knee stockings, or from the Achilles

tendon to the gluteal furrow for the thigh-high stockings. A tape measure is usually included with each package.

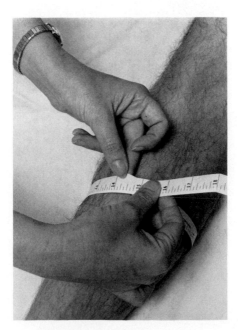

3 Measure the circumference of the midcalf (and the midthigh for the thigh-high stocking). Compare your measurements to the manufacturer's guidelines to make sure you have the correct size.

(Continued on p. 408)

Implementing

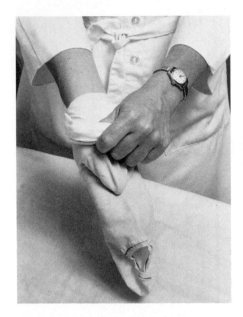

4 Make sure the stockings are "inside out." The manufacturer often packages them that way. Insert your hand through the top of the stocking deeply enough to grasp the stocking's toe.

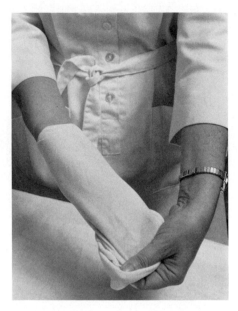

5 With your free hand, invert the stocking to its heel by pulling the stocking over the hand that is inside the stocking. Remove your hand from the inside of the stocking.

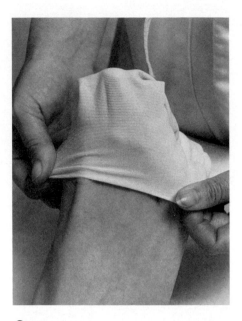

6 Grasp each side of the stocking and pull the inverted stocking foot over your client's toes.

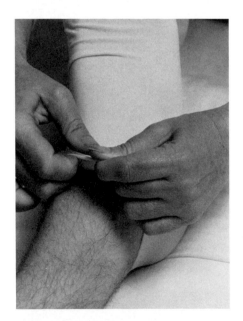

7 In one motion, pull the stocking past the client's heel so that the stocking will be anchored and not slip back.

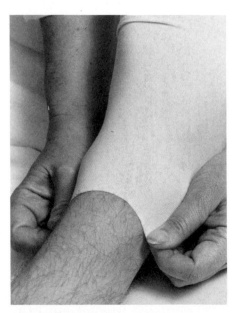

8 Grasp the fabric by the sides as you pull it up past the ankle.

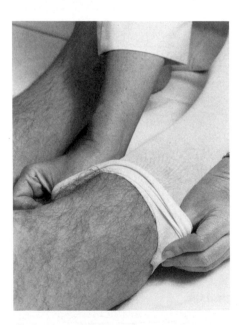

9 In increments of 2 inches at a time, continue to pull the stocking up in this manner until you reach the premeasured area. Apply the other stocking in the same way. <u>Because wrinkles can cause pressure areas, both stockings must fit smoothly</u>.

Evaluating

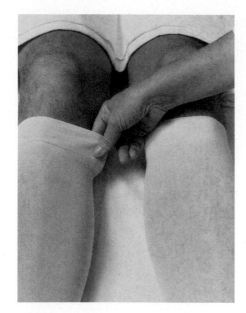

10 Periodically, check that the stocking does not roll at the top. Alert your client to watch for this, if he is able, explaining that rolling can produce a tourniquet effect. This can cause stasis to occur, predisposing thrombus formation and enhancing edema.

12 To minimize swelling proximal to the hose, and for client comfort, remove the stockings at least twice a day for 30 minutes at a time. Wash and dry the legs (or provide the client with the materials to do so) and reapply talc or corn starch. Always palpate peripheral pulses in the legs and feet before reapplying the hose, and observe for improvement or for an alteration in his circulatory system. Wash the hose with detergent and water as necessary.

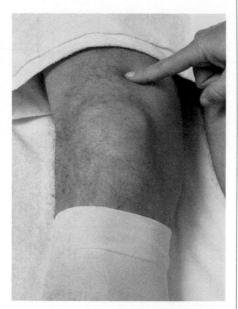

11 Monitor the client frequently for swelling proximal to the stocking top. To do this, press a finger into the flesh above the stocking. If you can see a dent after removing your finger, swelling has occurred and the stockings should be removed.

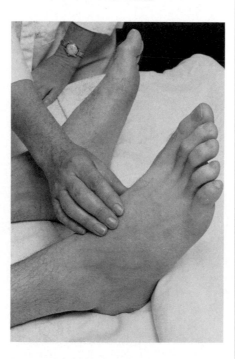

EMPLOYING BUERGER-ALLEN EXERCISES

Assessing and Planning

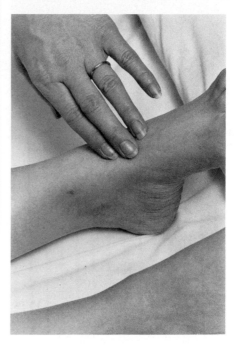

1 The physician may prescribe Buerger-Allen exercises for clients with occlusive arterial disorders—for example, arteriosclerosis obliterans, Buerger's disease, or Raynaud's disease. Explain to your client that these exercises will promote circulation in the lower extremities by the gravitational filling and emptying of the blood vessels. To evaluate the effectiveness of the exercises, you must first perform a baseline assessment of your client's legs and feet. While your client lies flat, palpate the femoral, popliteal, posterior tibial, and pedal pulses. Then assess for the presence or absence of pain and ulcerations and the temperature and color of the extremities.

(Continued on p. 410)

Implementing

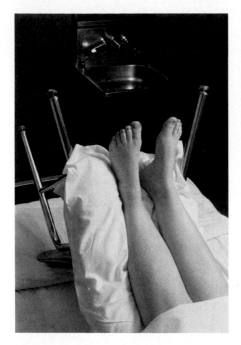

2 Initially, the client should recline with her legs elevated above the level of her heart for a minute, or until blanching occurs in the legs and feet. You may raise the foot of the hospital bed, but it is a good idea to show the client how to implement the procedure at home. In this photo, the back of a straight-back chair is cushioned with a pillow so that the chair's back supports the client's legs. Make sure you keep the client warm because chilling will further diminish arterial circulation.

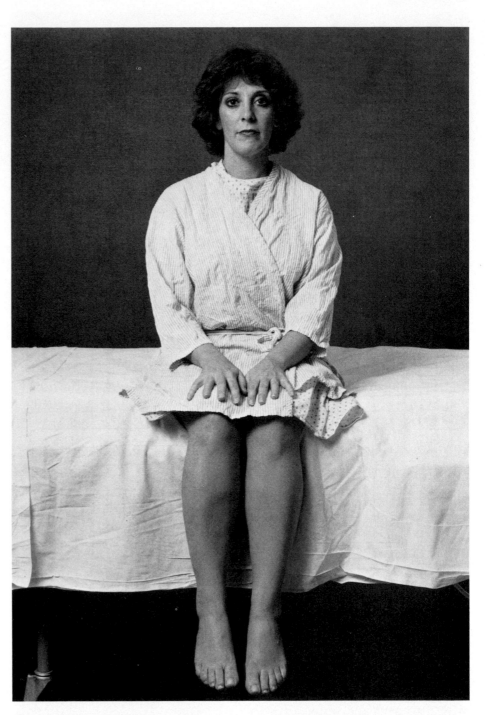

3 Once blanching has occurred, have the client sit on the side of the bed and plantarflex her feet. This is the first of six leg-stretching positions that are employed to promote blood flow and minimize stasis. This and the following five positions should be maintained for 30 seconds each. *Note: Instead of the six leg-stretching positions, the physician may prescribe one in which the client's legs dangle over the side of the bed for 3 minutes, or until they are pink.*

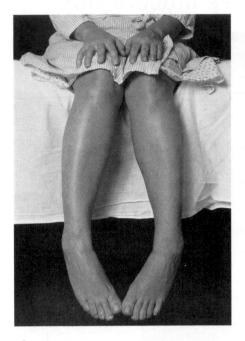

4 For the second position, the client plantarflexes and inverts her feet.

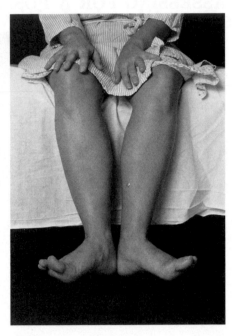

5 For the third position, the client dorsiflexes and everts her feet.

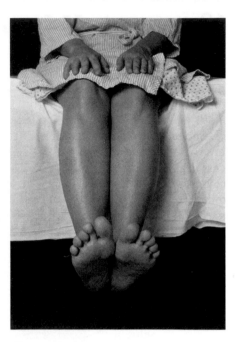

6 For the fourth position, the client dorsiflexes her feet.

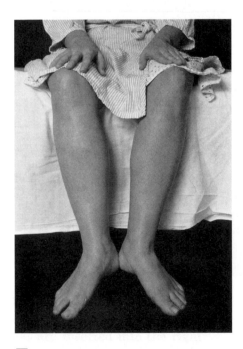

7 For the fifth position, the client plantarflexes and everts her feet.

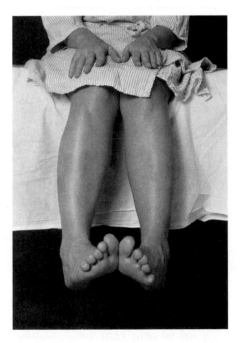

8 For the sixth position, she dorsiflexes and inverts her feet. Observe her feet and legs at this time. Optimally, they will be red or pink to indicate that adequate circulation has occurred.

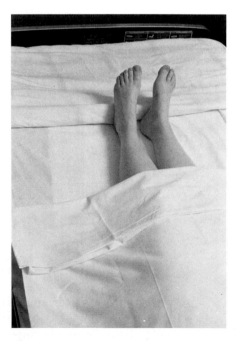

9 Finally the client should lie flat in a supine position. Usually, this position is maintained for 3–5 minutes. Depending on the physician's orders, the set may be repeated another four or five times. Buerger-Allen exercises are usually prescribed for three or four times daily.

1 The following are materials you may need for Hickman catheter management: sterile syringes for blood drawing and irrigation; a sterile syringe with an attached needle; 23-gauge, 2-cm sterile needle; sterile injection cap; alcohol swabs; tape; cannula clamp (or a rubber-shod hemostat); and an irrigant, either a dilute heparin solution or injectable normal saline. Generally, the catheter is flushed with heparin when it is routinely capped and/or clamped and after blood withdrawal; it is flushed with saline when it is routinely connected to a continuous intravenous infusion.

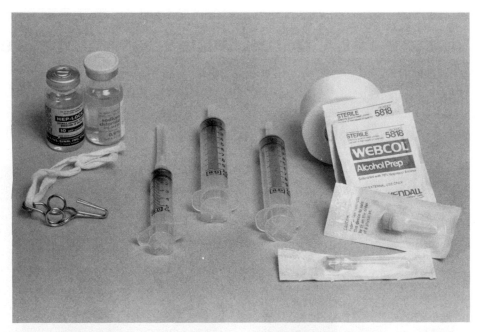

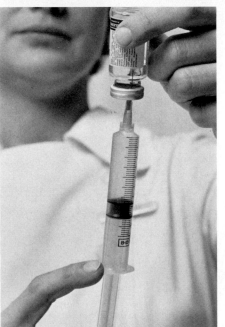

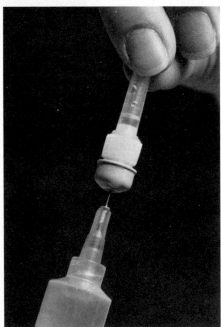

2 Attach the sterile needle to the 10-mL syringe and aspirate the irrigant in preparation for blood withdrawal or routine irrigation, and set it aside. *Caution: Ensure that all air bubbles are removed because the catheter is a direct line into the heart.*

3 The injection cap should be changed on a regular basis. If your client is scheduled for an injection cap change, remove the cap from the package. To prevent its contamination, grasp it by the protective cap (as shown) and inject the irrigant directly through the rubber diaphragm until you can see the return of the irrigant in the protective cap. This will ensure that all air has been removed from the injection cap. Set the cap aside.

Drawing Blood from the Hickman Catheter

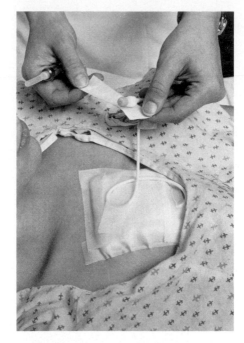

1 Wash your hands and explain the procedure to your client. Remove the tape that secures the injection cap to the catheter.

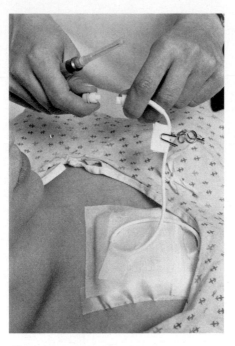

2 Separate the injection cap from the catheter.

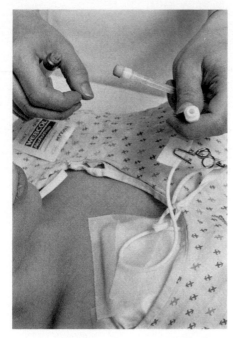

3 To prevent the contamination of the injection cap, remove the capped needle from the smaller syringe you will use to withdraw the blood, and attach it to the injection cap. Then set it aside, within reach. *Note: Many agencies change injection caps every 24 hours. If you will change the cap after this procedure, it will not be necessary to utilize this step. See step 3, p. 414.*

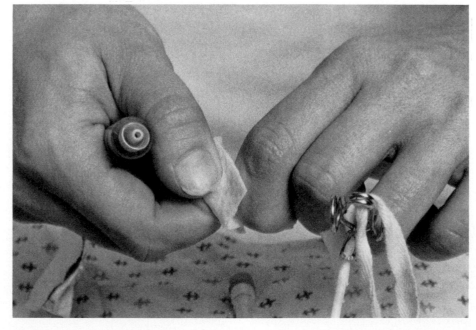

4 Clean the catheter's hub with an alcohol swab and let the alcohol dry.

(Continued on p. 416)

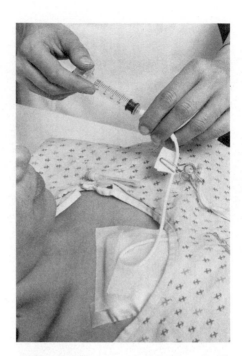

5 Attach the syringe to the catheter hub.

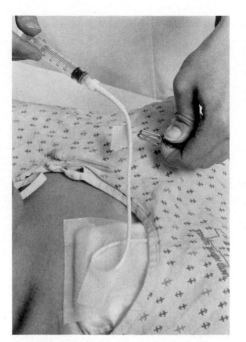

6 Remove the catheter clamp from the protective tape tab. *Note: To prevent puncturing the catheter, always place a tape tab over the catheter and attach the clamp only over the tape.*

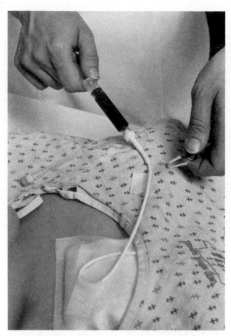

7 To clear the catheter of residual heparinized blood, withdraw 5 mL of blood (or the prescribed amount), and reclamp the catheter. Discard the blood later, following your agency's guidelines for blood disposal.

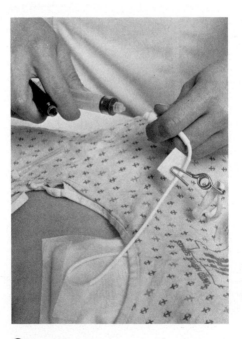

8 Remove the blood-filled syringe and attach a 10-mL syringe (or larger, depending on the amount of blood you are required to withdraw). Then remove the cannula clamp.

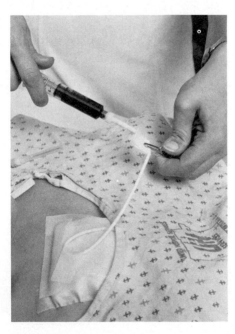

9 Withdraw the prescribed amount of blood and reattach the cannula clamp.

Flushing a Hickman Catheter after Blood Withdrawal

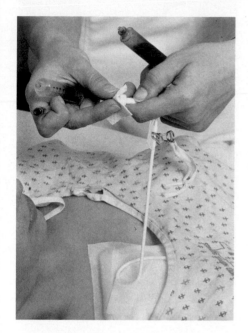

1 Remove the syringe containing the blood sample and clean the catheter hub with an alcohol swab, letting it dry.

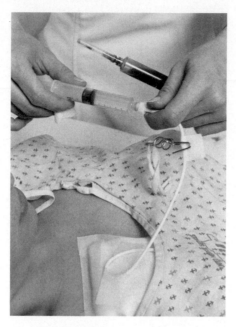

2 Cap the syringe containing the blood sample and attach the syringe containing the heparinized solution (or the prescribed irrigant).

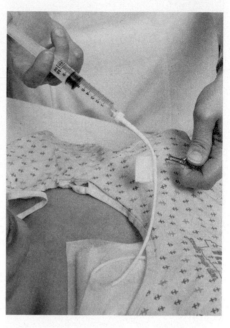

3 Remove the cannula clamp and inject the irrigant.

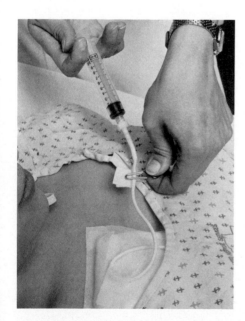

4 When you have injected all except the last 0.5 mL of the irrigant, clamp the catheter. Then inject the remaining irrigant. By producing positive pressure in the line, you will clear the line of blood and prevent its backflow into the line, thus deterring clotting.

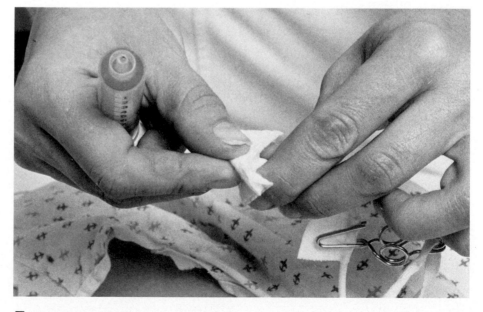

5 Remove the syringe, and clean the catheter hub with an alcohol swab; allow it to dry.

(Continued on p. 418)

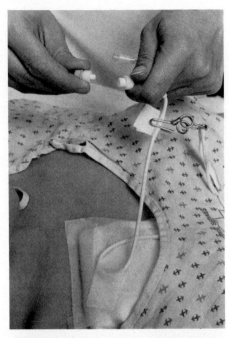

6 To replace the injection cap, first detach it from the capped needle.

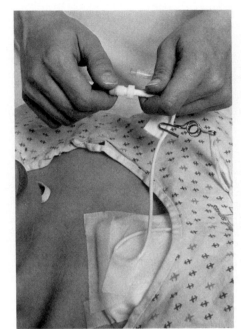

7 Reattach the injection cap to the catheter hub. →

8 Secure the connection at the catheter hub with a strip of tape.

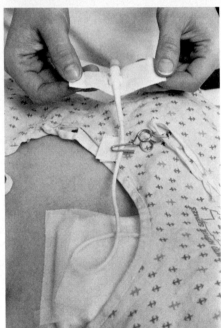

9 Fold the ends of the tape together to secure the connection. →

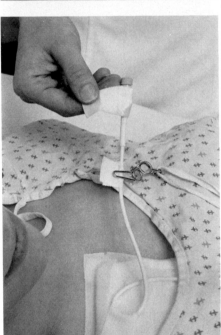

Performing a Routine Irrigation of a Capped Hickman Catheter

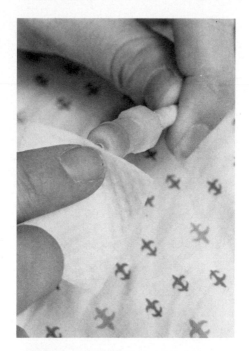

1 Generally, Hickman catheters are irrigated at least daily. Check your agency's policy for the frequency, amount, and type of irrigant. Catheters that are routinely capped and/or clamped are usually irrigated with a dilute heparin solution. After preparing 5.5 mL of the irrigant, cleanse the rubber port of the injection cap with an alcohol swab, and allow it to dry.

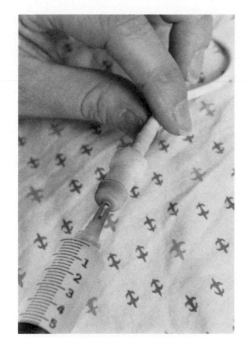

2 Insert the needle of the syringe into the rubber port of the injection cap.

3 Remove the cannula clamp, and infuse 5 mL of the irrigant.

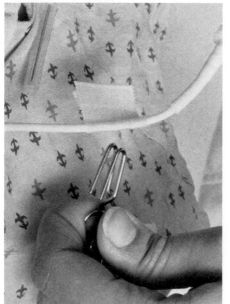

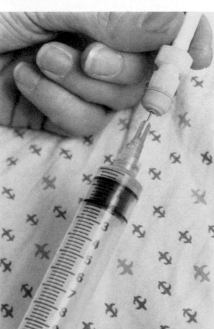

4 Reclamp the catheter, and inject the remaining 0.5 mL to establish positive pressure in the line.

Flushing a Hickman Catheter That Is Routinely Connected to a Continuous IV Infusion

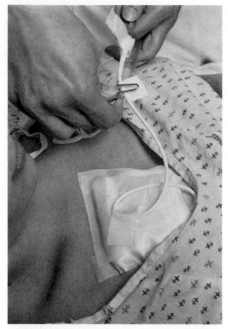

1 After preparing the prescribed amount of injectable normal saline, or the prescribed irrigant, clamp off the IV tubing to stop the infusion. Place the cannula clamp over the protective tape tab (as shown).

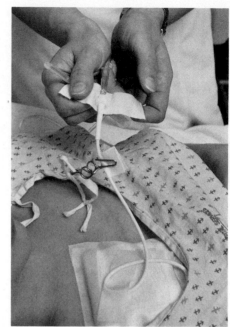

2 Remove the tape that secures the IV tubing to the catheter hub. →

3 Remove the capped needle from the syringe. After disconnecting the IV tubing from the catheter hub, attach the capped needle to the distal end of the infusion tubing to prevent its contamination.

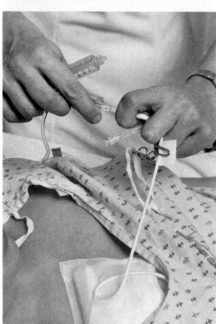

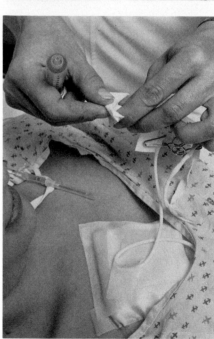

4 Clean the catheter hub with an alcohol swab, and allow it to dry. →

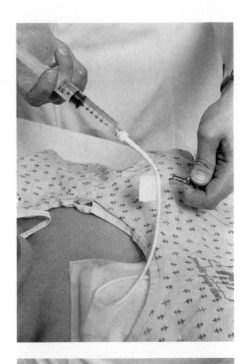

5 Attach the syringe to the catheter hub and remove the cannula clamp.

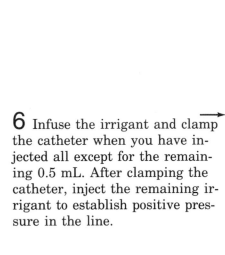

6 Infuse the irrigant and clamp the catheter when you have injected all except for the remaining 0.5 mL. After clamping the catheter, inject the remaining irrigant to establish positive pressure in the line.

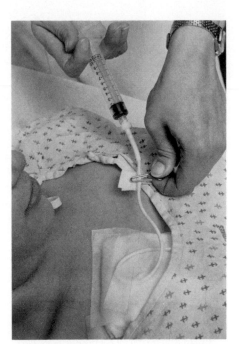

7 After removing the syringe, cleanse the catheter hub with an alcohol sponge, and allow it to dry. Remove the capped needle from the distal end of the IV tubing.

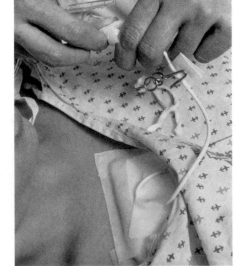

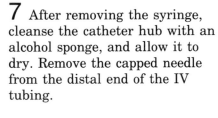

8 Insert the IV tubing into the catheter hub.

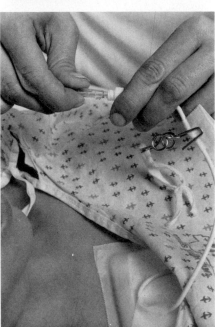

(Continued on p. 422)

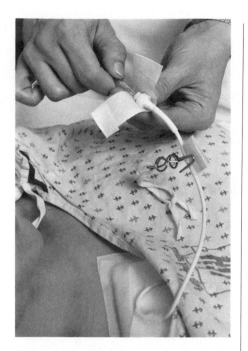

9 Attach a tape tab to secure the connection.

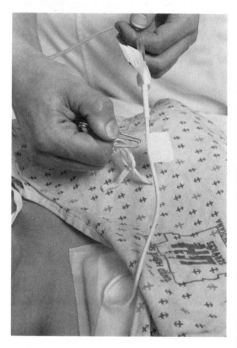

10 Remove the cannula clamp and adjust the roller clamp on the infusion tubing to achieve the prescribed rate of infusion.

CHANGING INTRAVENOUS TUBING ON CENTRAL LINES

Because a central venous catheter is inserted directly into the right atrium, it is imperative that you take every precaution to prevent infection and to minimize the risk of an air embolism. The Centers for Disease Control recommends that IV tubing and filters used for hyperalimentation solutions be routinely changed every 24–48 hours.

Assessing and Planning

1 When it is time to change both the tubing and solution container, wash your hands and assess the client's knowledge of the procedure. If she does not have a cardiac disorder, instruct her in the Valsalva maneuver. Explain that holding her breath and bearing down will prevent air from entering the catheter while you change the tubing. Then position her so that she is flat in bed, and remove her pillow. This will increase intrathoracic venous pressure, which will help prevent the development of an air embolism. *Note: If you assess that your client is noncompliant, obtain sterile gloves so that you can occlude the catheter hub with a sterile surface should your client inhale during the tubing change.*

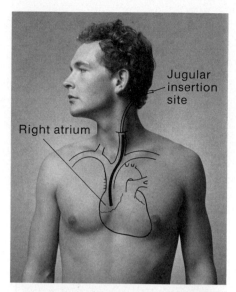

Jugular insertion site

Right atrium

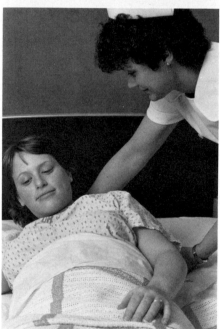

2 Inspect the container to ensure that it is intact and that the solution is clear and free of particulate matter. If your client is receiving hyperalimentation, carefully compare the contents on the fresh container's label to the physician's prescription, and ensure that the name and identification numbers on the prescription and container label match those on the client's identification band.

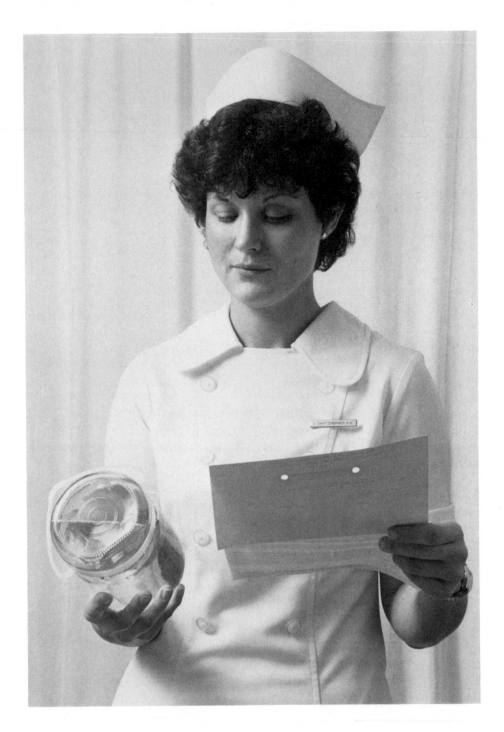

(Continued on p. 424)

Implementing

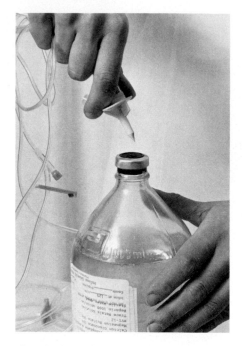

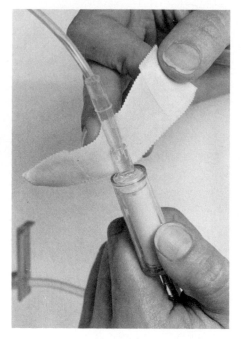

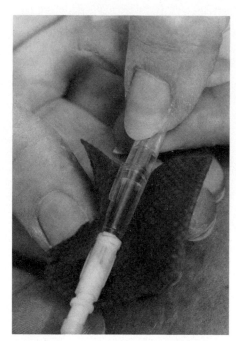

3 Spike the fresh solution container with sterile tubing. Attach a sterile filter and prime the tubing and filter, making sure you have flushed out all the air. Adjust the roller clamp to stop the infusion.

4 To ensure a closed system, tape the connection of the filter and tubing to prevent its separation.

5 Remove the tape that secures the connection between the catheter hub and IV tubing, and swab the connection site with an antimicrobial agent such as a povidone-iodine solution. Allow it to dry.

6 To minimize contamination, ask your client to turn her head away from the tubing, and insert a sterile gauze pad under the catheter hub to establish a sterile field. Just before you replace the tubing, ask her to perform a Valsalva maneuver. *Caution: If your client has a cardiac disorder, ask her to hold her breath, rather than to bear down.* Then quickly change the tubing.

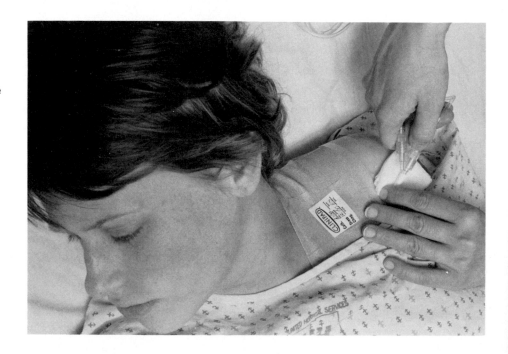

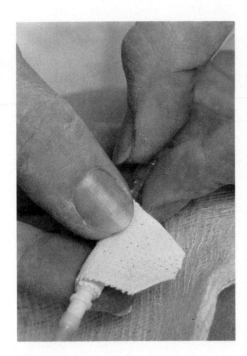

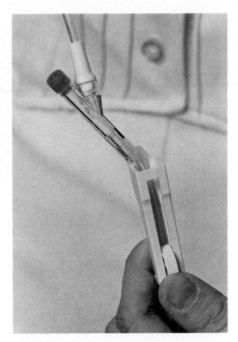

Evaluating

9 Monitor your client frequently to ensure that her vital signs are stable and that there is no evidence of an air embolism: hypotension, chest pain, cyanosis, confusion, weak pulse, and alterations in heart sounds. Also, inspect the tubing to ensure that the connections are intact and securely anchored with tape and that the solution container is replaced before it empties.

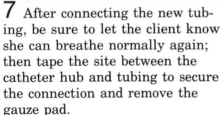

7 After connecting the new tubing, be sure to let the client know she can breathe normally again; then tape the site between the catheter hub and tubing to secure the connection and remove the gauze pad.

8 Adjust the roller clamp to infuse the solution at the prescribed rate. Label the tubing and solution container with the time, date, and your initials; reposition your client. Document the procedure. The dressing change procedure for central venous catheters is found on pp. 27–31.

ASSESSING AND INTERVENING FOR AN AIR EMBOLISM

1 All clients with IV lines are at risk for an air embolism. Rapid infusion rates compound the risk by producing high vascular pressure—for example, the administration of a unit of blood over a 10–15 minute period. Because an air embolism can be fatal, it is essential that you monitor and observe the client for the presence of chest pain, coughing, hypotension, cyanosis, and hypoxia. In addition, if the client does have an air embolism, auscultation over the right ventricle may reveal a churning "windmill" sound.

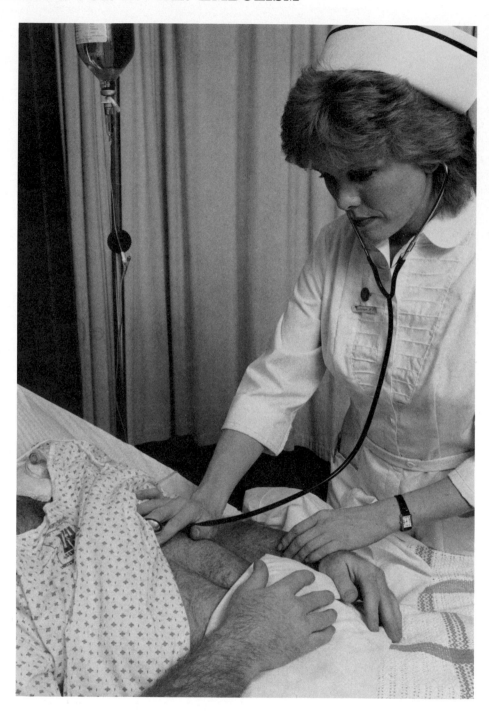

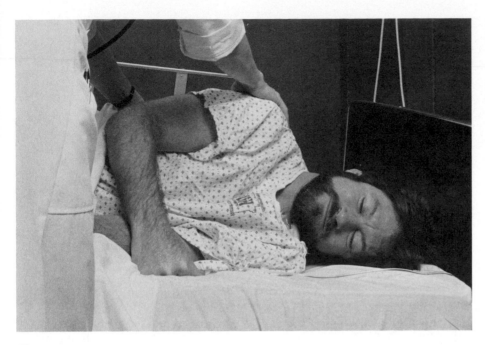

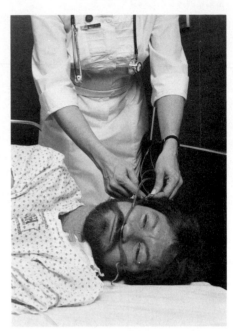

2 <u>Any indication of an air embolism necessitates an immediate intervention</u>. <u>Turn the client to his left side to displace the air into the apex of the heart</u> and to <u>help prevent its rapid movement into the pulmonary artery</u>. Then <u>remove the pillow and lower the head of the bed into Trendelenburg's position</u>. Lowering the head of the bed will increase intrathoracic pressure, decreasing the flow of air into the vein during inhalation.

3 Administer oxygen, if it is at the bedside, and notify the physician immediately. If the air has not slowly and safely dissipated into the pulmonary system, the physician may aspirate the air from the apical area. Stay with the client and continue to reassure him.

References

American Heart Association. 1980. Standards and guidelines for cardiopulmonary resuscitation (CPR) and emergency cardiac care (ECC). *JAMA* 244:453–509.

Andreoli, K.G., et al. 1979. *Comprehensive cardiac care*, 4th ed. St. Louis: C.V. Mosby.

Billings, D.M., and Stokes, L.G. 1982. *Medical-surgical nursing*. St. Louis: C.V. Mosby.

Bjeletich, J., and Hickman, R. Jan. 1980. The Hickman indwelling catheter. *AJN* 80:62–65.

Blumenthal, S., et al. 1977. Report of the Task Force on Blood Pressure Control in Children: recommendations of the Task Force on Blood Pressure Control in Children. *Pediatrics* 59 (supplement):797–820.

Brunner, L.S., and Suddarth, D.S. 1982. *The Lippincott manual of nursing practice*, 3rd ed. Philadelphia: J.B. Lippincott.

Cannon, C. Mar. 1980. Hands-on guide to palpation and auscultation. *RN* 43:20–27, 76.

Centers for Disease Control. 1981–1984. *Guidelines for the prevention and control of nosocomial infection.* Atlanta, Ga.: U.S. Department of Health and Human Services.

Crowley, M., and Baker, P. 1979. *Nursing care of the oncology patient with an indwelling silastic catheter—self-learning package.* Philadelphia: Hospital of the University of Pennsylvania, Department of Nursing.

Forshee, T., and Minckley, B. July 1976. How to put lumbar sympathectomy patients back on their own two feet. *RN* 39:18–23.

Grim, C.M. June, 1981. Nursing assessment of the patient with high blood pressure. *Nurs Clin North Am* 16:349–364.

Hirsch, J., and Hannock, L. 1981. *Mosby's manual of clinical nursing procedures*. St. Louis: C.V. Mosby.

Holloway, N. 1984. *Nursing the critically ill adult*, 2nd ed. Menlo Park, Calif.: Addison-Wesley Publishing.

Kirkendall, W.M., et al. 1980. *Report of a subcommittee of the Postgraduate Education Committee: recommendations for human blood pressure determination by sphygmomanometers.* Dallas: American Heart Association Communications Division.

Kirkis, E.J. Jan. 1983. "Hyperalimentation precautions" in *Tactics to hold microbes at bay. RN* 46:111.

Leutzinger, R., and Judson, A.L. Dec. 1981. Drawing blood from a Hickman catheter. *Nursing '81* 11:65–69.

The 1980 Report of the Joint National Committee on Detection, Evaluation and Treatment of High Blood Pressure. December, 1981. U.S. Department of Health and Human Services. NIH Publication No. 82–1088.

Nursing Photobook. 1981. Giving cardiac care. Horsham, Pa.: Intermed Communications.

Nursing Photobook. 1980. Using monitors. Horsham, Pa.: Intermed Communications.

Olds, S.B., et al. 1984. *Maternal–newborn nursing: a family-centered approach*, 2nd ed. Menlo Park, Calif.: Addison-Wesley Publishing.

Ostrow, L.S. Nov. 1981. Air embolism and central venous lines. *AJN* 81:2036–2038.

Schmidt, A.M., and Williams, D. Feb. 1982. The Hickman catheter: sending your patient home safely. *RN* 45:57–61.

Scordo, K. Aug. 1982. Taming the cardiac monitor. *Nursing '82* 12:58–63.

Smith, S.F., and Duell, D. 1982. *Nursing skills and evaluation.* Los Altos, Calif.: National Nursing Review.

Sorenson, K.C., and Luckmann, J. 1979. *Basic nursing: a psychophysiologic approach.* Philadelphia: W.B. Saunders.

Spence, A. 1982. *Basic human anatomy.* Menlo Park, Calif.: Benjamin/Cummings Publishing.

Thompson, J., and Bowers, A. 1980. *Clinical manual of health assessment.* St. Louis: C.V. Mosby.

Visich, M.A. Nov. 1981. A guide to assessing breath and heart sounds. *Nursing '81* 11:64–72.

Wilner, G.N. Nov. 1980. ECG accuracy without "buttering up" the patient. *Patient Care* 14:132.

Chapter 8

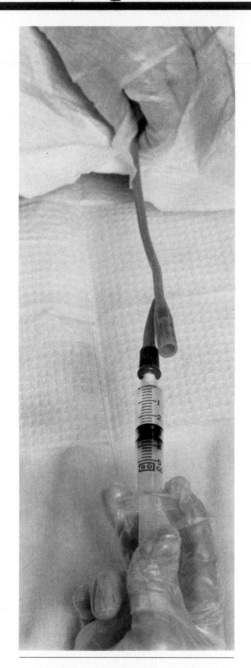

Managing
Renal-Urinary
Procedures

CHAPTER OUTLINE

ASSESSING THE RENAL-URINARY SYSTEM

The Renal-Urinary System

Nursing Assessment Guideline

Assessing the Bladder
    Inspecting
    Palpating
    Percussing

Palpating the Kidneys

Assessing Skin Turgor

Weighing the Client on a Bed Scale

Collecting a 24-Hour Urine Specimen

CATHETERIZING AND MANAGING CATHETER CARE

Performing Intermittent Catheterization
    Inserting a Robinson (straight) catheter into a female
    Inserting a Robinson (straight) catheter into a male

Managing a Foley Catheter
    General guidelines for Foley catheter management
    Performing a catheterization with a Foley (indwelling) catheter
    Making a catheter strap
    Obtaining a urine specimen
    Emptying the drainage bag
    Using a urine meter
    Irrigating the catheter
    Removing a Foley catheter

CARING FOR CLIENTS WITH RENAL-URINARY DISORDERS

Applying an External Urinary Device (with a Leg Drainage System)

Monitoring the Client Receiving Continuous Bladder Irrigation (CBI)
    Establishing CBI
    Nursing guidelines for the care of clients with continuous bladder irrigation

Nursing Guidelines for the Care of the Client with a Suprapubic Catheter

Nursing Guidelines for the Care of the Client with a Nephrostomy Tube

Administering a Sodium Polystyrene Sulfonate (Kayexalate) Enema

Performing the Credé Maneuver

CARING FOR CLIENTS WITH URINARY DIVERSIONS

Nursing Guidelines to Common Types of Urinary Diversions
    Ileal conduit
    Cutaneous ureterostomy
    Ureterosigmoidostomy

Performing a Postoperative Assessment

Managing Appliance Care
    Applying a postoperative (disposable) pouch
    Applying a reusable (permanent) pouch
    Connecting the pouch to a urinary drainage system

Catheterizing an Ileal Conduit

Assessing the Renal-Urinary System

THE RENAL-URINARY SYSTEM

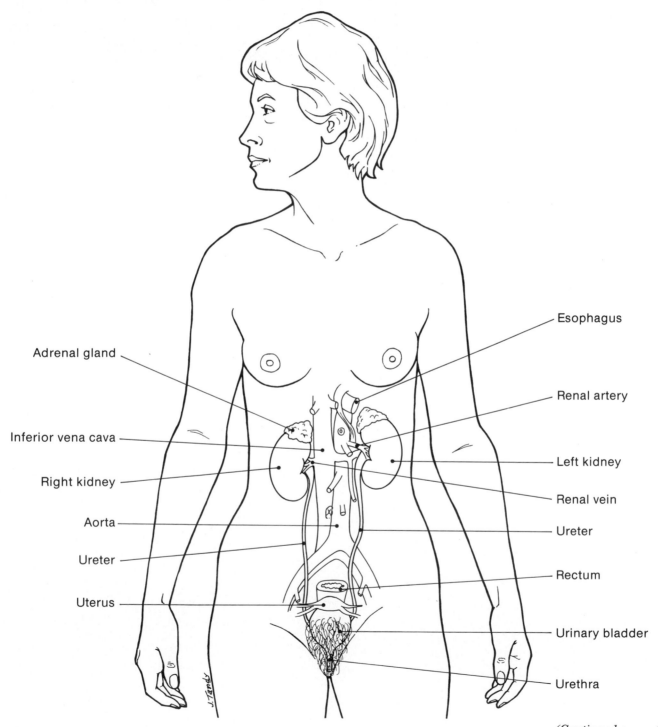

Esophagus

Renal artery

Adrenal gland

Left kidney

Inferior vena cava

Renal vein

Right kidney

Ureter

Aorta

Ureter

Rectum

Uterus

Urinary bladder

Urethra

(Continued on p. 432)

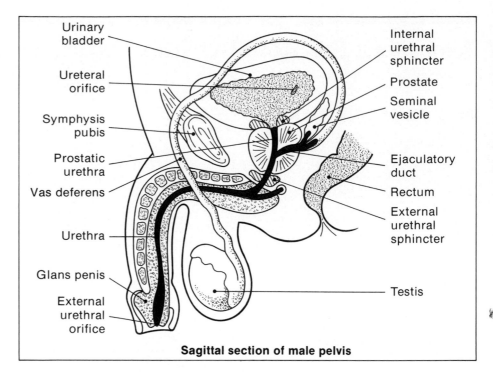

Sagittal section of male pelvis

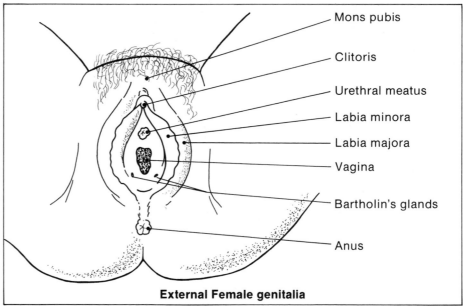

External Female genitalia

NURSING ASSESSMENT GUIDELINE

To assess your client's renal-urinary system, you need to interview him or her for subjective data, take vital signs, assess the bladder and kidneys, and obtain a urine specimen. A comprehensive nursing care plan includes a complete evaluation for the following subjective data:

Personal factors: for example, age, marital status, occupation, continued exposure to nephrotoxic substances such as carbon tetrachloride, use of recreational drugs

History or family history of: renal calculi, strictures, urinary tract disease and/or infections, incontinence, diabetes mellitus, renal transplants, dialysis, cardiac disease, or endocrine disorders such as diabetes insipidus

History of: renal/urinary trauma or surgery, blood transfusions, glomerulonephritis, autoimmune diseases

Dietary habits: intake in approximate amounts of sodium, calcium, protein, purines, potassium, phosphates, or acids; amounts consumed of coffee, tea, or alcoholic beverages; presence or history of polydipsia; food allergies

Risk factors: psychologic stressors, hypertension, pregnancy, smoking

Medications: diuretics, antispasmotics, anticholinergics, aspirin or acetaminophen; presence of drug allergies

Alterations in urinary elimination: frequency, urgency, retention, nocturia, dysuria, residual urine, hesitancy, burning during voiding, stress incontinence, presence of an ostomy

Amount and character of urine: polyuria, oliguria, anuria; changes in color, odor, clarity

Flow of urinary stream: high/low pressure, change in size

Fluid status: dehydration, thirst, presence of peripheral or periorbital edema

Pain: location—for example, lower back, flank, perineum, suprapubic area, groin; intensity; relieved by; intensified by

Urethral discharge: amount and character

Presence of genital sores or ulcers

ASSESSING THE BLADDER

Inspecting

Routine assessment of the bladder is essential when you are caring for clients with urinary tract disorders, as well as for those who have indwelling catheters. Be sure that you provide warmth and privacy for your client, and that you have washed your hands and explained the reason for the assessment. To facilitate the procedure, the client's gown should be raised to the umbilicus and the sheet or drape lowered to the symphysis pubis. Unless your client is obese, a distended bladder can usually be assessed visually while you are at eye level to the lower abdomen. Often you will be able to see a swollen mound just proximal to the symphysis pubis.

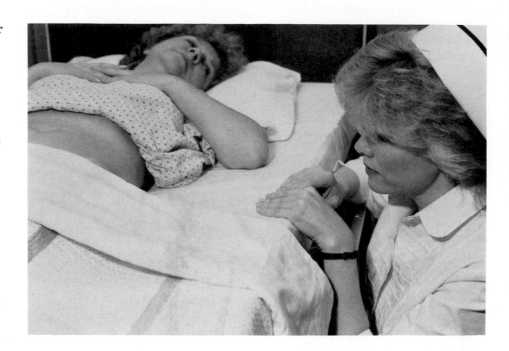

Palpating

If your client is oliguric or anuric and you need to assess for bladder retention to ensure that catheterization is indicated; if you are assessing your client for a potential catheter obstruction; or if you are assessing for residual urine in clients with neurogenic bladders, light palpation of the bladder can be employed to help determine bladder size. Palpate at the midline, approximately 5 cm (2 in.) above the symphysis pubis. If the bladder is distended, you should be able to feel its firm, rounded contour. *Note: For routine assessment, the client should void prior to bladder palpation to minimize the potential for discomfort.*

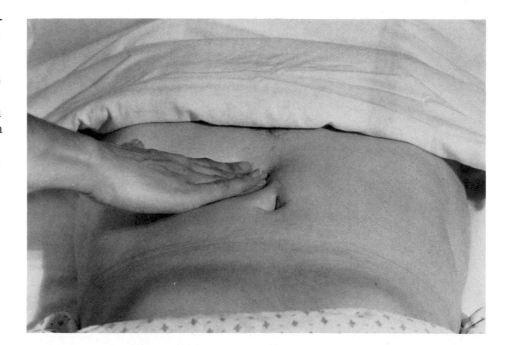

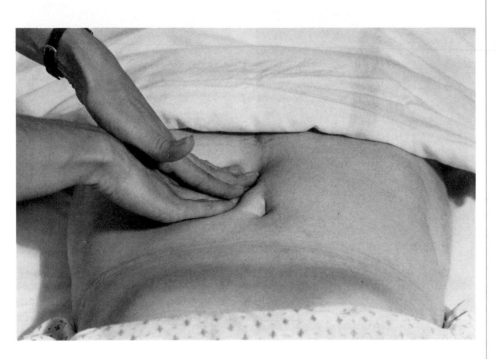

PALPATING THE KIDNEYS

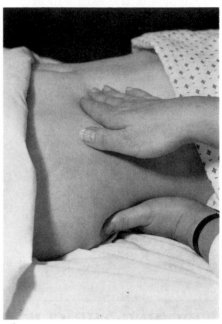

Deep Palpation: When the bladder is not distended, it may be necessary to deeply palpate to assess for location and size. To do this, press with the fingertips of both hands approximately 2.5–5 cm (1–2 in.) proximal to the symphysis pubis, near the midline. Assess for size and location of the bladder and for the presence of any masses. Be sure to note indications of client discomfort, as well.

Percussing

Percussion is another assessment tool that will help you determine whether the bladder is empty or if it contains urine. Place a middle finger at the midline, approximately 5 cm (2 in.) above the symphysis pubis. To elicit sounds, sharply strike that finger with the opposite middle finger. If the bladder contains urine, you should hear dull sounds as you continue to percuss downward toward the symphysis pubis. However, an empty bladder should produce tympanic (hollow) sounds.

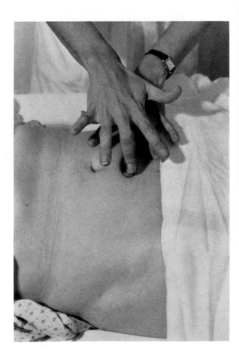

Although not always a routine assessment for the hospitalized urologic client, kidney palpation can be incorporated into a comprehensive assessment. Position your hands on both sides of the client's flank at the area between the iliac crest and lower costal margins (as shown). Instruct the client to inhale, and increase the pressure between your hands with each inhalation until you feel you have achieved the maximum depth. As the client inhales deeply a final time, you should be able to feel the lower edge of the kidney between your hands. This will be more difficult if your client is obese. Compare your assessment of the left kidney to that of the right kidney. Assess for differences in size, an absence of a kidney, masses, nodules, and for discomfort you may potentially elicit in the client.

(Continued on p. 436)

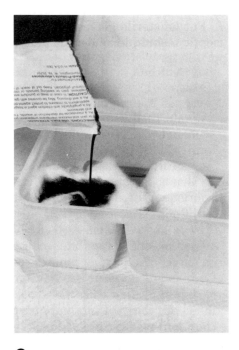

9 Set one or two of the cotton balls aside, and pour the antimicrobial solution over the others.

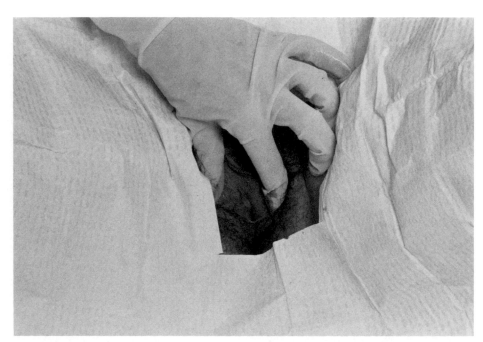

11 You are ready to prepare the urethral meatus and its surrounding area. With your nondominant hand, separate the labia to expose the urethral meatus. Use your thumb and index finger to apply slight upward and backward tension. This hand is now considered contaminated.

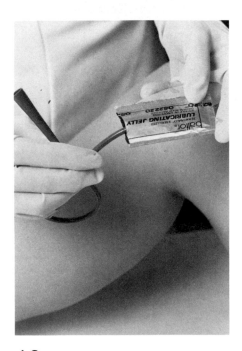

10 Open the sterile lubricant and either place the catheter's tip into the package (as shown) or squeeze the lubricant onto the sterile field and generously lubricate the tip of the catheter.

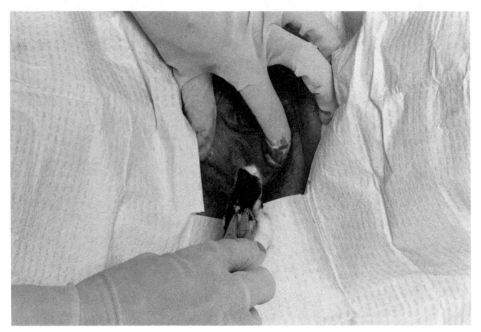

12 With your dominant hand, grasp a saturated cotton ball with the sterile forceps. With one downward stroke per cotton ball, cleanse on each side of the meatus. After each stroke, discard the used cotton ball into a waste container. Cleanse the meatus (as shown) with one downward stroke. Continue to separate the labia until you have completed the catheterization. *Note: If the labia are allowed to fall together, repeat the cleansing process.*

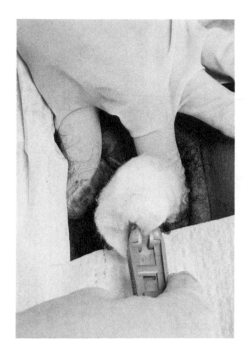

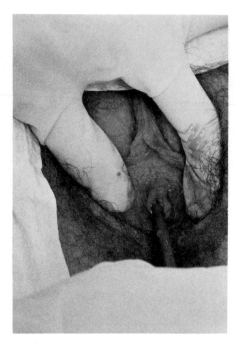

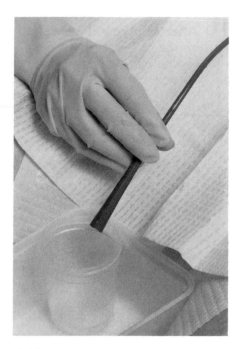

13 After preparing the area, wipe the meatus with a dry cotton ball, using one downward stroke. Discard the cotton ball.

14 Gently insert the catheter into the meatus, and ask the client to breathe deeply and slowly and to bear down with her pelvic muscles. If you meet resistance, slightly angle the catheter toward her symphysis pubis, but do not force the catheter. If urine has not returned after you have inserted the catheter 7.5–10 cm (3–4 in.), it is possible that your client is dehydrated or has recently voided. It is more likely, however, that you have inserted the catheter into the vagina, rather than into the urethra. Use the extra pair of sterile gloves and a new catheter and repeat the catheterization. Keep the original catheter in place to avoid making the same mistake.

15 When you have successfully catheterized the client, obtain a urine specimen if one has been ordered. Place the sterile specimen cup at the distal end of the catheter. After obtaining the specimen, allow the urine to drain into the empty catheterization tray. Follow agency policy regarding the amount of urine you should allow to drain. Some experts feel that a rapid decompression of the bladder, resulting from a quick release of large amounts of urine (quantities greater than 800–1000 mL), can lead to shock.

(Continued on p. 444)

Performing a Catheterization with a Foley (Indwelling) Catheter

Assessing and Planning

1 Follow the steps for assessing and planning in the procedure, pp. 438–444, for performing intermittent catheterization. In addition to the catheterization kit, you will also need the following sterile supplies: drainage collection bag with tubing, a syringe and sterile water for inflating the catheter balloon, and two Foley catheters and an extra pair of sterile gloves in the event either becomes contaminated during the procedure. In addition, you might wish to keep an extra drainage tubing protector and an antimicrobial wipe at the bedside to help prevent contamination of the opened system during subsequent interventions such as an irrigation or instillation.

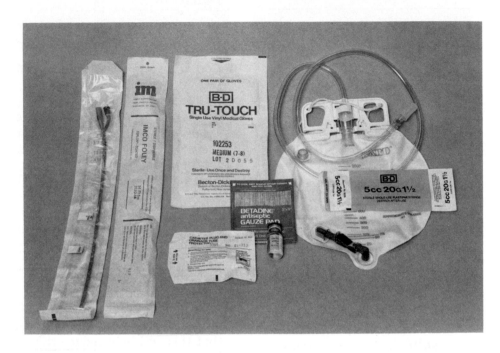

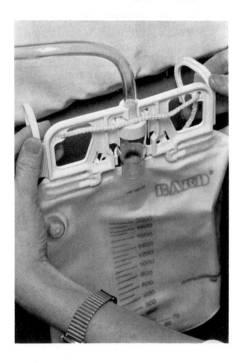

2 Attach the drainage collection bag to the bed frame and bring the drainage tubing up onto the bed so that it will be readily accessible. Make sure the end of the tubing remains covered by the drainage tubing protector.

3 After opening the sterile catheterization kit, aseptically open one of the sterile packages containing the Foley and drop the catheter onto the sterile field. Do the same for the sterile syringe if it is not prepackaged with the catheterization kit. Cleanse the urethral meatus and surrounding area, following the appropriate steps for preparing the female or the male found in the preceding procedures.

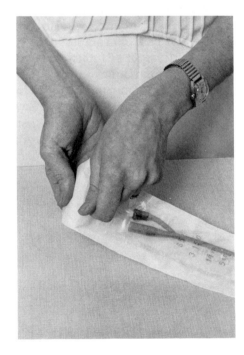

Implementing

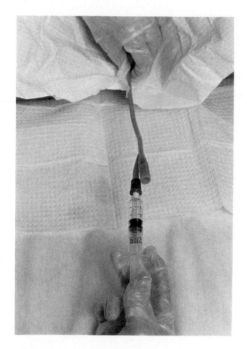

4 Following the steps in the previous two procedures for intermittent catheterization of the male or the female, insert the catheter.

To make sure the catheter is in the bladder, advance it another 2.5 cm (1 in.) beyond the distance at which urine begins to flow. For the adult female, the total distance of the insertion will be approximately 7.5–10 cm (3–4 in.). The total distance for the adult male, however, can be as much as 25 cm (10 in.), and the bifurcation of the catheter might be quite close to the urethral meatus. If the syringe for balloon inflation does not already contain the sterile water, aseptically aspirate the appropriate amount. The usual amount is 5 mL, but this can vary depending on the brand and size of catheter used. The appropriate amount is always stamped on the lumen of the balloon portal. Slowly inject the water as you assess the client for discomfort. If the client complains of pain, immediately aspirate the water because the balloon may be incorrectly positioned in the urethra. After inflating the balloon,

pull back gently on the catheter to check for resistance, a sign that the balloon is correctly positioned against the proximal wall of the bladder.

5 Remove the drainage tubing protector and connect the drainage tubing to the open lumen of the catheter. This often requires manipulation and because your gloves can no longer be considered sterile, it might be necessary to use the antimicrobial wipe at the connection site. Secure the tubing to the bed linen with the attached clip (below). Be certain to keep the tubing looped on the bed rather than hanging on the floor.

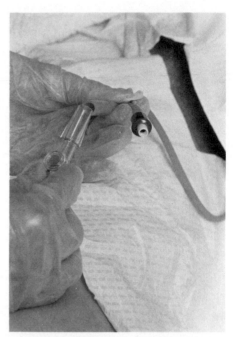

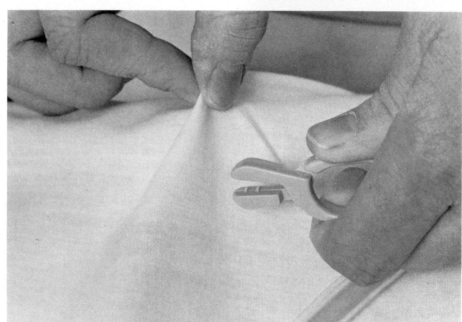

(Continued on p. 450)

Evaluating

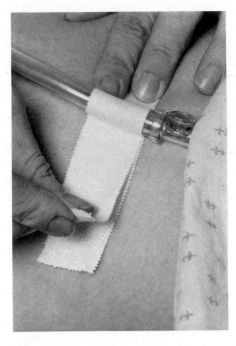

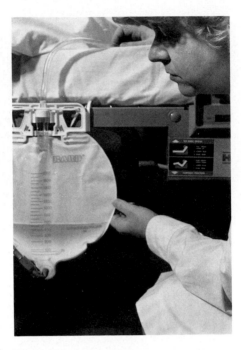

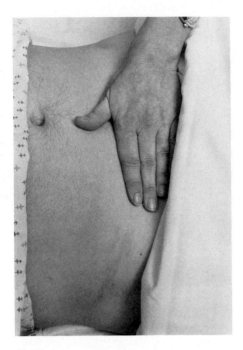

6 Tape the drainage tubing (not the catheter) to your client to help prevent it from becoming dislodged. For female clients, tape the tubing to the medial thigh. For the male client, tape the tubing either to the anterior thigh or the lower abdomen. It is thought that the latter position especially minimizes urethral pressure that would occur at the normal penoscrotal angle. For more secure taping, place a strip of tape on your client's skin; then tape the catheter to the tape (as shown). Allow some slack in the tubing. If the catheter will be left indwelling for an extended period of time, protect your client's skin by making a dressing similar to a Montgomery strap (see the next procedure). Label the drainage bag with the time and date so that it can be changed periodically according to agency protocol.

7 Document the procedure, noting the time and date of catheterization as well as the size and type of catheter used. Periodically check the drainage tubing for patency and ensure that the output of urine is adequate when compared to the client's intake. Assess the urine for the presence of blood, cloudiness, or a foul odor, which are indications that the client may have a bladder infection.

8 If the client has a diminished urinary output, inspect the lower abdomen and palpate or percuss the bladder to assess for urine retention, which can occur with an occluded catheter. Obtain an order for an irrigation, if indicated. Also, assess the client for the presence of fever, chills, or discomfort, which are indicators of a bladder infection. Ensure that the perineum is washed daily.

Making a Catheter Strap

Instead of using tape to anchor your client's Foley catheter, consider making a catheter strap, which is similar to a Montgomery strap. This will eliminate the need for repeated removal and reapplication of tape when frequent repositioning of the Foley is necessary. To make the catheter strap, you will need two pieces of tape 10 × 10 cm (4 × 4 in.) and a 25-cm (10-in.) piece of twill tape.

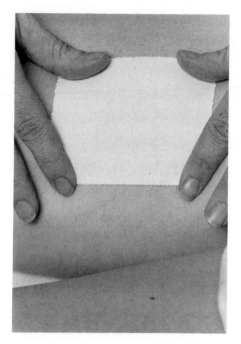

1 For a female client, adhere one of the tape squares to the medial thigh. Attach the tape to the anterior thigh or lower abdomen for male clients. Be sure to shave the site first, if necessary.

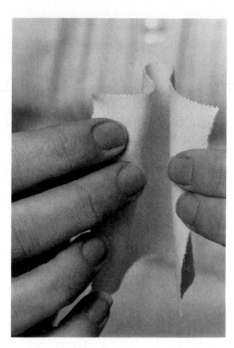

2 Fold the other square in half, so that the nonadhering surfaces face one another.

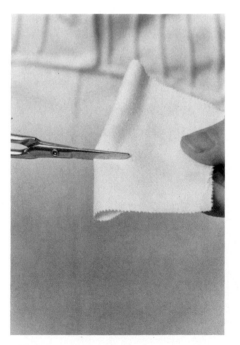

3 Cut two slits along the folded edge, 6 mm (¼ in.) in width and approximately 2.5 cm (1 in.) apart.

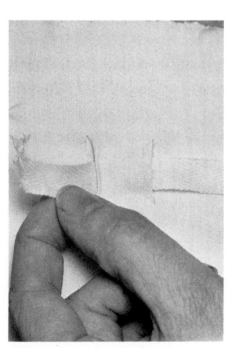

4 Unfold the tape and pull the twill tape through the slits.

(Continued on p. 452)

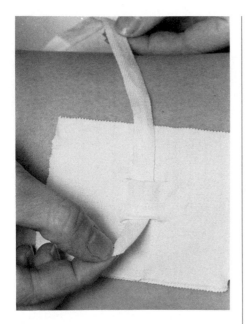

5 Adhere the second tape to the first, and pull the twill tape until it is at equal lengths on each side.

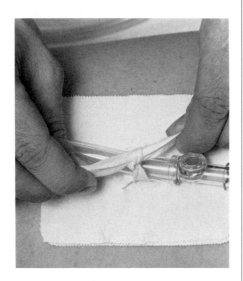

6 Position the drainage tubing over the twill tape and tie the tape around the tubing. When the outer tape square becomes soiled, you can easily replace it without removing the inner square, thus saving your client discomfort.

Obtaining a Urine Specimen

As you know, urine in the drainage bag is considered contaminated; disconnecting the catheter from the drainage tubing opens the system and increases the potential for infection. Therefore, urine samples for diagnostic testing must be obtained through a closed system, either through a sampling port or directly through the urinary catheter.

1 To obtain the specimen, you will need to clamp the drainage tubing for a few minutes (usually around 15) to allow the urine to collect in the catheter.

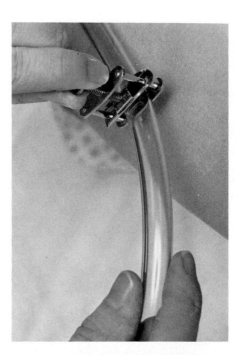

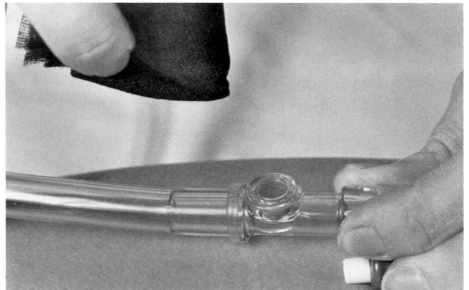

2 Wash your hands and cleanse the sampling port with an antimicrobial wipe. Allow it to dry.

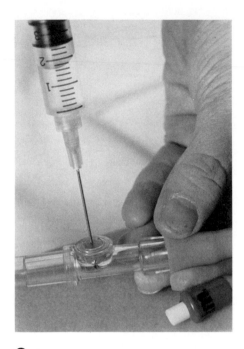

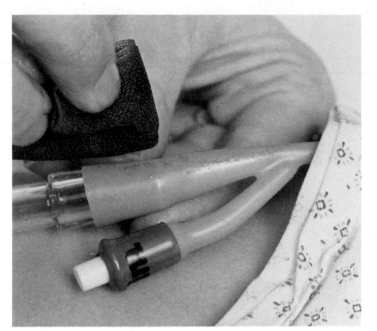

3 Aspirate the urine directly through the port, using a sterile needle and syringe. Usually, 2–3 mL will be adequate for a diagnostic test. Cleanse the sampling port again with an antimicrobial wipe.

4 If the catheter does not have a sampling port, cleanse the catheter just distal to the bifurcation.

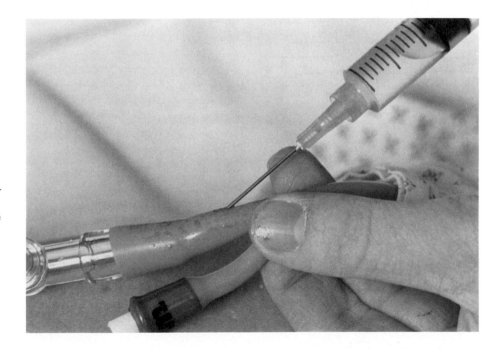

5 Using a 21–25-gauge needle and a sterile syringe, aspirate the urine through the catheter wall. Point the needle away from the bifurcation to prevent puncturing the balloon port and aspirating the balloon's contents. Remove the needle and cleanse the site again.

(Continued on p. 454)

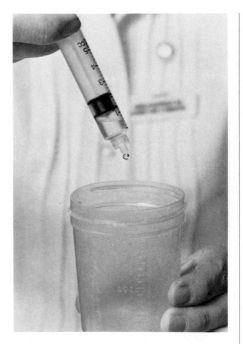

6 Inject the urine into a sterile specimen cup unless the syringe itself is to be sent to the laboratory. Label the specimen with the client's name, the time and date of collection, and note that it was obtained from the catheter. If you cannot send the specimen to the laboratory immediately, refrigerate it. Be sure that you have unclamped the catheter.

Emptying the Drainage Bag

The urinary drainage bag should be emptied every 8 hours, or more frequently during periods of large urinary output. This is essential in reducing the infection risk because urine that is allowed to stagnate is an excellent medium for bacterial growth.

1 To empty the bag, wash your hands; then position the client's measuring container under the spout. Detach the spout from its protective sleeve.

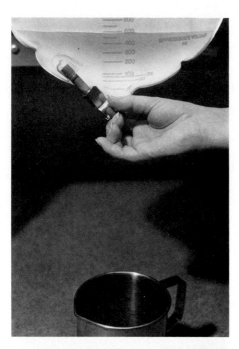

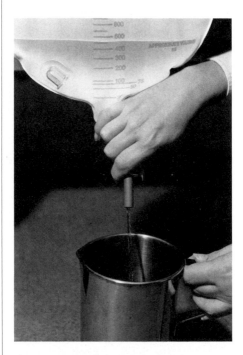

2 Open the clamp, allowing the entire contents to drain into the measuring container. To prevent contamination, do not touch the spout with your fingers or with the measuring container.

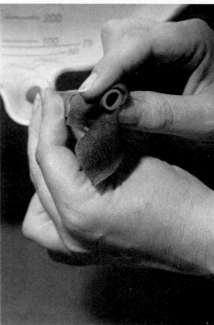

3 After emptying the drainage bag, clean the spout with an antiseptic wipe and reinsert it into its sleeve on the drainage bag. Measure and record the amount of urine. Empty and wash the measured container. Wash your hands.

Using a Urine Meter

When close and accurate monitoring of urinary output is necessary, for example, with clients in acute renal failure, obtain a urine meter with a drainage bag and attach it to your client's Foley catheter. The urine meter will enable you to measure minute quantities of urine, either hourly or during specified time intervals.

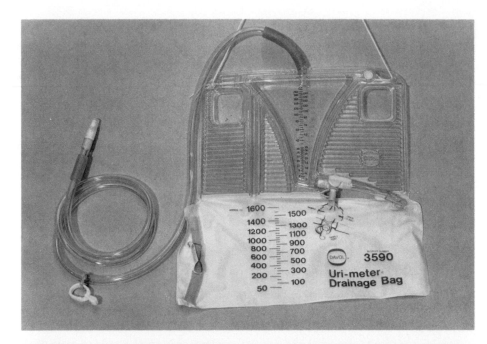

1 Wash your hands and explain the procedure to your client. Place a bed-saver pad under the catheter, and attach the urine meter to the bedside frame next to the Foley drainage bag. Secure the drainage tubing to the bed linen so that it will be readily accessible.

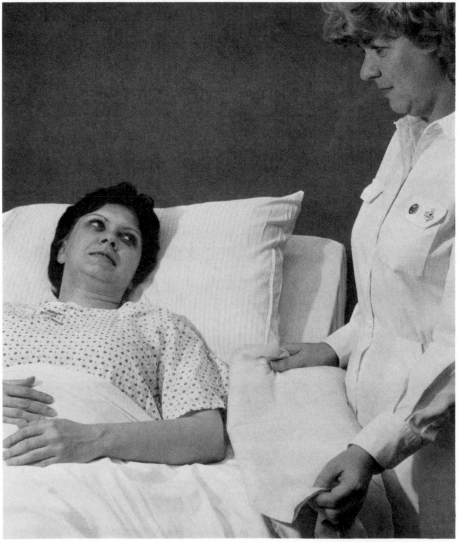

(Continued on p. 456)

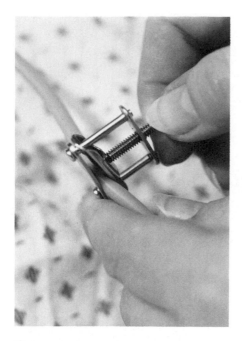

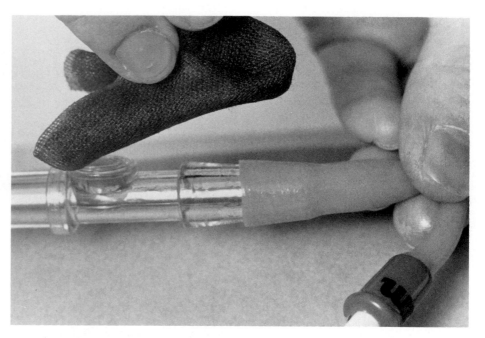

2 Straighten the drainage tubing to drain the urine into the drainage bag, and then clamp the catheter.

3 Thoroughly cleanse the connection site of the catheter and drainage tubing with an antiseptic wipe. Because it is sometimes difficult to manipulate the tubing without touching the ends, it may be a good idea to apply sterile gloves.

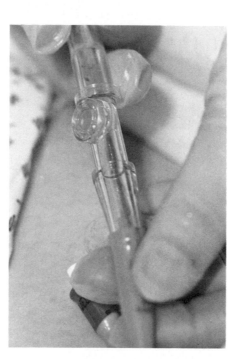

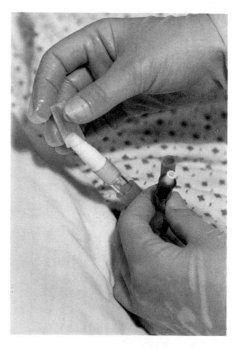

4 Aseptically detach the Foley drainage tubing from the catheter.

5 Remove the protective cap on the end of the urine meter drainage tubing, and aseptically insert the tubing into the catheter lumen. Unclamp the catheter and tape the drainage tubing to your client's thigh or abdomen. After measuring the output, discard the Foley drainage system.

6 Hourly, or during specified time intervals, straighten the drainage tubing and inspect the collection chamber to assess the amount of urine that has collected. Record the amount and open the stopcock to allow the urine to drain into the drainage bag. *Note: When the client no longer requires hourly urine checks, just keep the stopcock open to allow the urine to drain into the drainage bag. This will prevent reopening the system to attach a regular drainage bag, which could potentially contaminate both the system and the client's urinary tract.*

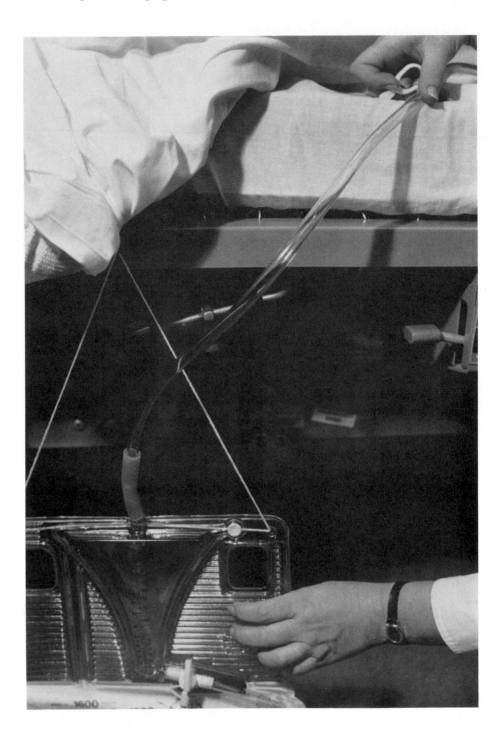

Irrigating the Catheter

Assessing

1 Because irrigating a catheter can greatly increase the risk of infection by opening a closed system, irrigation should not be performed unless you are certain the catheter is obstructed. Diminished urinary output is an unacceptable rationale for irrigation, unless it is accompanied by additional indications of obstruction (see step 2, facing page). Evaluate the integrity of the collection system by inspecting the drainage tubing for kinks or exterior obstructions. Evaluate your client's intake and compare it to the output. If you assess that your client might be dehydrated, increase the fluid intake and re-evaluate the output after 30–45 minutes. Because hypotension can also reduce urinary output, be sure to check the client's blood pressure.

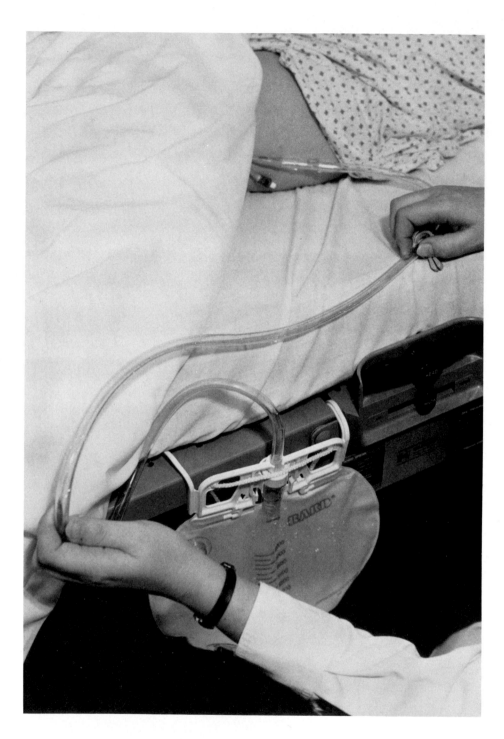

Planning

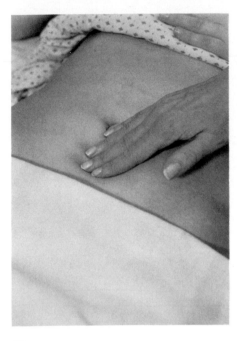

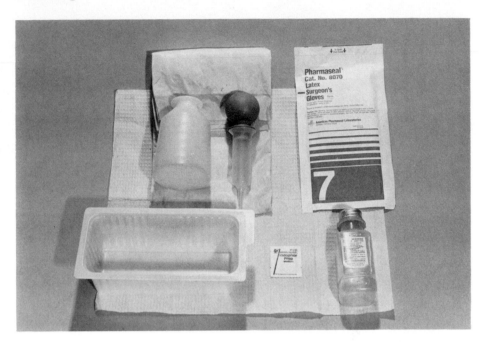

2 Inspect the suprapubic area and palpate or percuss your client's bladder. If the bladder is distended, the urinary output minimal (less than 30 mL/hr), blood clots are noted, urine is leaking around the catheter, or the client is experiencing bladder spasms, obtain an order for an irrigation.

3 Obtain a catheter irrigation kit or assemble the following *sterile* materials: underpad, for use as a sterile field and bed protector; drainage tray; graduated container; 50–60-mL bulb (*not* piston) syringe; gloves; an antiseptic wipe; and normal saline or the

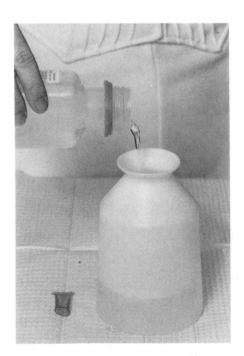

prescribed irrigant warmed to room temperature. You will also need a bedsaver pad. Remember to keep the following items sterile at all times: the open ends of both the drainage tubing and the catheter, the irrigant, and the syringe.

4 Wash your hands and explain the procedure to your client. After the client assumes a dorsal recumbent position, place a bedsaver pad under the Foley catheter. Aseptically open the irrigation tray, and place the underpad over a clean, dry surface to make a sterile field. Pour the sterile irrigant into the graduated container, and position the empty tray close to the client's perineum.

(Continued on p. 460)

Implementing

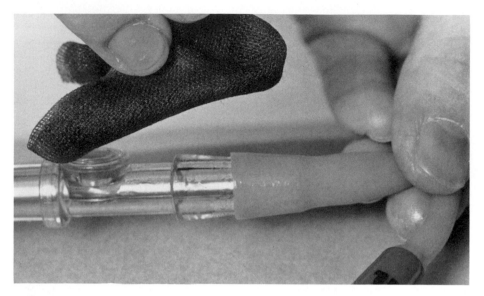

5 Clean the connection of the drainage tubing and catheter with an antiseptic wipe.

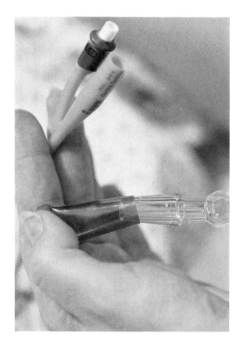

6 Disconnect the drainage tubing from the Foley. Keep the end of the drainage tubing sterile by capping it with a tube protector (as shown) or by attaching a sterile gauze pad and securing it with a rubber band. To keep the end of the catheter sterile, place it over the drainage tray so that it will be protected as you apply sterile gloves.

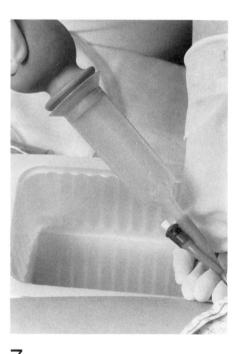

7 Put on sterile gloves and aspirate 30–50 mL of the sterile irrigant into the bulb syringe. Attach the syringe to the end of the catheter, and inject the irrigant gently by slowly squeezing the bulb of the syringe.

Evaluating

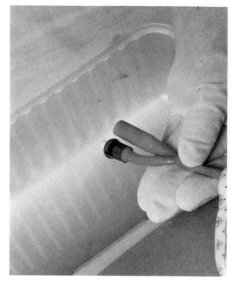

8 Remove the syringe and allow the irrigant to return into the drainage tray by gravity. After the irrigant has returned, and if it is indicated, repeat the irrigation process until the returns are clear. If the fluid fails to return, gently rotate the catheter between your fingers, press gently on the suprapubic area, or ask the client to perform a Valsalva maneuver or turn from side to side. If these measures fail to return the irrigant, apply gentle suction with the bulb. This might be necessary if blood clots are obstructing the catheter. Unless absolutely necessary, avoid aspiration with a piston syringe because vigorous suctioning can damage the bladder wall. Follow agency protocol for further intervention if you still are unable to return the irrigant. It may be necessary to reconnect the drainage tubing and closely observe the client for the next hour or two, assessing for continued indications of obstruction as well as for eventual gravity drainage, which may occur once bladder spasms cease. If the obstruction continues, notify the physician for further intervention such as changing the catheter.

Removing a Foley Catheter

When the physician has ordered the discontinuation of your client's Foley catheter, you will first need to deflate the balloon to allow the catheter to pass through the urethra.

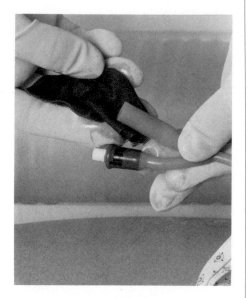

9 After completing the irrigation, clean the open end of the catheter with an antiseptic wipe.

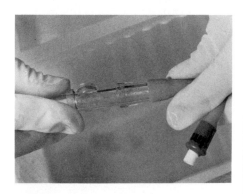

10 Grasp the drainage tubing, remove the protective cover, and aseptically connect the drainage tubing to the open end of the catheter. Assist the client into a comfortable position and remove the used equipment from the bedside. Measure the amount of the return and compare it to the amount that was instilled. Document the procedure, noting the amount and character of the return. Be certain to note the amount of residual irrigant on the intake and output record, as well. Continue to assess the client to ensure that there are no indications of bladder distention, spasms, or diminished urinary output.

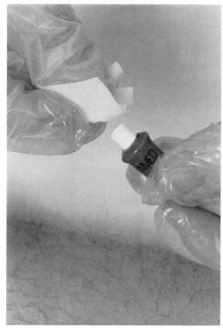

1 Place a bedsaver pad under your client's catheter and cleanse the balloon port with an antiseptic wipe. Untape the catheter from your client's thigh or abdomen.

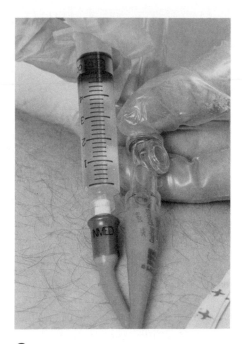

2 Attach a sterile syringe to the balloon port (some catheters may require both a syringe and a needle). Then aspirate the water. The amount required to inflate the balloon should be imprinted on the lumen of the balloon port. Be certain to aspirate the same amount of water that was injected after the catheter's insertion. When the water has been aspirated, pinch the catheter between your thumb and index finger to prevent urine from filling the urethra during the removal. Gently pull on the catheter to remove it from your client's bladder and urethra. If you are unable to withdraw the catheter, do not use force. Notify the physician, instead, for further intervention. Remove the catheter and drainage bag from the bedside and provide your client with povidone-iodine or soap and water for cleansing the meatus and perineum. Measure and document the output and record the procedure. During the first 24 hours following the removal of the Foley catheter, or according to agency protocol, document the time, amount, and character of each voiding.

Caring for Clients with Renal-Urinary Disorders

APPLYING AN EXTERNAL URINARY DEVICE (WITH A LEG DRAINAGE SYSTEM)

Assessing and Planning

When caring for male clients for whom the prolonged use of indwelling catheters may be contraindicated, you might assess the need for an external collection device such as the Hollister™ Male Urinary Collection System. Exdwelling catheters, also known as condom and Texas catheters, usually require a physician's order. Be sure to read manufacturer's instructions carefully before applying the exdwelling catheter used by your agency.

1 If an external urinary device has been prescribed for your client, explain the procedure and, if appropriate, prepare to instruct him in the application technique. Assemble the following equipment: leg drainage bag, extension tubing, leg straps, skin protector, and the exdwelling (condom) catheter.

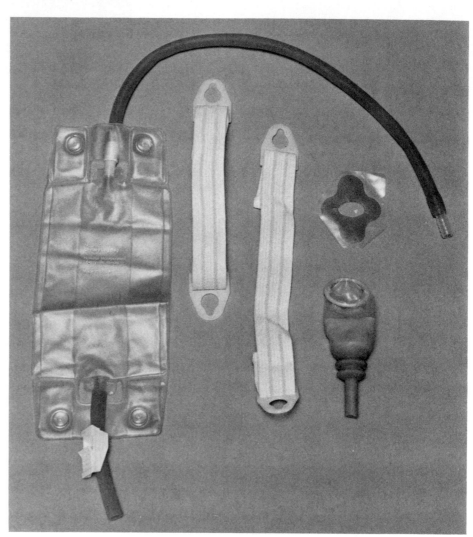

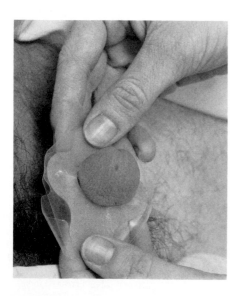

2 Wash your hands and begin the procedure by trimming or pushing the pubic hair away from the penis. It is seldom necessary to shave the hair, because hair that adheres to the sticky surface of the adhesive skin protector can be carefully pulled away. Gently pull the glans penis through the opening of the skin protector. The skin protector will stretch and yet rapidly retain its original shape without constricting the penis or losing its elasticity.

Implementing

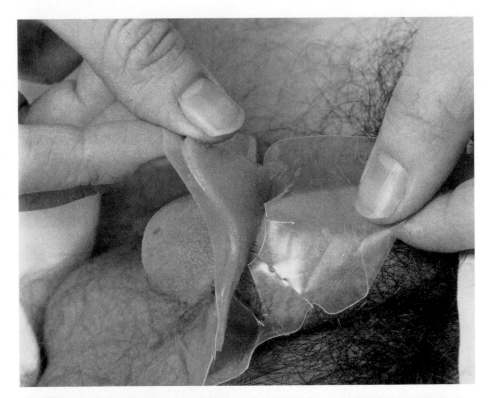

3 Pull off the protective film on the underside of the skin protector. Adhere the posterior surface of the skin protector to the shaft of the penis. Be certain that the pubic hair is pushed away first.

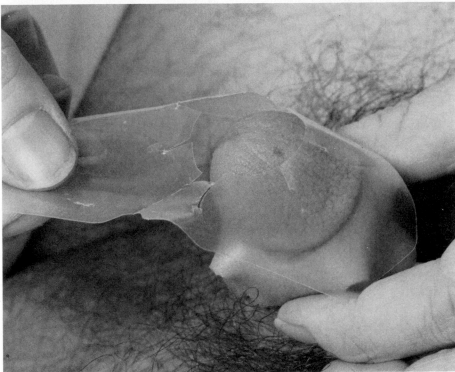

4 Remove the protective film from the anterior surface of the skin protector.

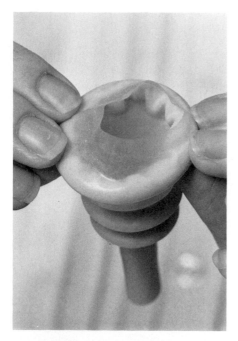

5 Roll the catheter until the inner flap is exposed. This is important because it is this flap that prevents the reflux of urine.

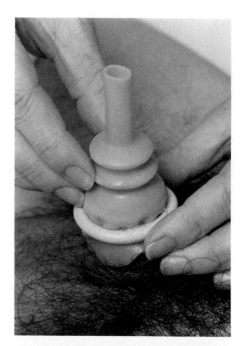

6 Position the catheter over the 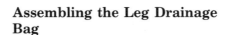 glans penis so that the opening of the inner flap surrounds the urethral meatus.

7 Carefully unroll the catheter with as little wrinkling as possible until it covers the skin protector. Gently press along the exterior of the catheter to adhere it to the skin protector. *Note: If more than a few wrinkles occur, do not attempt to reposition the catheter on the skin protector. See step 11 for removal instructions.*

Assembling the Leg Drainage Bag

8 After removing the drainage bag from its container, close the drain clamp at the bottom of the bag.

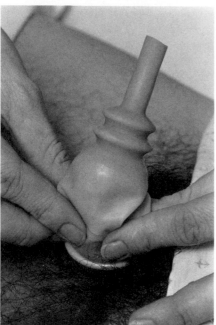

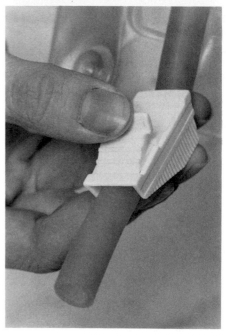

9 Position the bag at the medial aspect of the lower leg, and bring each strap around the leg, attaching them to the buttons on the drainage bag. Adjust each strap so that it securely attaches the drainage bag to the leg yet does not constrict circulation.

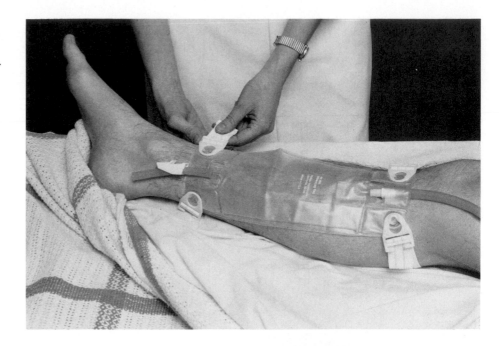

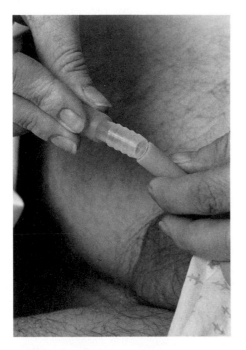

10 Attach the extension tubing to the external urinary device via the connector. The tubing should have enough slack so that it does not tug on the external catheter. For shorter clients, the tubing can be cut to ensure a good fit. Explain to the client that the drainage bag can be emptied by opening the drain clamp. Document the procedure. *Note: For nonambulatory clients, a closed drainage collection bag can be used instead.*

Evaluating

11 Periodically assess the skin under the straps for pressure areas or irritation, and ensure that the straps are not too tight by placing two fingers between the client's skin and the straps (as shown). Alert, mobile clients should be shown how to adjust the straps and to assess for the presence of leakage or irritation.

It is recommended that the catheter be changed daily. To remove the catheter, unroll it off the penis together with the skin protector. After removal, warm water can be used to remove any residue left by the skin protector.

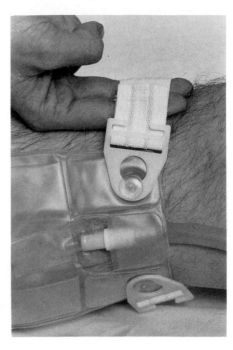

MONITORING THE CLIENT RECEIVING CONTINUOUS BLADDER IRRIGATION (CBI)

Establishing CBI

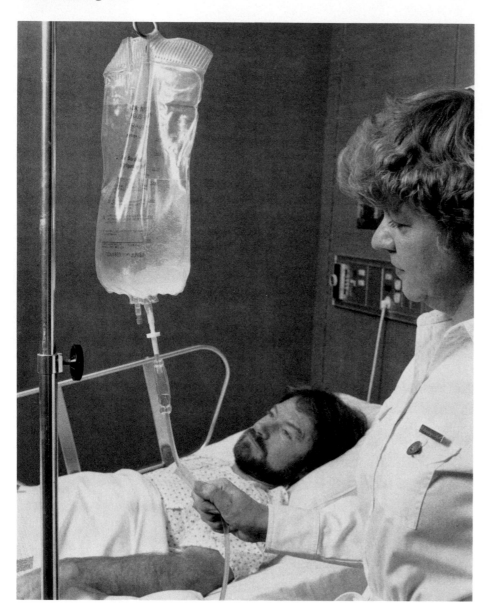

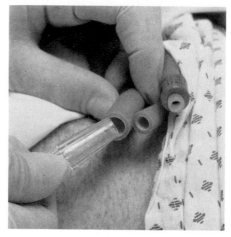

2 If the three-way catheter is not already attached to a large collection bag, you may need to detach the regular-sized collection bag and replace it with the large bag. To do this, briefly clamp the catheter, cleanse the large out-flow lumen with an antiseptic wipe, and aseptically attach the tubing for the large collection bag (as shown). Unclamp the catheter.

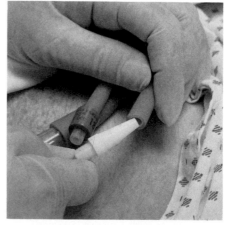

3 Cleanse the inflow lumen with an antiseptic wipe and aseptically insert the connector for the primed infusion tubing. Establish the prescribed flow rate and refer to the following guidelines for client care. Document the procedure.

1 If your client has had a transurethral prostatectomy, he might return from surgery with a three-way Foley catheter, which allows closed continuous bladder irrigation. The irrigation is usually performed for a 24-hour period, during which the client remains on bed rest. If the irrigation solution and drainage bag were not already connected in surgery, it might be your responsibility to assemble the equipment and establish the irrigation. Explain the procedure to your client and wash your hands. Obtain the prescribed irrigation solution (usually a glycine preparation), its special irrigation tubing, and a large (3000–4000 mL) collection bag (optional). Spike the solution container, hang it on an IV pole, and prime the tubing as you would an intravenous infusion set. Be certain to flush out all the air, and then clamp off the tubing.

Nursing Guidelines for the Care of Clients with Continuous Bladder Irrigation

- Unless otherwise prescribed, keep the client on bedrest during CBI (usually 24 hours).
- Moderate bleeding (pink to deep-pink returns) is normal. Bright red returns containing numerous blood clots are indicative of hemorrhage, and the physician should be alerted immediately.
- With normal hematuria, maintain the infusion rate of the irrigant at 40–60 drops/min. Increase the rate if the returns are a brighter red, and decrease the rate when the returns become more clear.
- Monitor the vital signs at least every 4 hours during the irrigation (every 15 minutes if they are unstable). Assess for these indicators of impending shock if the returns are bright red: hypotension, pallor, diaphoresis, and rapid pulse and respirations.
- To ensure that there is no obstruction, which can occur with blood clots, inspect the catheter for patency and assess the client's suprapubic area for distention. In addition, question the client regarding the presence of severe discomfort or recurring bladder spasms.
- Keep careful records of intake and output, subtracting the amount of irrigation solution from the total output to determine the true amount of urine production.
- Irrigate only if the catheter is obstructed and if you have a physician's order to do so.
- If the physician orders traction on the balloon portion of the catheter, maintain traction with tape or a gauze strip. The traction will keep the balloon wedged against the prostatic fossa to minimize bleeding.
- If it is not contraindicated, encourage a fluid intake of 2–3 L/day. Dilute urine has less potential for the growth of bacteria and the formation of encrustations.
- Provide the client with cranberry juice and other fluids high in ascorbic acid. Organisms do not grow well in acidic urine.
- When a glycine irrigating solution is used, assess for these signs of hyponatremia: muscle twitching, confusion, convulsions.

Nursing Guidelines for the Care of the Client with a Suprapubic Catheter

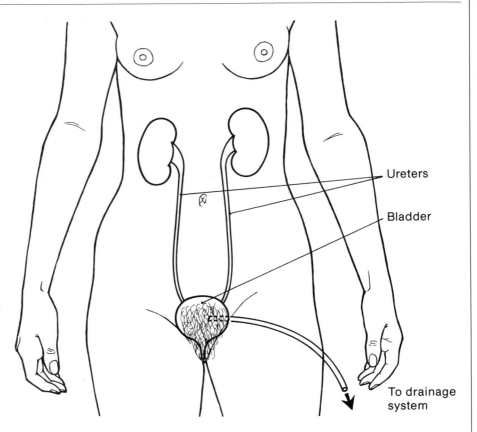

Ureters

Bladder

To drainage system

If your client is having bladder or prostatic surgery, a vaginal hysterectomy, or if the urethra is impassable, the physician might drain the bladder via an incision through the suprapubic area into the bladder. The catheter is then attached to a closed drainage collection container.

- To prevent dislodging, tape the tubing securely to the lateral abdomen.
- Should the catheter become dislodged, cover the site with a sterile dressing and inform the physician at once for immediate replacement.
- To prevent contamination from the backflow of urine, keep the drainage collection container below the level of the client's bladder.
- Slight hematuria is normal during the first 24–48 hours postinsertion. Bright red drainage is abnormal and should be reported immediately. Be sure to document the character and amount of drainage. It should normally have a characteristic urine odor. Foul-smelling, cloudy urine or drainage is indicative of an infection.
- Keep drainage records from the suprapubic catheter separate from those of other indwelling catheters or tubes.
- Inspect the catheter for patency, and prevent external obstruction. Irrigate only if an internal obstruction is noted, following the procedure, pp. 458–461.

- Assess the dressing for drainage and change it as soon as it becomes wet, using aseptic technique. Because it contains urine, a saturated dressing can lead to skin breakdown. Consider applying a pectin wafer skin barrier around the catheter insertion site to protect the skin.
- Encourage a fluid intake of at least 2–3 L/day. Dilute urine minimizes the potential for infection and encrustations.
- Promote cranberry juice and fluids high in ascorbic acid. An acidic urine minimizes the potential for bacterial growth.
- Prior to removal, the physician will order the catheter clamped for 3–4 hours at a time to test the client's ability to void spontaneously. After the client has voided, unclamp the catheter and measure the residual urine in the collection container. Notify the physician when the residual urine is less than 100 mL after each of two successive voidings. Usually the catheter then can be removed safely.

Nursing Guidelines for the Care of the Client with a Nephrostomy Tube

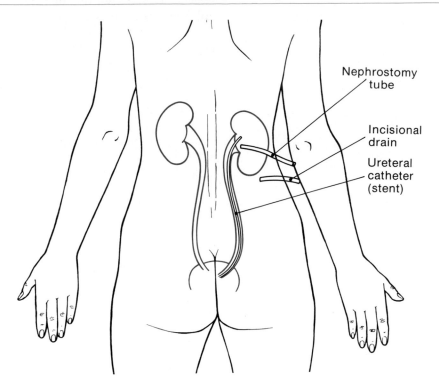

Nephrostomy tube

Incisional drain

Ureteral catheter (stent)

A nephrostomy tube might be inserted for your client who has a ureteral obstruction, a nephrolithotomy, pyeloplasty, or nephrostomy. The tube is either inserted under fluoroscopy, eliminating any incision, or it is inserted directly into the renal pelvis via an incision in the flank and anchored in place with one or more sutures. The tube is then connected to a closed drainage collection container. Ureteral catheters (stents) and drains might also be inserted (as shown).

■ To prevent the tube from becoming dislodged, tape it securely to the client's flank. Elastic tape works especially well. Unless otherwise ordered, keep the client on bed rest.

■ Should the tube become dislodged, cover the site with a sterile dressing and notify the physician at once for immediate replacement.

■ To prevent infection from reflux, keep the drainage collection container below the level of the client's kidney at all times.

■ Monitor and record the character and amount of drainage in the collection container. Some hematuria is normal during the first and second day postinsertion; bright red drainage is abnormal and should be reported to the physician immediately. An abrupt cessation in urine is indicative of a dislodged catheter.

■ During the first 24 hours postinsertion, monitor the client for indications of hemorrhage: decrease in blood pressure, rapid pulse and respirations, and copious amounts of bright red drainage. Also assess for these indicators of infection: increase in temperature, chills, foul-smelling and cloudy urine in the collection container.

- To reduce the risk of infection, keep the drainage system closed at all times unless you have a physician's *specific* order for irrigation.
- If irrigation has been prescribed, instill a maximum of 5 mL of irrigant at one time into the tube. The average renal pelvis can hold no more than 5 mL of fluid. Greater amounts, resulting in overdistention, can damage the kidney. To instill the irrigant into the tube, it may be necessary to attach a male adaptor to a 5-mL syringe (as shown).

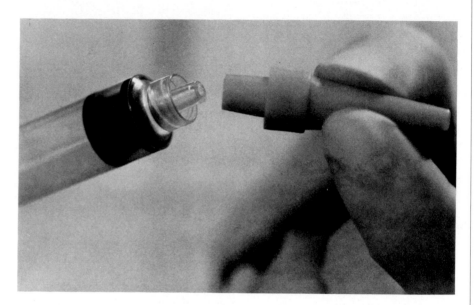

- Assess the dressing for excessive drainage and the insertion site for leakage around the tube. Either problem is indicative of a tube that is dislodged or obstructed. To prevent skin breakdown from the highly irritating urine, change the dressing before it becomes saturated.
- Because pyelonephritis can result from an infection, *always* use aseptic technique for dressing changes and irrigation.
- If a urethral catheter is also indwelling, monitor and record the drainage from the nephrostomy tube separate from that of the urethral catheter.
- To minimize the potential for infection and the formation of calculi, encourage a fluid intake of at least 2–3 L/day.
- Promote the intake of cranberry juice and other fluids high in ascorbic acid. An acidic urine is less likely to promote bacterial growth.
- Once ureteral patency has been determined, the physician might order the nephrostomy tube clamped before removal to ensure client tolerance. During the clamping period, assess the client for the presence of flank pain, fever, or for a diminished urinary output. These are indications of ureteral obstruction.

ADMINISTERING A SODIUM POLYSTYRENE SULFONATE (KAYEXALATE) ENEMA

Sodium polystyrene sulfonate is a sodium resin, which exchanges sodium for potassium in the gastrointestinal tract for clients with hyperkalemia. It is frequently given with sorbitol, which because of its hypertonicity induces diarrhea. This facilitates expulsion and prevents reabsorption of the potassium.

1 If your client has hyperkalemia, which could be caused by a diminished urinary output, acid–base imbalance, or cellular breakdown, the physician might prescribe sodium polystyrene sulfonate. However, if the client is unable to tolerate it orally because of nausea and vomiting or diminished bowel sounds, it will be necessary to administer it rectally. Assemble the following materials to administer the enema: the prescribed amounts of sodium polystyrene sulfonate and sorbitol; one or more 50-mL piston syringes, depending on the prescribed amounts to be administered; water-soluble lubricant; a hemostat or tubing clamp; clean glove; a container for mixing the enema solution; a rectal tube with an inflatable balloon; a device for inflating the balloon such as a sphygmomanometer bulb; and a kit for administering a cleansing tap water enema after the client has expelled the sodium polystyrene sulfonate. In addition, you will need a bedsaver pad and a bedpan at the client's bedside, unless your client is able to walk to the bathroom. Mix the prescribed amounts of sodium polystyrene sulfonate with the sorbitol and aspirate or pour the solution into the piston syringe(s). If it is too thick for an easy administration, dilute it slightly with water.

Assessing and Planning

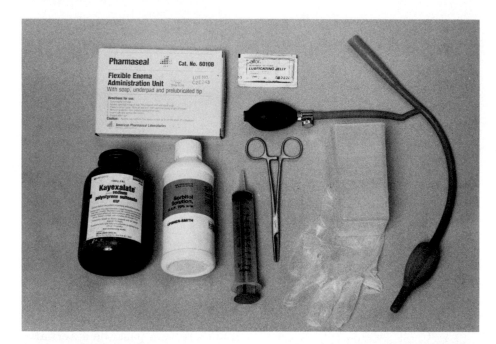

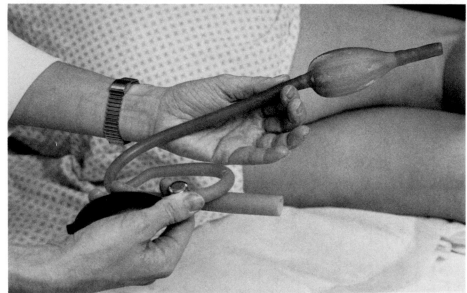

2 Review the procedure in Chapter 5 for administering a retention enema. Wash your hands and explain the procedure to the client. Assist her into a left side-lying (Sim's) position and place a bedsaver pad under the buttocks. Assess the integrity of the balloon at the end of the rectal tube: compress the inflating bulb and count the number of compressions that are needed to inflate the balloon to two-thirds of its capacity. Make a note of that number. *Caution: To prevent injury to the rectal tissue, never inflate the balloon more than two-thirds of its capacity once it is in the rectum.*

Implementing

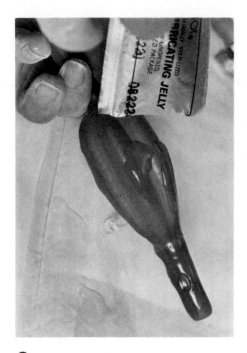

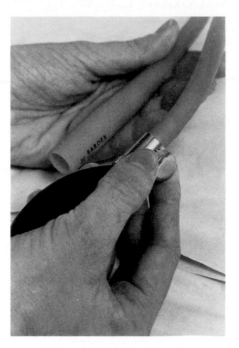

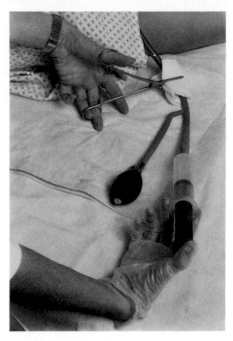

3 Generously lubricate the tip and balloon of the rectal tube with water-soluble lubricant. Be sure that the balloon is completely collapsed.

4 Put on a clean glove and insert the deflated balloon into the client's rectum past the external and internal sphincters. Inflate the balloon, compressing the bulb the same number of times required to inflate it to two-thirds of its capacity (see step 2, p. 472). Inflating the balloon will help the client retain the solution. Pull back gently on the rectal tube to ensure that the balloon is properly inflated and cannot be pulled past the sphincters.

5 Attach the piston syringe containing the solution to the open end of the rectal tube. Position the opened hemostat around the area you will later clamp. Administer the medication in a bolus, clamp the tubing, and remove the empty syringe. Either attach another syringe containing the solution or maintain the clamped tubing for 30–45 minutes, or the prescribed amount of time, until the client is allowed to expel the solution. Be reassuring and periodically advise the client of the time remaining until the solution can be expelled.

Evaluating

6 When the retention time has expired, unclamp the tubing, deflate the balloon, and remove the tube from the client's rectum. The client may then expel the solution. If the client is ambulatory, ask to see the returns in the toilet. Otherwise, assist the client onto the bedpan. After the expulsion, administer cleansing tap water enemas until the returns are clear and no longer brown. Provide materials for cleansing the rectal area, and assist the client into a position of comfort. Document the procedure and its results. Continue to assess the client for indications of hyperkalemia: weakness, cramps, twitching, diarrhea.

PERFORMING THE CREDÉ MANEUVER

Manual pressure applied to the bladder, the *Credé* maneuver, can be employed to facilitate the removal of urine for clients whose bladders are irreversibly flaccid, for example clients with hypotonic neurogenic bladders. The procedure should not be performed without a physician's order. It is contraindicated for clients with especially strong sphincter resistance because the high intravesical pressure it produces can potentially result in ureteral reflux and infection (Lerner and Khan 1982:424).

Assessing and Planning

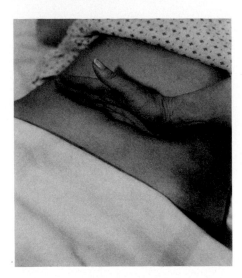

1 Usually the procedure is performed every 4–6 hours to prevent the bladder from becoming overly distended. However, you should periodically assess your client's bladder for distention during the interim periods. When the bladder is full, provide privacy and assist a female client onto a bedpan or provide a urinal for your male client. Clients with arm and hand strength and mobility should be taught to use the maneuver as an alternative to self-catheterization. When the client is in a comfortable position, place the ulnar surface of your hand at the umbilicus.

Evaluating

3 Percuss the client's bladder to ensure that all the urine has been removed. If you elicit dull sounds, you must repeat the procedure until all urine has been expressed. This will help prevent urinary tract infections caused by residual urine. If you elicit tympanic, hollow sounds, assume that the bladder is empty. Remove the urinal or bedpan and assist the client into a position of comfort. Document the procedure.

Implementing

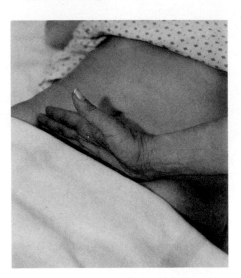

2 Instruct the client to bear down with the abdominal muscles, if possible. Press downward and sweep your hand onto the suprapubic area, using a kneading motion to initiate urination. Continue the maneuver every 30 seconds until urination ceases.

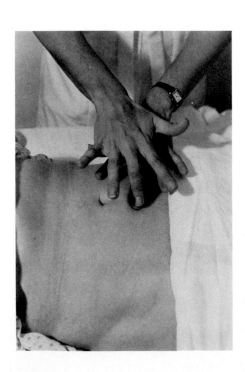

Caring for Clients with Urinary Diversions

Nursing Guidelines to Common Types of Urinary Diversions

Ileal Conduit (Also Called Ileal Loop, Bricker's Loop, Ileal Bladder)

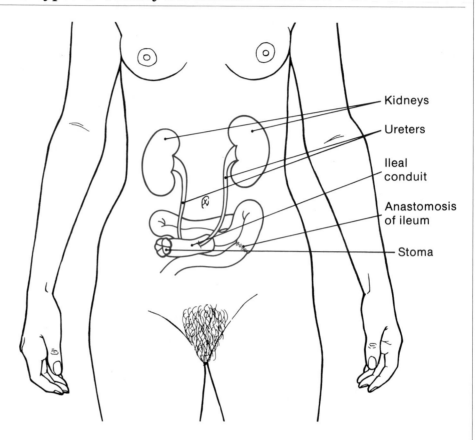

Kidneys

Ureters

Ileal conduit

Anastomosis of ileum

Stoma

Description	A 15–20-cm (6–8-in.) segment of the ileum is removed to function as a pipeline for the urine. The ureters are then detached from the bladder, shortened, and anastomosed to the ileum. The ileal segment is brought out through the abdomen where it forms a stoma. Urine then flows from the kidneys through the ureters and out through the ileal conduit and stoma. The intestine is anastomosed and it continues to function normally.
Indications	Bladder malignancy, congenital anomalies, intractable incontinence, chronic urinary tract infections, neurogenic bladder.
Nursing Considerations	*Note: You can also follow these guidelines for clients who have had colon conduits.*

- The continuous flow of urine requires the constant use of an appliance.
- Mucus can normally be found in the urine because of the nature of the ileal segment that is used.
- If the client has had bladder cancer, a cystectomy will also have been performed, as well as a prostatectomy for the male client.

(Continued on p. 476)

- An indwelling urethral catheter (drain) might be inserted to drain mucus and to minimize the potential for infection. When the client has had a cystectomy, do *not* irrigate the catheter because doing so could result in peritonitis.
- Ureteral stents might also be inserted temporarily to anchor the ureteral-ileal attachment and to prevent the leakage of urine. These stents also drain into the appliance (pouch), and are usually removed on the fifth to seventh postoperative day.
- Inspect the incisional dressing at least every 4 hours and change it as soon as it is wet, using aseptic technique. Change the dressing carefully to prevent disruption of the drains.
- Assess for indications of a urinary tract infection: chills, increased temperature, flank pain, hematuria.
- See the following procedures for more information on the care of clients with ileal conduits.

Cutaneous Ureterostomy

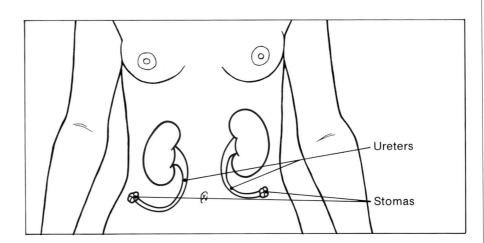

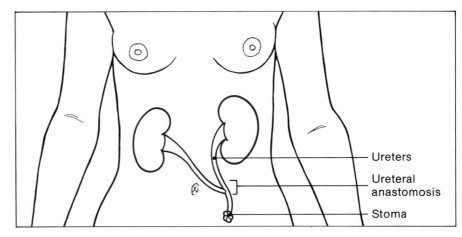

Description

The ureters are resected from the bladder and one or both then are brought directly through the abdominal wall. Although it is more common for the client to have two stomas requiring the use of two appliances, one ureter might be joined to the other inside the body, resulting in one stoma. Usually the ureters are sutured flush with the skin without a protruding stoma.

Indications:	This is an older method of urinary diversion and one that is employed less frequently than the ileal conduit. It is indicated for clients with intractable incontinence, bladder malignancies, and other urinary conditions in which the more complicated surgeries involving intestinal resections are contraindicated. This is often a temporary procedure, for example, with the child for whom later reversal is intended, or it is employed for clients whose life expectancy is minimal.
Nursing Considerations	(Also see the guidelines for the ileal conduit)

- Because the stoma is small and flush with the skin, fitting the appliance will be difficult. Extra care must be taken to prevent urine leakage and skin breakdown.
- Mucus particles in the collection system are abnormal because an intestinal segment is not used.
- If the client has an indwelling urethral catheter for draining blood and mucus from the diseased bladder, hand irrigate *only* if ordered.
- Carefully assess the client for these indicators of ureteral and stomal stenosis: oliguria, anuria, and/or a stomal retraction. If stenosis does occur, irreversible damage to the urinary tract may result.

Ureterosigmoidostomy

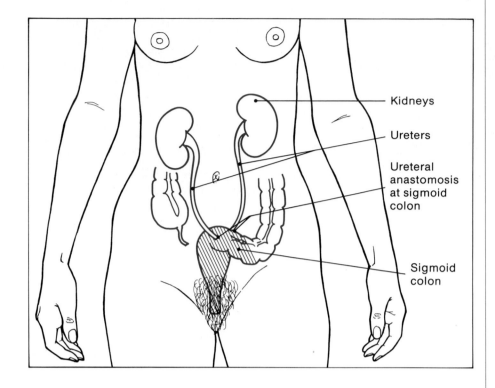

Kidneys

Ureters

Ureteral anastomosis at sigmoid colon

Sigmoid colon

Description

The ureters are resected from the bladder and anastomosed to the sigmoid colon for drainage through the rectum so that both stool and urine will be evacuated from the rectum.

Indications

Same as for an ileal conduit or cutaneous ureterostomy; however, this procedure is used more frequently for children or for adults who are psychologically incapable of accepting a stoma.

Nursing Considerations

- Be especially alert to the following indicators of urinary tract infection, which are more frequently seen with this procedure because of potential reflux of fecal material into the urinary tract: chills, increase in temperature, flank pain, hematuria.
- Keep the various drainage tubes separate and well labeled to facilitate careful monitoring of the amount and character of the drainage from each—for example, "left ureteral catheter," "right ureteral catheter," "rectal tube," and "urethral catheter," if appropriate.
- Assess for problems such as gross hematuria and a sudden decrease in drainage from each tube. Expect to see clear to amber urine from the ureteral catheters (stents) and fecal-stained and/or blood-tinged drainage from the rectal tube.
- Hand irrigate the rectal tube *only* with a specific order to do so, instilling not more than 30 mL of normal saline under gentle pressure. Only a physician should change the rectal tube during the first 4 postoperative days.
- After the removal of the rectal tube and ureteral catheters, encourage the client to evacuate the rectum at a minimum of every 4 hours to prevent the absorption of urinary electrolytes through the colonic mucosa. Failure to evacuate the urine could result in

hyperchloremic acidosis or hypokalemia, as evidenced by nausea, vomiting, increased temperature, lethargy, and weakness.

■ Prior to discharge, instruct the client in rectal tube self-insertion for the drainage of urine during the night. *Caution: Never insert the tube more than 10 cm (4 in.) because the ureteral attachment to the colon is usually 15–20 cm (6–8 in.) from the anus.*

■ Meticulous perianal care is crucial to prevent skin breakdown from the drainage of both urine and feces.

■ Assess for indications of leakage of urine at the attachment of the ureters to the colon: abdominal distention, paralytic ileus, abdominal discomfort, oliguria. The physician should be notified immediately if these occur.

■ Teach the client about diets free of gas-forming foods to minimize flatulence, which can result in fecal and urinary incontinence.

■ Encourage an intake of a minimum of 2–3 L/day to keep the urinary tract well irrigated.

PERFORMING A POSTOPERATIVE ASSESSMENT

1 Regardless of the type of urinary diversion surgery that was performed, the postoperative assessment of your urostomy client will be basically the same. Explain to the client that you will be assessing his stoma and the area surrounding it (the peristomal area), the amount and character of the urine, and the integrity of the stomal sutures. Remember that your positive and reassuring attitude is crucial both to the client's acceptance of the surgery and to his altered body appearance and function.

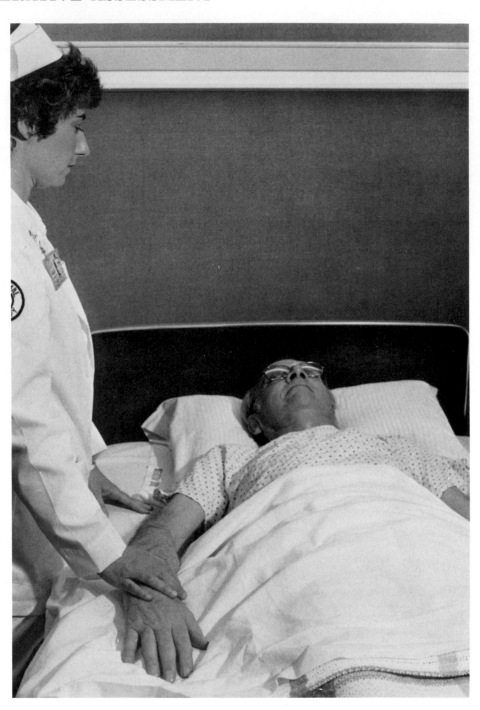

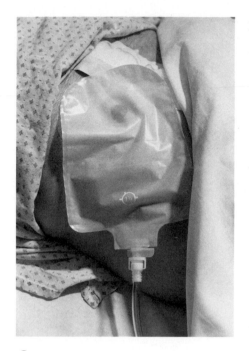

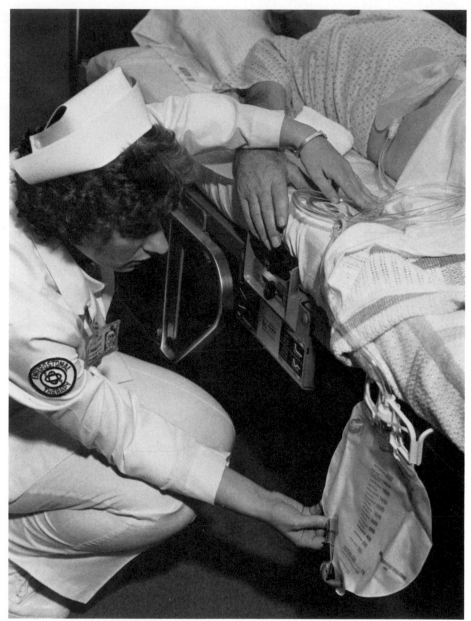

2 Raise the client's gown to expose the pouch, and place a bedsaver pad under the involved flank to protect the bed linen. As you do this, place your hand under the client's back to check for dampness, which could indicate that the pouch is leaking urine. Note that the postoperative pouch angles toward the side of the bed. This makes it accessible to the nurse and enterostomal therapist and facilitates its connection to a urinary drainage bag while the client is on bed rest. Inspect the area around the pouch's attachment to the faceplate to ensure that leakage has not occurred. Ask the client if he is experiencing itching or burning, which are signs of leakage. If either has occurred, the pouch must be changed and replaced with one that fits correctly. Otherwise, your client can continue to wear the same pouch for 3–4 days.

3 Inspect the drainage bag to ensure that urine is flowing adequately and that the output is comparable to the client's intake of fluids. Optimally, the output will be around 1500 mL/day. A diminished production of urine might be caused by reduced intake, urinary blockage, or kidney failure. An absence of urine can be indicative of a leak in the conduit system or a blockage of the ureters, and could necessitate a return to surgery. Also note the character of the urine. If your client has an ileal conduit, the urine might contain mucus because of the nature of the intestine that was used to form the conduit. This is normal. The urine may be dark in color if the client is taking antibiotics, is dehydrated, or has impaired liver function. Be sure to report immediately abnormal quantities of blood. Some postoperative hematuria is not unusual, but it should gradually decrease.

(Continued on p. 482)

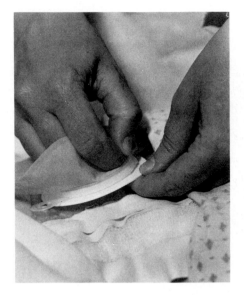

4 To inspect the stoma, slip your fingers under the faceplate to anchor it in place, and grasp the tab with your other hand. Be sure to have a clean cloth or gauze pad available to absorb the urine after the pouch has been opened.

5 To detach the pouch from the faceplate, lift up on the tab. When the area has been dried, assess the stoma. It should be pink or red, similar in color to the mucosal lining of the mouth. Slight bleeding may be normal due to the large number of capillaries in the area. Note whether the stoma is flush with the skin or protruding; assess the degree of edema, if present. Explain to the client that the stoma will continue to decrease in size over the next 6–8 weeks, and this will necessitate frequent stomal measurements to ensure a properly fitting pouch and skin barrier. Make sure the opening in the skin barrier is the exact measurement of the stoma. It should touch the stoma on all sides. Finally, inspect the sutures to make sure they are intact. Replace the pouch, wash your hands, and document your observations.

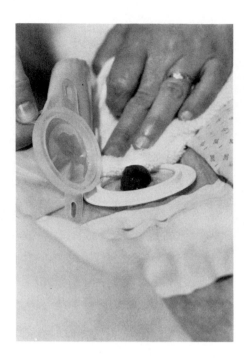

MANAGING APPLIANCE CARE

Applying a Postoperative (Disposable) Pouch

Assessing and Planning

1 A disposable pouch is usually applied on the client's third or fourth postoperative day. Many clients choose to wear disposable pouches after their discharge rather than change to reusable (permanent) pouches, which are described in the next procedure. The materials used for disposable pouches will vary from agency to agency. The following is a general procedure for pouch application and it should include these materials or a variation of the same: a measuring guide, a disposable pouch, tape (optional), a skin barrier such as a pectin wafer, a skin preparation to protect the skin from a reaction to

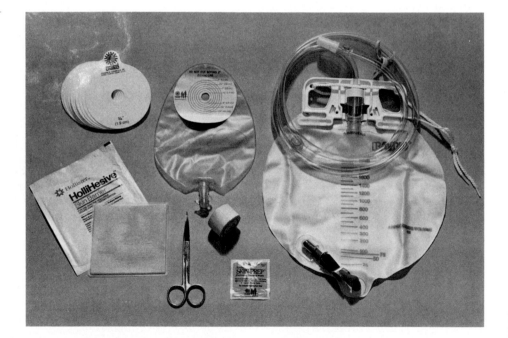

the tape if it is used, and scissors. In addition, a urine collection bag can be used during the night, or while the client is on bed rest. Be sure to stock the client's bedside stand with plenty of clean cloths or gauze pads, and bed-saver pads. If you will use tape to reinforce the seal of the pouch, cut four strips approximately 10 cm (4 in.) in length.

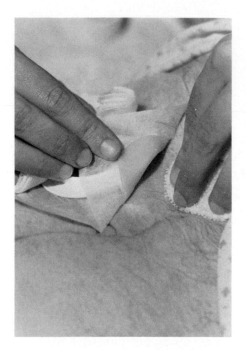

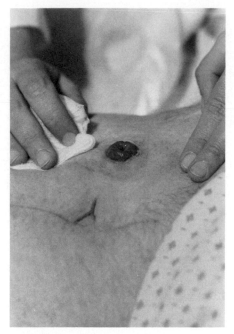

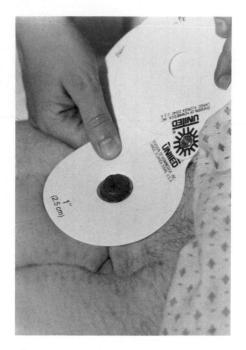

2 Explain the procedure to the client and lower the head of the bed to decrease the angle at the peristomal area, but do encourage the client to inspect the stoma and ask questions during the procedure. This procedure can also be used for client teaching. Place a bed-saver pad under the involved flank to protect the bed linen, and have clean cloths, gauze pads, toilet paper, or tampons accessible for absorbing the urine. Remove the pouch by following steps 4–5 in the preceding procedure. Then moisten a cloth with warm water and lift up the uppermost inside corner of the skin barrier. Place the moist cloth at the loosened corner and gently depress sections of the skin as you peel back the adhesive material. The moist cloth will help loosen the adhesive and facilitate its removal as quickly and painlessly as possible.

3 When you have removed the skin barrier and faceplate, inspect the stoma and peristomal area. Assess for irritation, allergic reactions to the tape or adhesive, weeping, or inflamed hair follicles (folliculitis). If the opening of the skin barrier is too large and allows seepage of urine onto the peristomal area, you might see an alkaline encrustation that consists of white crystalline deposits. Hyperplasia, which is a very tender area of thickened skin, can also result from prolonged exposure to urine, especially if the urine is alkaline. Clean the skin with a warm, wet cloth. If you use soap, it must be nonoily, (for example, Ivory), because oily soaps will leave a residue, which can prevent the proper adherence of the pouch. Ask the client to hold a rolled gauze pad, toilet paper, cloth, or tampon over (but not in) the stoma to absorb the urine.

4 Measure the stoma with the measuring guide.

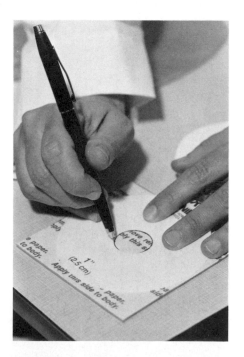

Implementing

5 Trace the outline of the measured stoma on the back of the pectin wafer skin barrier. If the stoma is irregular in shape, you will need to customize the pattern to fit the shape of the stoma.

(Continued on p. 484)

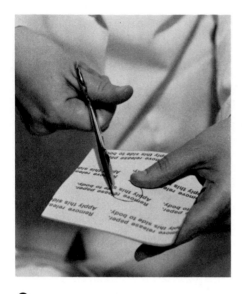

6 Cut out the circle (or shape) you have traced.

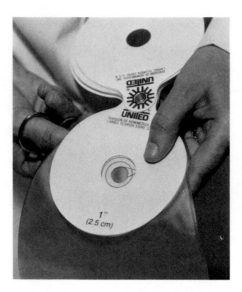

7 Place the same measuring guide over the adhesive paper backing on the pouch and add another ¼ in. to the stomal measurement. By making the pouch opening slightly larger than that of the skin barrier, you will ensure an adequate seal to prevent leakage.

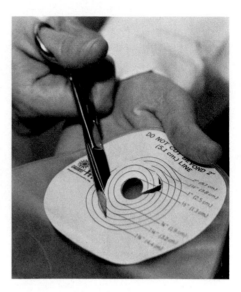

8 Carefully cut along the outline on the adhesive backing, making sure you do not puncture the pouch. *Note: To avoid cutting the pouch, place a small finger through the hole in the adhesive backing, and lift up on the area to be cut.*

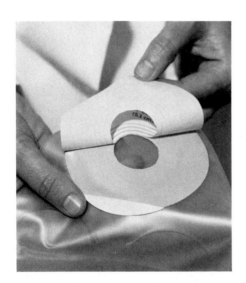

9 Remove the protective paper backing from the pouch.

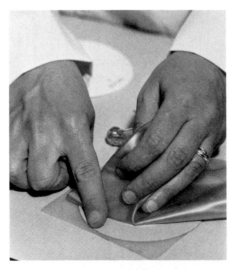

10 Adhere the sticky surface of the pouch to the front surface of the skin barrier (the side that is *not* covered by the protective paper backing). Press around the attached surfaces in a circular fashion.

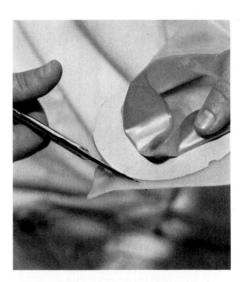

11 Once the pouch has been securely anchored to the skin barrier, trim the skin barrier to the exact size and shape of the adhesive disk on the back of the pouch. This will allow a smaller and neater adhesive area, reducing the potential for irritation.

Ap

Ass

1

disp
the
ity
sha
how
cate
the
hel
assi
othe
ton
adh
resu
Jac
pou
exp
age
que
com
app
cha
foll
ing.

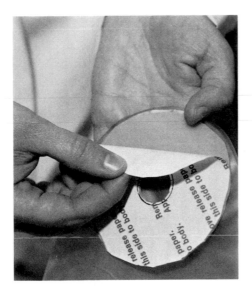

12 Remove the protective paper backing from the skin barrier.

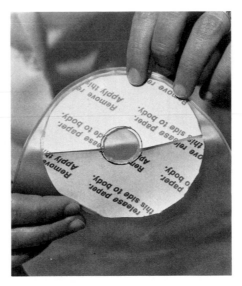

13 Cut the paper in half and reattach it to the skin barrier. This will enable you to attach the skin barrier to the client's skin in two steps, which will help to ensure a smoother, more secure fit.

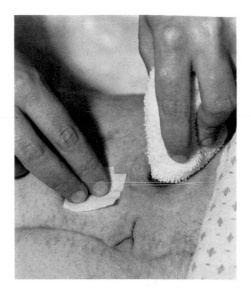

14 If you plan to reinforce the pouch with tape, prepare the periphery of the peristomal skin with a skin preparation before applying the skin barrier and pouch. This will help to prevent a skin reaction to the tape. Be sure to let the skin dry thoroughly before applying the skin barrier and pouch. *Caution: Do not apply a skin protector to skin that is broken or irritated.*

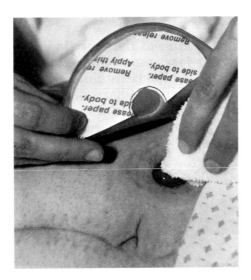

15 Remove the bottom half of the protective paper backing and position the pouch so that the opening is directly over the stoma. While the client is on bed rest, angle the tail of the pouch toward the side of the bed (as shown). Then adhere that section of the barrier and pouch to the client's skin.

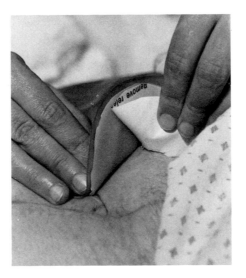

16 Remove the top half of the protective paper backing.

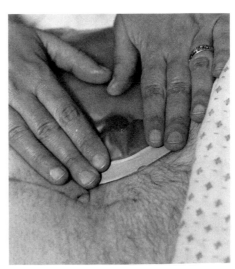

17 Securely adhere that section to the client's skin by gently pressing around the periphery with your fingertips. The warmth of your hands will enhance the seal.

(Continued on p. 486)

9 Another exercise for evaluating both wrist and hand flexors is to have the client tightly grip your index and middle fingers. Assess the strength of both hands and compare the strength of one to the other. The dominant hand might normally be stronger.

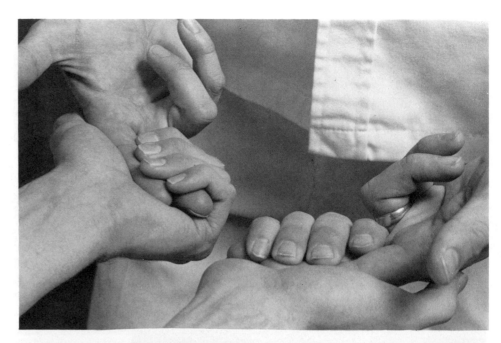

10 When the client has assumed a supine position, closely observe his ability to flex each hip. Instruct him to alternately pull each bent knee in toward his chest. Optimally, the opposite hip will remain extended as the other flexes.

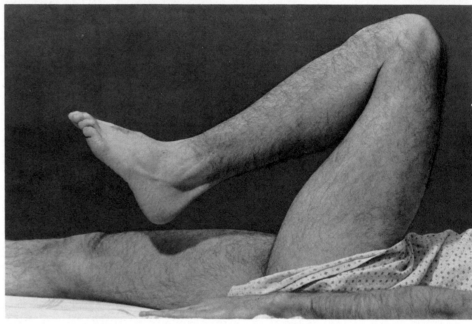

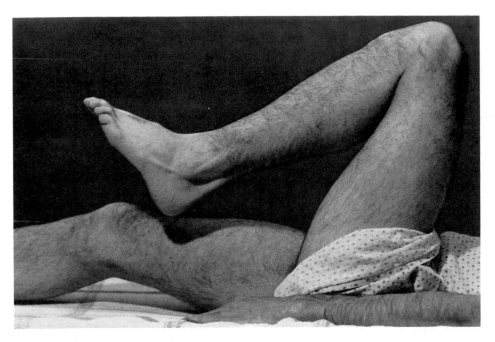

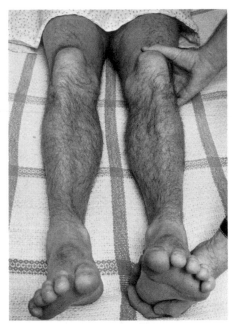

11 If the opposite hip also flexes (as shown) the client has a positive Thomas test, which is indicative of a flexion contracture of that hip. *Note: With the client in this position, you can easily test* *the strength of the knee extensors (quadriceps) by holding the client's knee into his chest as he attempts to extend his hip*. Repeat the assessment on the client's opposite side.

12 If it has been necessary for you to perform passive ROM on the hip joints, evaluate the strength of the hip abductor muscles by holding the client's leg at the midline as he attempts to abduct it.

13 Evaluate the hip adductor muscles by holding the client's leg in the abducted position as he attempts to adduct the leg back to the midline.

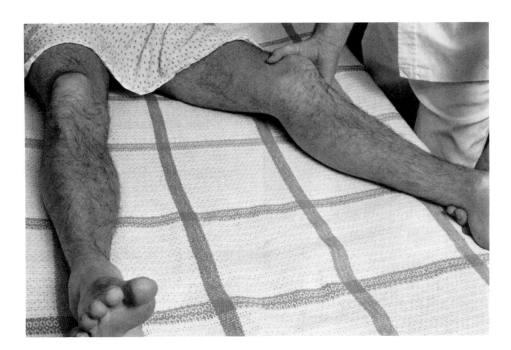

(Continued on p. 516)

Wrapping a Joint

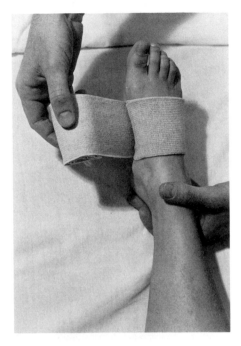

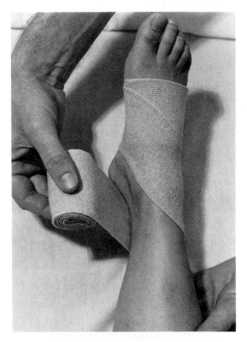

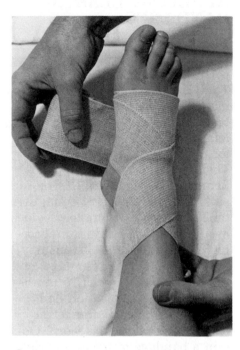

1 Some joints can be properly immobilized or supported with a figure-eight turn. First, anchor the bandage in place by making a double circular turn on the area of the limb distal to the joint.

2 Begin a figure-eight turn by making an ascending turn and wrapping the bandage around the joint.

3 Finish the figure-eight turn by making a descending turn.

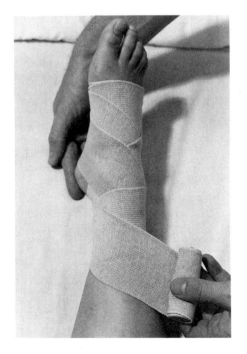

4 Continue the turns by overlapping the bandage in an alternately ascending and descending fashion.

5 When the joint has been →
wrapped in an even and wrinkle-free manner, secure the end of the bandage to the rest of the wrapped surface with tape or clips. *Caution: If the bandage is to be applied to decrease edema rather than to support the joint, it is essential that the heel also be wrapped or fluid will collect in the heel, potentially resulting in pressure necrosis.*

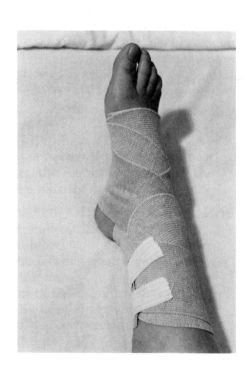

Wrapping a Residual Limb (Stump)

Postoperatively, a residual limb is wrapped with an elastic bandage to reduce swelling and to mold the stump for eventual prosthetic fitting. One effective way to wrap a residual limb is to employ a modified figure-eight turn. Be sure to include client teaching in this procedure.

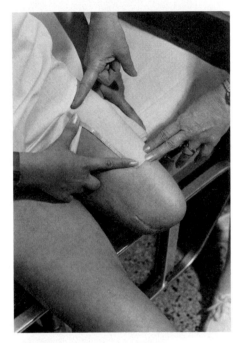

1 It is essential that you position the end of the elastic bandage high on the groin, and that this area is properly wrapped without bulging fatty tissue. If the fatty tissue is not contained by the wrapped bandage, the prosthesis will not fit properly.

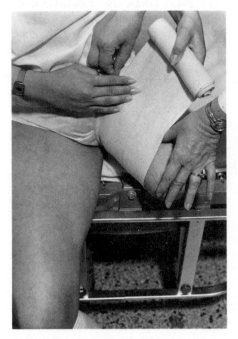

2 Make a circular turn to anchor the bandage in place.

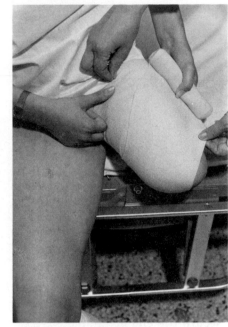

3 Make a spiral turn that overlaps the circular turn, and wrap the distal end of the residual limb.

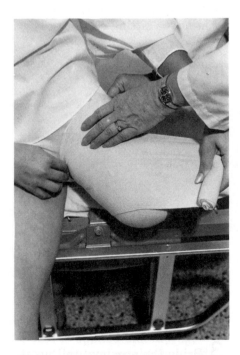

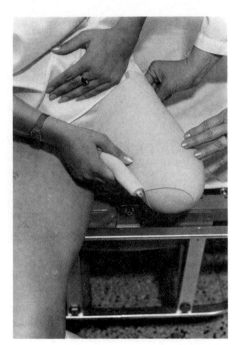

4 Make alternately descending turns and ascending turns (right) until the residual limb has been completely wrapped.

(Continued on p. 532)

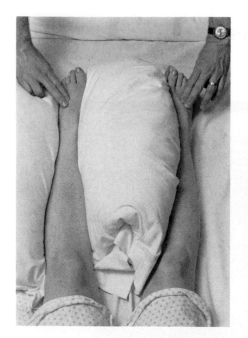

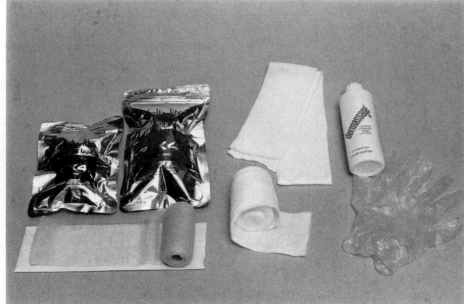

2 Assess the client's neurovascular status by following the procedures, pp. 518–519. Establish the client's baseline in both extremities prior to cast application. Evaluate and record: color, temperature, sensation, edema, capillary refill, and pulsations.

3 The materials used for cast application will vary, depending on whether a plaster or synthetic cast will be applied. The following are materials that are typically used when a synthetic cast is applied: rolls of cast material; stockinette, padding, or sheet wadding; a lubricant, either massage cream or one that is water-soluble; and two pairs of disposa-

ble gloves. In addition, you will need a plastic-lined bucket filled with fresh water. The water temperature will be determined by the brand of synthetic cast material used. Use a water thermometer to attain the desired temperature. Generally, lukewarm water is used when a plaster cast is applied.

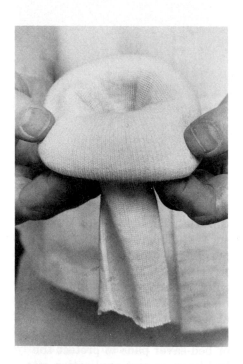

4 After the stockinette has been measured and cut to fit the extremity, ensure that it is rolled to facilitate its application onto the extremity.

5 Hold the limb erect as the →
physician applies the stockinette, supporting the extremity in the neutral or prescribed position. The physician will smooth out all the wrinkles after the stockinette has been applied.

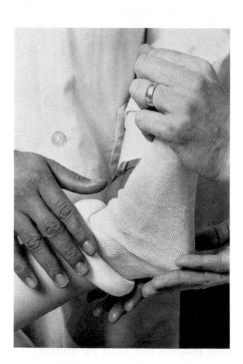

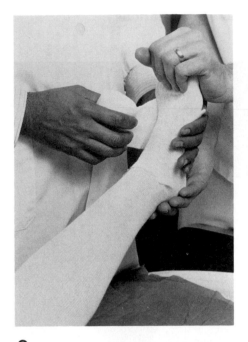

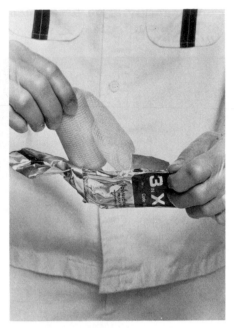

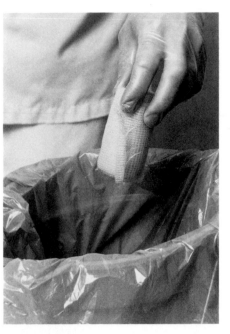

6 Continue to support the limb in the neutral or desired position as the physician wraps padding around the extremity. One to three layers of padding will be used, and extra padding may be applied over bony prominences or the injured area. It should not, however, cover the edges of the stockinette. Be certain to maintain the extremity in the same prescribed position throughout the entire procedure. A failure to do so could produce wrinkles inside the cast, potentially resulting in pressure areas that can lead to neurovascular impairment.

7 When a synthetic cast is applied, usually both the physician and the assistant apply gloves, and the synthetic casting material is then removed from its package. Opening the package earlier could affect the chemical composition of the cast material.

8 The roll of cast material is then immersed in water for the required amount of time, usually 7–12 seconds, but this will vary depending on the type of cast material that is used. Typically, the roll is then gently squeezed to remove the excess water.
Note: Some synthetic cast materials are activated by compression or by special lights and might not require water.

9 Support the limb by grasping → the client's toes (or fingers for arm casts) as the physician applies the cast material. If possible, you should also support the limb in areas on which the physician has not yet applied the cast material. Depending on the size and desired thickness of the cast, one to several rolls of cast material may be applied. The physician takes tucks or twists the cast material to ensure conformity to the limb. The stockinette is then pulled over the cast material to cover proximal and distal opening edges, and it is secured in place by another layer or two of the cast material.

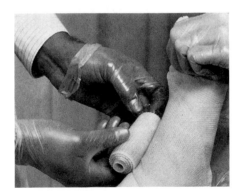

(Continued on p. 536)

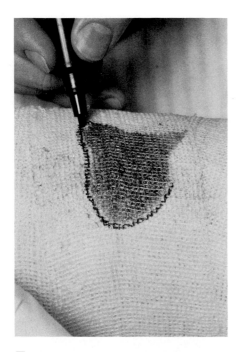

5 Monitor postsurgical or post-traumatic drainage by inspecting the entire cast. Encircle—or simply measure—the drainage stain after every shift (depending on agency policy) to provide a baseline for subsequent evaluation of the amount of exudate. Inform the physician of daily amounts and/or changes. It is also essential that you inspect both the sheet and underside of the cast to ensure that drainage has not also seeped into these areas. A foul-smelling odor from the cast or cast openings should be noted and promptly reported, because it can be indicative of an infection.

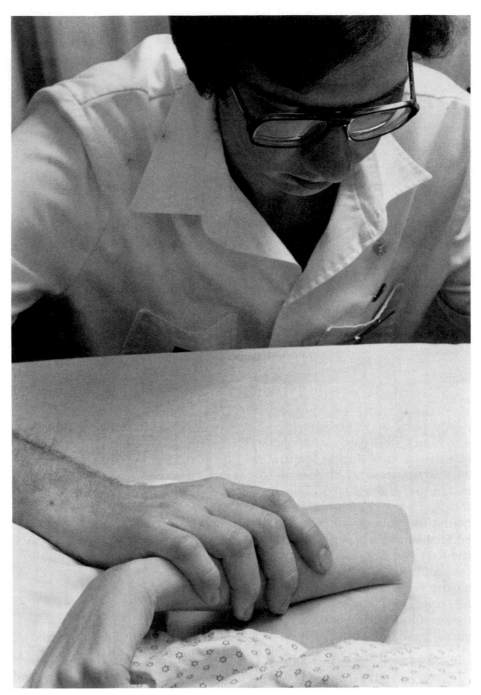

6 Because your client might be immobilized for several hours or even days, assess the skin integrity on an ongoing basis, especially around bony prominences and cast edges, which have greater potential for skin irritation or breakdown. Massage these sites with alcohol to toughen the skin. Before using alcohol, make sure the skin is unbroken.

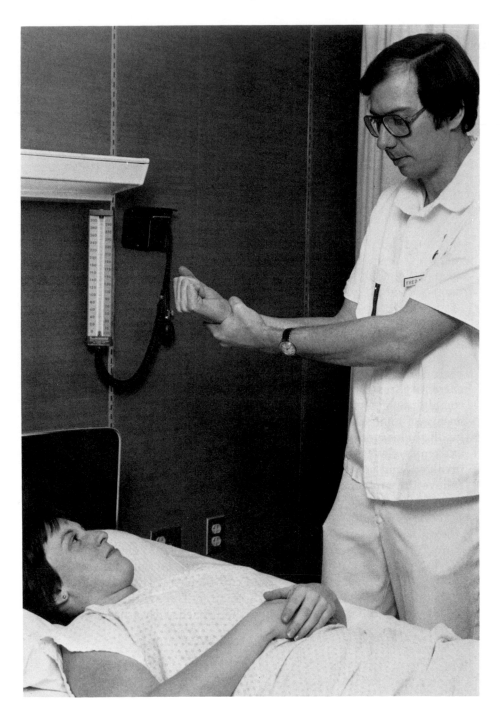

7 Ensure that the client receives full ROM exercises on the unaffected extremities, as well as on the joints distal and proximal to the cast unless it is medically contraindicated. Teach your client active ROM exercises for the unaffected extremities, and assisted ROM for the casted extremity, which can be implemented with physician approval once healing has occurred. Also, explain that moving the fingers or toes of the casted extremity will enhance peripheral circulation to minimize edema and pain. With physician approval, isometric exercises can be taught to the client to minimize muscle atrophy in the affected limb. Teach the isometric (muscle-setting) exercises on the unaffected limb so that the client can adapt the exercise to the casted limb. Demonstrate muscle palpation so that the client can feel the changes that occur with muscle contraction and relaxation.

Managing Routine Traction Care

MAKING A BOWLINE TRACTION KNOT

There are several types of knots that are used for traction. The bowline knot is one that will not slip, and we therefore recommend its use over others.

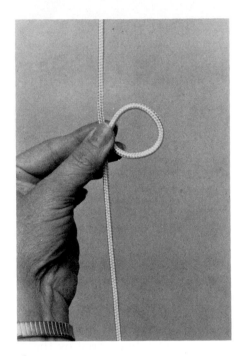

1 Make a loop in a traction rope that is both intact and unfrayed.

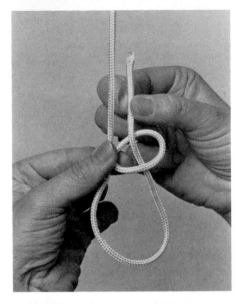

2 Bring the end of the rope up through the loop.

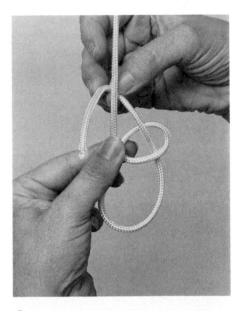

3 Wrap the end behind and around the rope that is proximal to the loop.

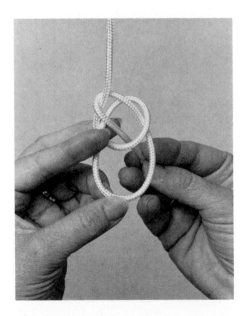

4 Thread the end down through the original loop.

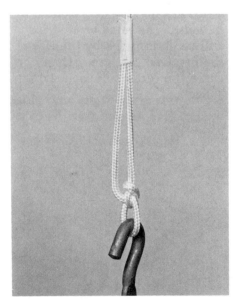

5 Tighten the knot and attach the weight to the loop that is below the knot. To prevent the end from fraying, wrap it with a small strip of tape. It is also a good idea to tape the end to the rope to discourage others from tampering with the knot.

General Guidelines for the Care of the Client in Traction

■ Perform and document neurovascular assessments prior to application of the traction apparatus to provide a baseline for subsequent assessments. For nonadhesive skin traction (for example, Buck's boot, cervical collar, or pelvic belt) perform a neurovascular assessment every 4 hours, and 30–45 minutes after every reapplication of the traction. For adhesive skin traction (for example, Buck's with adhesive straps or Bryant's) and skeletal traction, perform the assessments hourly during the first 24 hours, and every 4 hours thereafter if they are normal for the client and remain stable. Assessments should be repeated 30–45 minutes after the extremities are rewrapped with adhesive skin traction.

■ Unless the traction involves the neck or upper extremities, provide the client with a trapeze and instruct her or him in its use.

■ For clients receiving continuous traction, the use of sheepskin pads or pressure-relief mattresses is essential to the integrity of the skin.

■ To provide the prescribed line of pull, ensure that the client maintains proper alignment and that the ropes and pulleys are in alignment, as well.

■ Because the immobilized client is at risk for the development of thrombi secondary to venous stasis, secure an order for antiembolic stockings and apply them following the procedure in Chapter 7.

■ Make sure the client exercises the uninvolved extremities and joints, using ROM, ankle circling, and isometric (muscle-setting) exercises. Unless contraindicated, isometric exercises should be employed on the involved extremity as well.

■ For the immobilized client, monitor and document bowel status and evaluate the diet. Increase roughage and obtain an order for a stool softener or cathartic if indicated. Ensure an adequate fluid intake (at least 2–3 L/day) to prevent urinary tract infections, retention, and renal calculi.

■ To prevent respiratory complications, encourage coughing and deep breathing exercises and/or the use of incentive spirometry; auscultate the chest for lung sounds daily to identify and avert the development of hypostatic pneumonia or atelectasis. For further detail, see Chapter 6.

CARING FOR CLIENTS IN SKIN TRACTION

Applying Cervical Traction

Cervical traction is applied for clients with cervical spine disorders, "whiplash," muscle spasms in the neck, or neck pain. Generally, nurses can apply cervical traction for the client who does not have a significant fracture or subluxation.

1 Review a traction manual before entering the client's room so that you are familiar with the setup, and then assemble the cervical traction apparatus. Explain the procedure to the client and perform a baseline neurologic assessment on the upper extremities. It is essential that the client and family members be informed about the importance of maintaining the prescribed position; avoiding the adjustment or removal of the traction apparatus unless it is approved; and reporting the presence of pressure, pain, parasthesia, or weakness in the neck or upper extremities immediately. The client should remain supine for this therapy, with the shoulders relaxed and level, and the back flattened against the bed.

Assessing and Planning

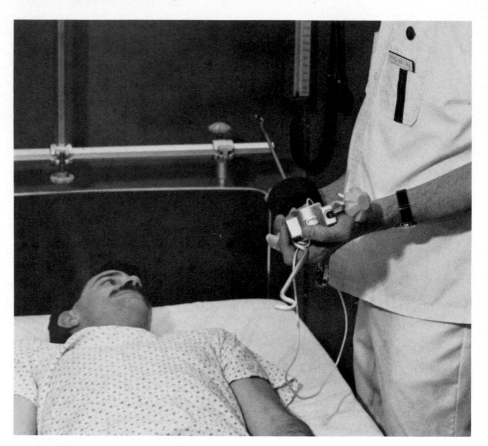

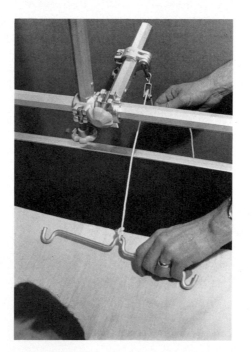

2 Attach the prescribed traction frame to the bed. Ensure that the spreader bar is of an appropriate size. It should be wide enough so that once the cervical collar is attached, the straps will neither touch the sides of the client's head nor pinch his ears. The client should also be positioned far enough down in bed so that there is ample room for the spreader bar and rope. The rope should then be tied to the spreader bar and threaded through the pulley, with the prescribed weight (usually no greater than 5 pounds) attached to the opposite end.

Implementing

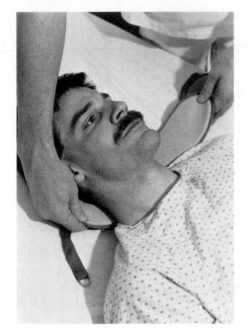

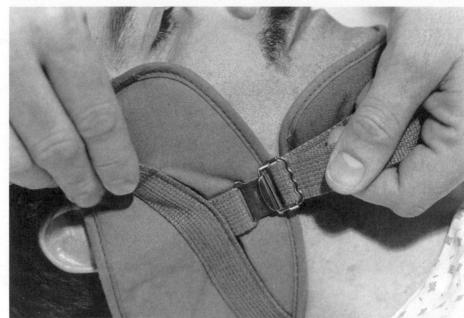

3 Insert the cervical collar carefully under the client's neck; then buckle the straps (right).

4 Adjust the collar if the strap is not centered over the chin, and make sure that the strap does not touch the client's throat. When the client is comfortable in the collar, attach the ends of the spreader bar through each of the collar rings (far right). Use slow, even motions to avoid jerking the weights and injuring the client. When the weights are connected, make sure that the traction pull is over the occiput rather than the chin, and that it is bilaterally equal. Ask the client if it pulls more on one side than the other. Document the procedure.

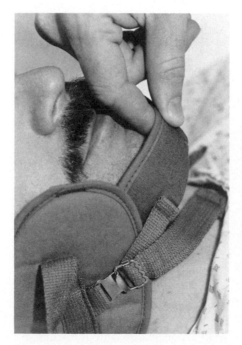

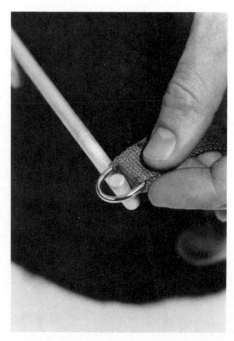

(Continued on p. 546)

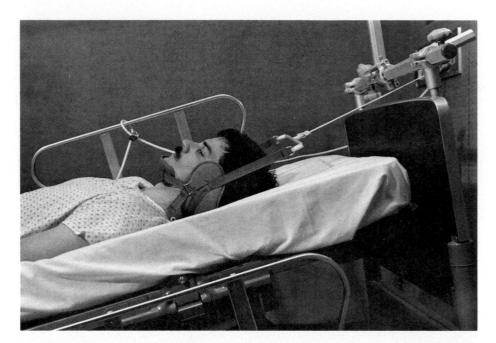

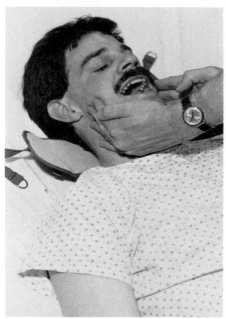

5 The physician may request that the head of the bed be elevated to provide countertraction. If this is the case, ensure that the pulley system can be raised and lowered independent of the bed so that the direction of the traction force can be altered to accommodate the client's position.

6 If intermittent rather than continuous traction has been prescribed, perform thorough client assessments after removing the collar and discontinuing the traction. Palpate the client's temporomandibular joint (see p. 510) to assess for discomfort or limited range of motion. Pain in this area, headaches, and neck pain are indications that the weight might be too much for the client's tolerance, and the physician should be informed of the problem. Also, evaluate skin integrity at this time by inspecting the ears, chin, and occipital areas for the presence of skin irritation or pressure from the collar. Inspect and massage the skin over the elbows, heels, sacrum, and other bony prominences as well, to enhance local circulation. Remember to perform neurologic assessments on the upper extremities 30 minutes after the traction has been reapplied.

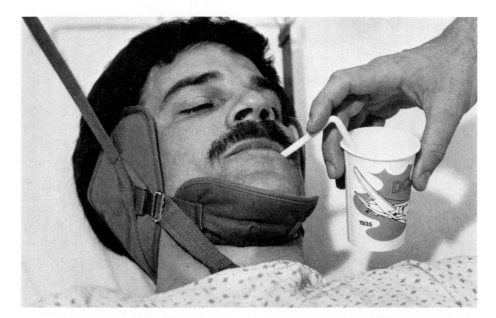

7 Evaluate the client's oral intake. If continuous traction is prescribed, it may be necessary to modify the diet to one that is soft or liquid to facilitate the client's chewing and swallowing. If the client must be immobile for prolonged periods of time, encourage a fluid intake of 2–3 L/day to minimize the potential for a urinary tract infection, retention, and renal calculi. Be sure to keep a glass containing fluids and a straw within the client's reach.

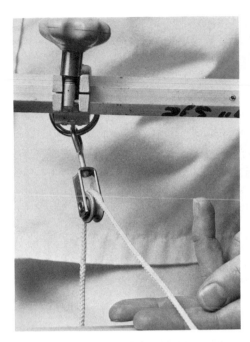

8 During routine assessment of the client, also evaluate the traction apparatus. The weights should hang freely, and the ropes must be unfrayed and centered over the pulley tracks. Check the client's alignment in relation to the traction apparatus to ensure that he receives a direct line of pull.

Applying a Pelvic Belt

Pelvic traction is applied for clients with sciatica, low back pain, and muscle spasms in the lower back.

Assessing and Planning

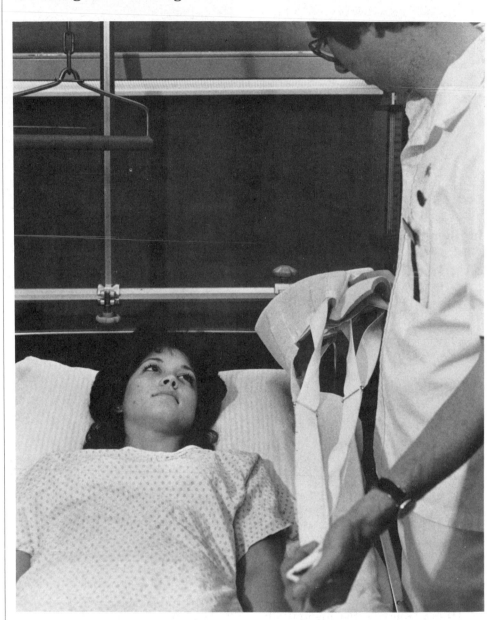

1 Obtain the prescribed traction apparatus and a pelvic belt sized to fit your client. Review a traction manual to assist you with assembling the traction apparatus used by your agency. Explain the procedure to your client, and obtain and record the client's baseline neurologic assessments. In addition, evaluate the strength of both legs by instructing the client to press her feet against both your hands (see step 12, p. 550). Explain the importance of maintaining the prescribed position, keeping the traction uninterrupted, and reporting immediately any prolonged discomfort, weakness, or paresthesia of the lower extremities.

(Continued on p. 548)

Evaluating

5 Unless the client alerts you sooner, assess the client and evaluate the temperature of the pack after approximately 10 minutes. Assess the client for potential complications such as diaphoresis, hypotension, and tachycardia. Unwrap the pack and inspect the skin for excess erythema, and then rewrap the pack. Question the client about her comfort level. When the treatment time has elapsed, remove the pack, evaluate the client's skin, and obtain posttreatment vital signs. Document the procedure and the client's response.

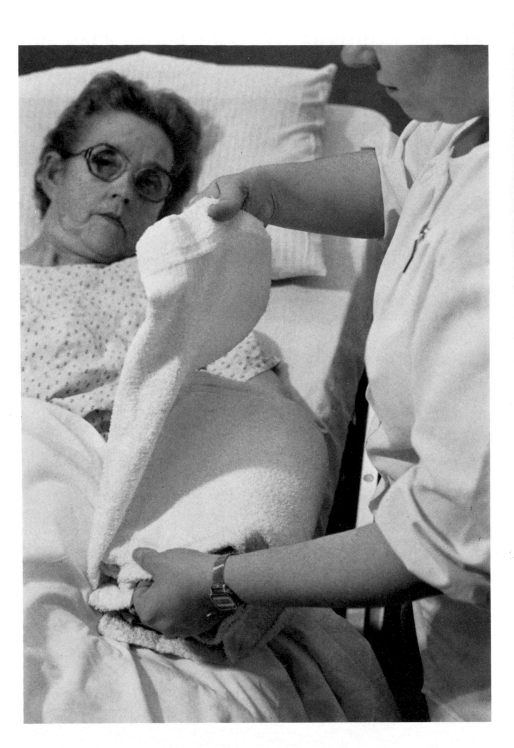

TRANSFERRING THE CLIENT WITH A TOTAL HIP REPLACEMENT

When hip adduction and hip flexion are contraindicated, for example for a client with a total hip replacement, follow these steps to transfer the client from the bed to the wheelchair. Be sure that the client has enough upper body strength and mobility in the uninvolved leg to assist you with this procedure. Explain the procedure to the client and ensure that he understands each step and his role during the transfer.

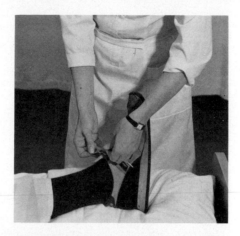

1 Put a sturdy rubber-soled shoe on the client's uninvolved foot so that he can safely pivot during the transfer.

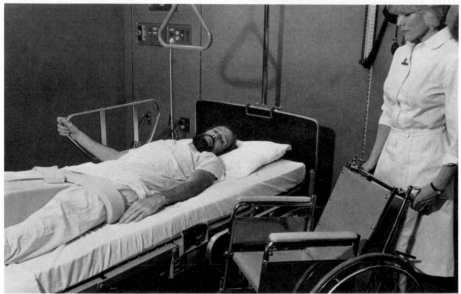

2 Position a wheelchair at a 45° angle to the head of the bed on the side opposite the client's involved hip. Lock both the wheelchair and the bed to keep them stable during the move. Either swing away or remove the foot rests so that they will not obstruct the move. If the wheelchair has an adjustable backrest, tilt it back to minimize the hip flexion for the client once he sits in the chair. However, if the chairback does not recline, place a pillow in the seat to help keep the client's hip in as much extension as possible.

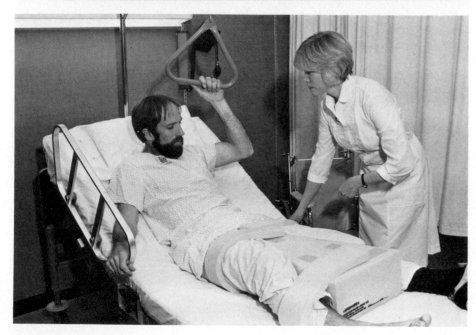

3 Raise the head of the bed to a level the client can tolerate, but no greater than 45°. Remember to keep the client's hips in minimal flexion to prevent the dislocation of the involved hip. Although it is not possible to keep the client's hips in full extension during this procedure, by keeping them constantly abducted with an abduction pillow, the potential for dislocation is minimized.

(Continued on p. 580)

4 To begin the transfer, grasp both the client's involved leg and the abduction pillow, and ask the client to lift his upper body into a slight sitting position as you do. Remember to bend your knees, keep your back straight, and separate your feet to provide a wide base of support.

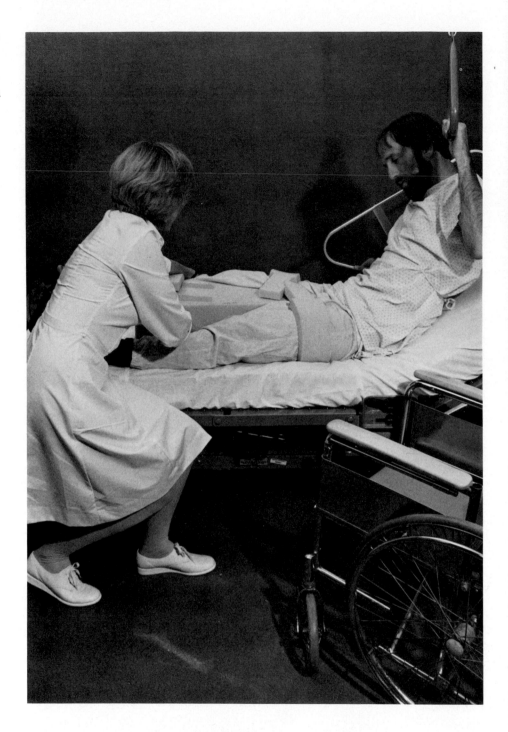

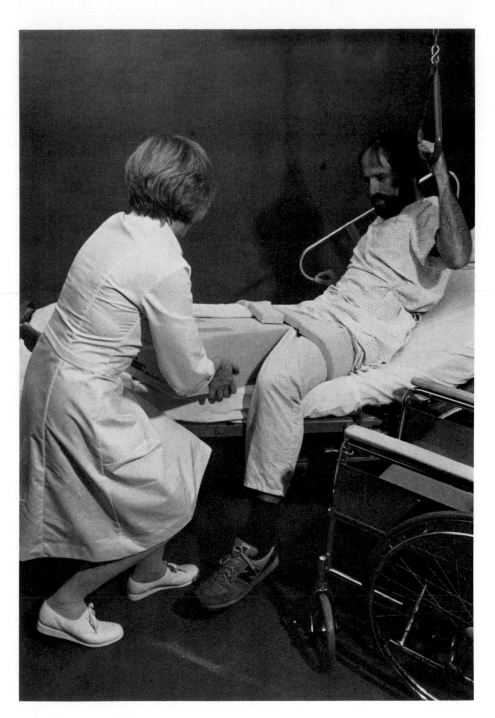

5 Pivot onto your forward foot as you move the client's involved leg and abduction pillow to the side of the bed.

(Continued on p. 582)

6 Shift your weight onto your back foot as you move the pillow and leg off the bed. At the same time, instruct the client to slide his buttocks toward the edge of the bed.

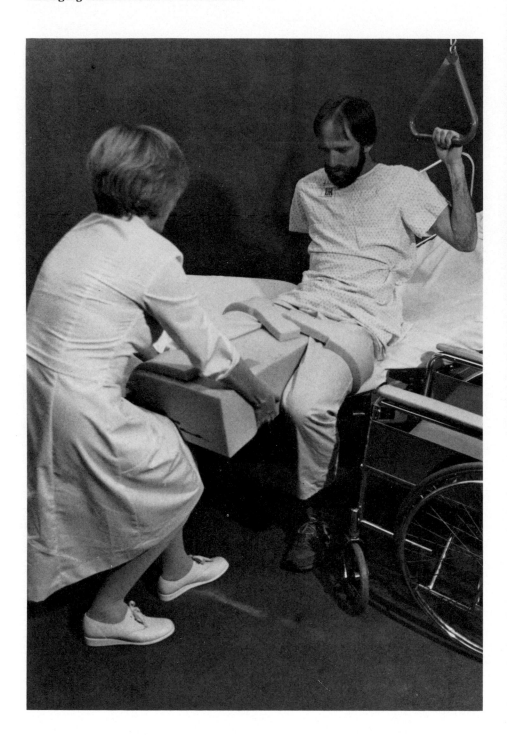

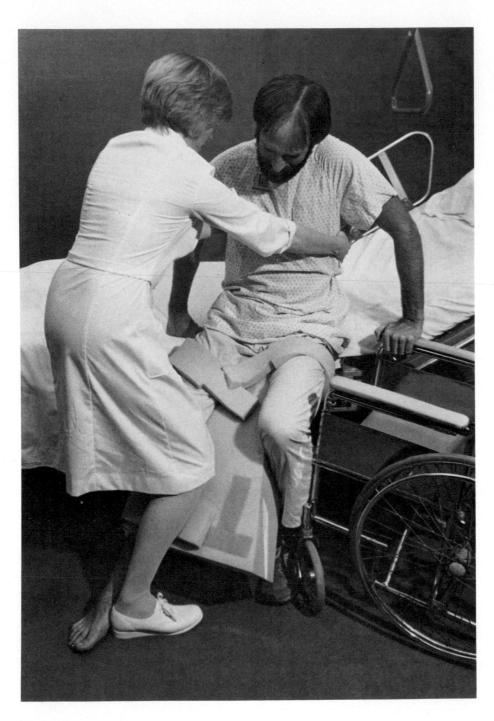

7 Once both of the client's legs are off the bed, instruct him to grasp the wheelchair armrest that is closer to him, and to stand and bear weight on his uninvolved leg unless the physician has allowed weight bearing on the involved extremity also. Position your hands under his axillae as you guide him into a standing position. *Note: If the client is more dependent, you should place a transfer belt around his waist and grasp him at waist level by holding onto the belt.*

(Continued on p. 584)

8 Once the client is standing, instruct him to grasp the opposite armrest and to pivot on his uninvolved foot until the backs of his legs are positioned against the seat of the wheelchair.

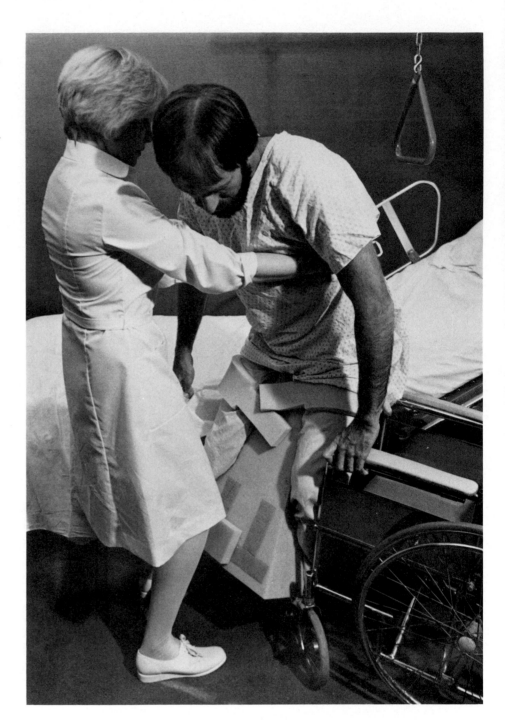

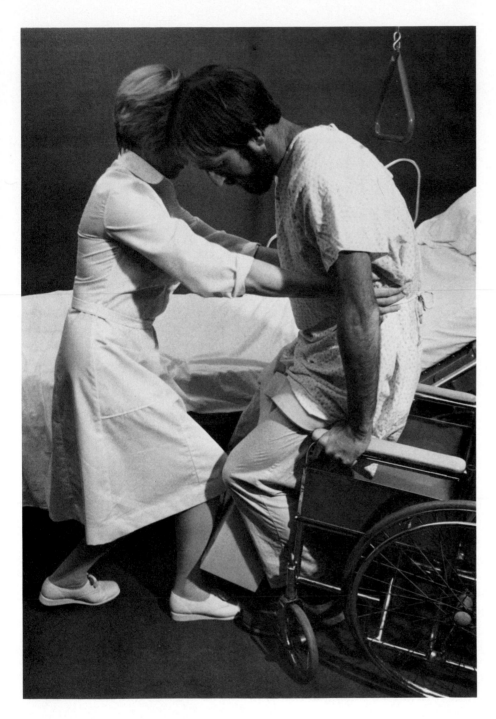

9 When the client attains the position described on the facing page, instruct him to grasp both armrests and to prepare to sit, avoiding bending over at the waist as he begins his descent. Although the abduction pillow will prevent you from keeping your body close to the client's, you should position your forward knee against the client's uninvolved knee to help keep him stabilized.

(Continued on p. 586)

10 As the client lowers his body into the wheelchair, bend your knees and lower your body as you continue to guide him.

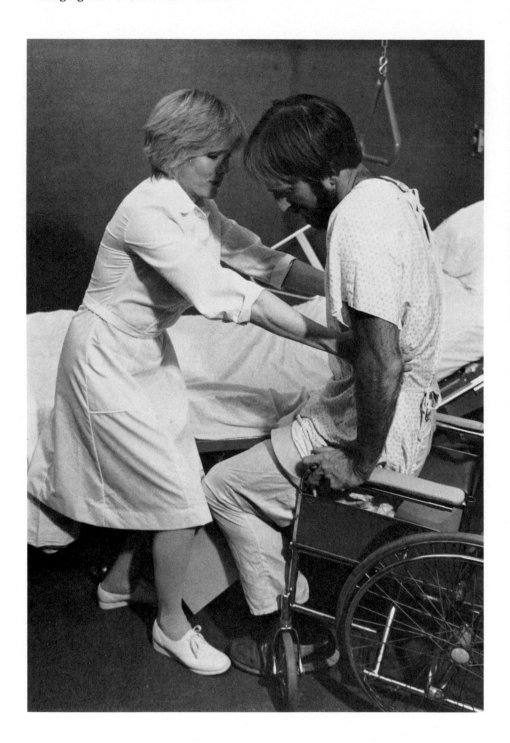

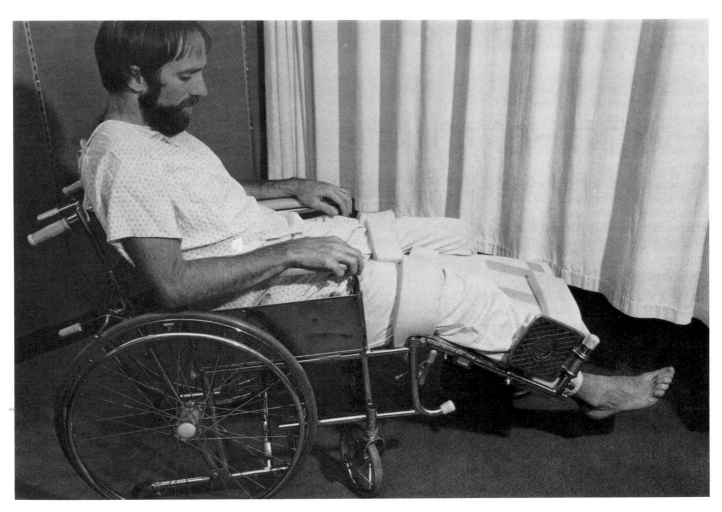

11 Support the client's involved leg with his knee in slight flexion by repositioning the legrest. Ensure that his hips are minimally flexed and that they remain in abduction. To return the client to the bed, reverse these steps.

Alert/Awake: responds promptly and appropriately to verbal and tactile stimuli

Lethargic: drowsy, responds slowly yet appropriately

Obtunded: somnolent, may be disoriented when awake

Stuporous: arouses with difficulty, may be combative, might respond to simple commands

Semicomatose: responds to painful stimuli only

Comatose: unresponsive even to painful stimuli, hypotonic

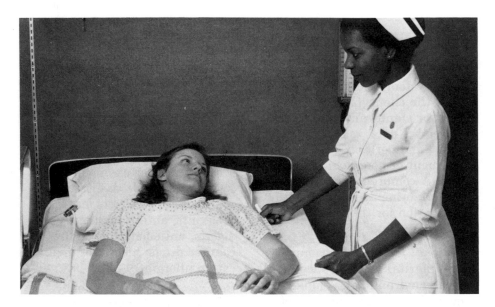

1 Evaluate your client's level of consciousness using the above scale, and take vital signs. Assess the client for a slowed or rapid pulse rate concomitant with a rising systolic blood pressure, which can occur with increasing intracranial pressure. Count the respirations, noting the rate, depth, and rhythm. Be especially alert to Cheyne-Stokes respirations, which are distinguished by periods of hyperventilation followed by periods of apnea. This is one type of breathing pattern that can occur with a brain dysfunction. Because wide fluctuations in temperature can occur with the neurologically impaired client, monitor the client's temperature closely.

If your client does not awaken easily to your voice or touch, painful stimuli should be *cautiously* applied. For example, exert pressure with your knuckles on the sternum or pinch the sternocleidomastoid muscle, being certain to avoid causing any harm to the client. Either stimulus should elicit a response. If the client is comatose, observe the posture after a painful stimulus has been applied. Posturing can be indicative of neurologic damage or disease. *Decerebrate* posturing, which can occur with upper brainstem injury, is the extension of the extremities after a stimulus. *Decorticate* posturing is upper extremity flexion with lower extremity extension, and it can occur with an injury to the cortex.

Observe and test the client's orientation to time, person, and place; behavior; mood; knowledge; memory; and speech patterns. Are the responses prompt and appropriate to the questions asked, and does she respond correctly to simple commands? Note the facial expression and the ability to maintain eye contact with you, and assess whether her mood is appropriate to the situation. One way to test abstract reasoning is to ask the client to interpret a simple proverb. Long-term and short-term memory can be evaluated during a health history. Finally, note whether the client's speech patterns are appropriate for her educational, socioeconomic, and ethnic background. It is wise to avoid asking questions that can be responded to with "yes" or "no" answers.

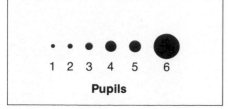

Pupils

As you evaluate mental status, inspect the client's eyes. They should open spontaneously, and both eyes should move together in unison. Evaluate the size and shape of the pupils and note whether they are bilaterally equal. Use a pupil gauge (as shown above) to assist you with documenting their size.

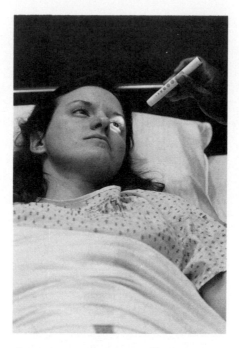

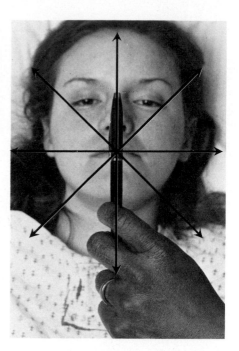

2 Check the pupillary response to light. Dim the lights and instruct the client to focus her gaze on an object in her direct line of vision. Move your penlight from outside the client's field of vision toward the pupil and shine the light into the left eye, observing for a pupillary reaction. Repeat the test on the right eye. Optimally, both pupils will react equally (and at the same rapid rate) and constrict to the same size. Evaluate the client's consensual light reflex by observing each pupil as the light is shined into the opposite eye. The right pupil should constrict as the light is shined into the left eye, and vice versa. If this response does not occur, the client might have brainstem dysfunction.

3 In some clinical situations, the physician may request that you test the client's extraocular eye movements during the neurologic check. To do this, position a pen 30–37.5 cm (12–15 in.) from the client's nose. Instruct the client to focus her eyes on the pen but to avoid moving her head. Slowly move the pen up and down, to each side, and then on the diagonals, as depicted by the arrows in the photo. If her third (oculomotor), fourth (trochlear), and sixth (abducens) cranial nerves are intact, she should be able to follow the movements of the pen with her eyes moving in unison. Describe any deficit, if present. Observe for involuntary, rapid movements of the eyeball (nystagmus), which can occur with neurologic impairments such as a cerebrovascular accident (CVA), cerebellar tumor, or with multiple sclerosis. Nystagmus can also occur with diphenylhydantoin (Dilantin) toxicity.

(Continued on p. 596)

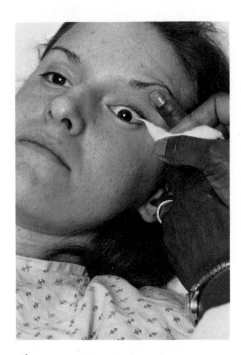

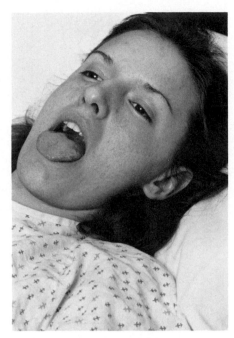

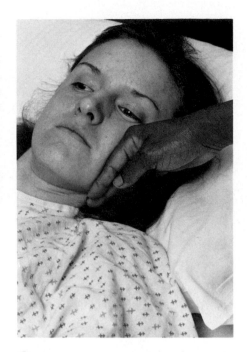

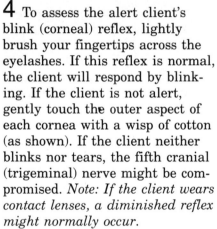

4 To assess the alert client's blink (corneal) reflex, lightly brush your fingertips across the eyelashes. If this reflex is normal, the client will respond by blinking. If the client is not alert, gently touch the outer aspect of each cornea with a wisp of cotton (as shown). If the client neither blinks nor tears, the fifth cranial (trigeminal) nerve might be compromised. *Note: If the client wears contact lenses, a diminished reflex might normally occur.*

5 Evaluate the ability of the client to extend her tongue. Note whether the tongue quivers excessively or deviates to one side, and document accordingly. Your client's inability to perform this task, or excessive quivering or a weakness on one side of the tongue, suggests an impairment of the twelfth cranial (hypoglossal) nerve, which can occur with a CVA.

6 The eleventh cranial (spinal accessory) nerve mediates the sternocleidomastoid and upper trapezius muscles. To test its integrity, place your hand against the client's cheek and instruct her to turn her head toward your hand. Repeat the assessment on the opposite side. With a neurologic impairment such as a CVA or a brain tumor, the client may have a unilateral deficit in strength.

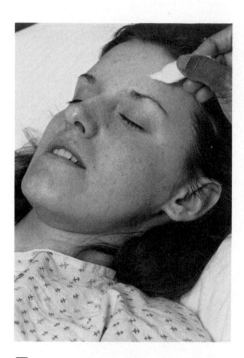

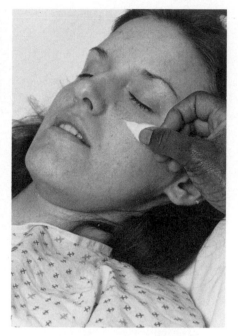

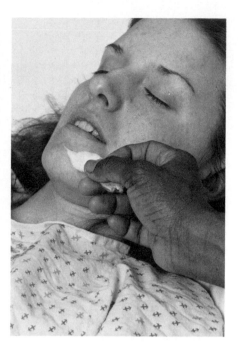

7 Test the client's nerve sensory function next. Explain that she is to describe both the sensation and location of the sensation while her eyes are closed. Be sure to show her the cotton wisp so that she does not become alarmed, expecting a painful process. Touch the client's forehead.

8 Touch her cheek and then her chin (right). Repeat the test on the opposite side of the client's face. She should describe a tickling sensation on all three areas of the face and the sensations should be felt equally on both sides. If the response is abnormal,

you can use a pin to assess other areas of the body. However, a pin should be used judiciously, and never on the face. See the procedure, pp. 601–603, for assessing sensory function using a dermatome chart.

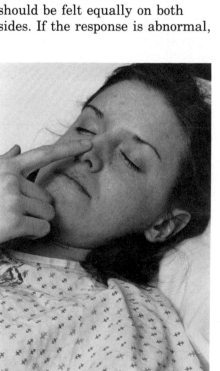

9 To test coordination (cerebellar function), instruct the client to close her eyes and to alternately touch her nose with the index fingers of her right hand and then her left hand, gradually increasing the speed of the movements. With a normal response, the movements will be smooth and accurate.

(Continued on p. 598)

10 To evaluate the motor function of the client's upper extremities, ask her to grip and squeeze your index and middle fingers. Document the strength of each hand, noting whether the grip is bilaterally equal or unequal. Remember, however, the client's dominant hand may normally be stronger than the nondominant hand. *Note: To quickly recall which of the client's hands is stronger, cross your hands so that your right hand is grasped by the client's right hand and your left hand by the client's left hand. By recalling which of your hands was gripped more tightly, you can readily document which of your client's hands is stronger.* Other tests for upper extremity motor function are found in Chapter 9.

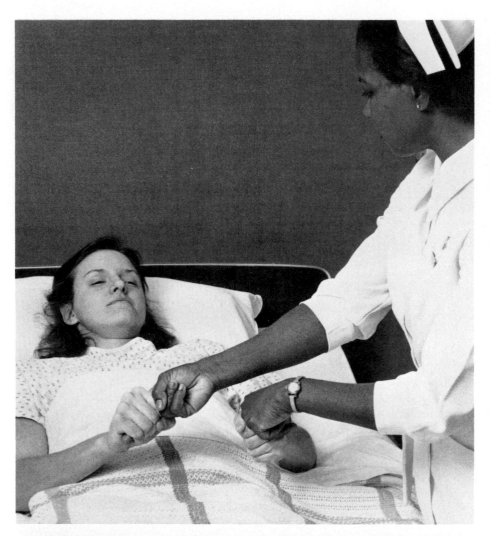

11 To evaluate the coordination (cerebellar function) of the lower extremities, instruct the client to slide her left heel down her right shin and to repeat the procedure on her left shin using her right heel. She should be able to do this smoothly and accurately. Document any deficit.

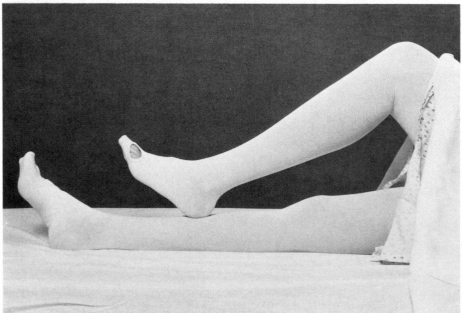

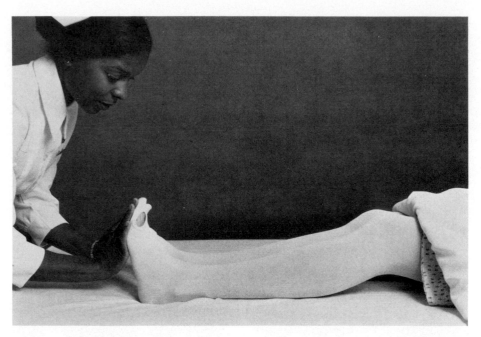

12 To evaluate the motor function of the lower extremities, push your hands against the soles of the client's feet. Instruct her to resist the pressure. Document the response, noting whether it is bilaterally equal or unequal. Note also whether the tone of the muscles is normal, hypotonic, or hypertonic. Other tests for lower extremity motor function are found in Chapter 9.

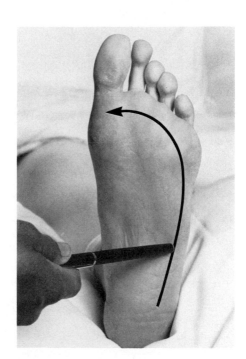

13 To test the client's plantar reflex, stroke along the lateral surface of the sole of each foot, as shown by the arrow on the photograph. If the toes curl downward, her response is normal. However, if the smaller toes fan apart and the large toe dorsiflexes toward the client's head, this is called the Babinski reflex. A positive Babinski is considered normal in the infant under 12–18 months, but it is a sign of motor nerve dysfunction in the adult.

14 To help orient the neurologically impaired client to the month and date, keep a brightly colored calendar within sight. Also, photographs of family and friends are important constants in the client's life and should be used in the hospital environment whenever possible.

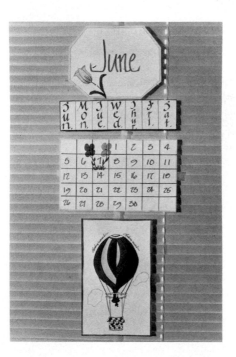

Testing Cerebellar and Motor Function

If your client is ambulatory, you can perform gross motor and balance testing to evaluate cerebellar function. See steps 9–12 in the preceding procedure for motor and cerebellar testing for the client who is on bed rest.

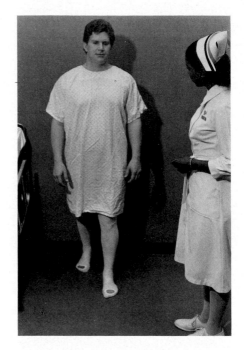

1 Instruct the client to walk across the room in a straight line. Observe the gait and posture. Normally, movements will be smooth and even, and the arms will swing slightly in opposition to the gait. Be alert to an unsteady gait, rigid or flaccid arm movements, and swaying, which can occur with a cerebellar dysfunction.

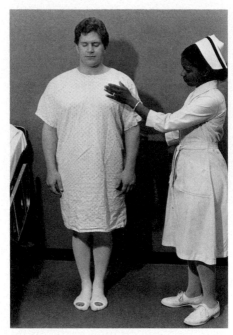

2 Evaluate the client for a positive Romberg's sign. Instruct him to stand still, with his arms at his sides and his feet together. He should first perform the test with his eyes shut, maintaining the stance for a full minute, and then repeat the test with his eyes open. Without touching him, guard him with your hands as you observe him in this position. Normally, you can expect to see slight swaying. Excessive swaying or an inability to maintain the stance without widening his foot base (whether the client's eyes are open or shut) occurs with a positive Romberg's sign. If he has trouble maintaining his balance only when his eyes are shut, he has a loss of position sense referred to as *sensory ataxia*. If he can not maintain his balance whether or not his eyes are open or shut, the condition is referred to as *cerebellar ataxia*.

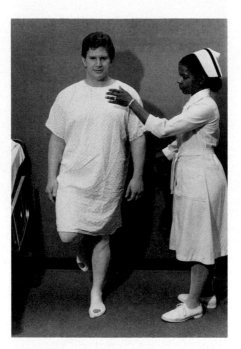

3 Instruct the client to stand first on one foot and then on the other. Guard him as you observe his stance. Normally, the stance can be maintained for at least 5 seconds. An inability to maintain the stance occurs when the equilibrium is disturbed. Document the results of the testing.

Assessing Sensory Function Using a Dermatome Chart

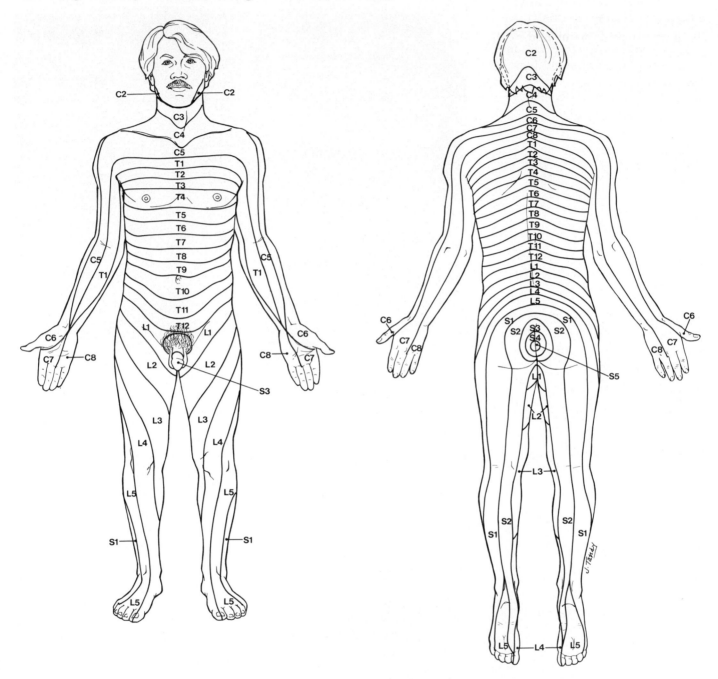

If you are assessing a neurologically impaired client who is alert and cooperative, you can evaluate sensory function by testing dermatome zones. Dermatome zones, which are divided into segmental skin bands as depicted by these overlays, compare anatomically to the innervation by a dorsal root to a cutaneous nerve. These nerves deliver the sensations of pain, temperature, touch, and vibration to the spinal cord and, ultimately, to the brain. The *spinothalmic* tract transmits the sensations of pain, temperature, and crude touch; the *dorsal column* tract transmits the perceptions of light touch and vibrations. Even though there is usually a great deal of overlap in nerve distribution, a knowledge of the dermatome zones can help you locate the approximate level of the neurologic lesion or injury. For example, a diminished or heightened response at the client's thumb can alert you to a potential disorder at level C6 of the spinal cord.

(Continued on p. 602)

1 Explain the procedure to the client, and display the instruments that will be used during the assessment. A safety pin and cotton wisp are commonly used to test sensation.

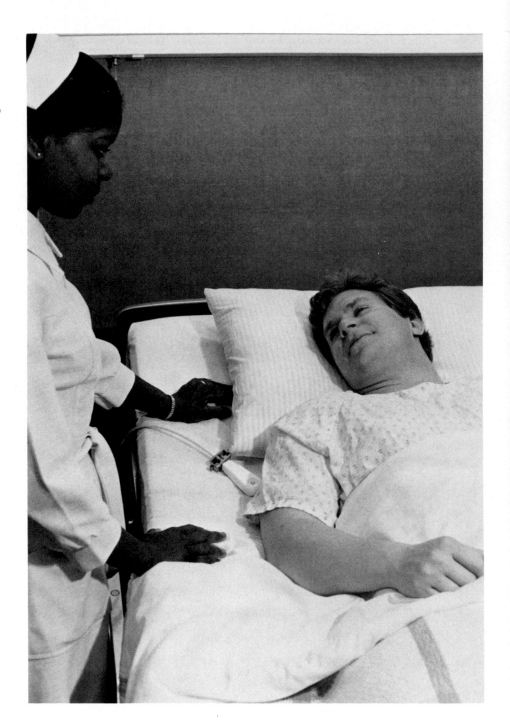

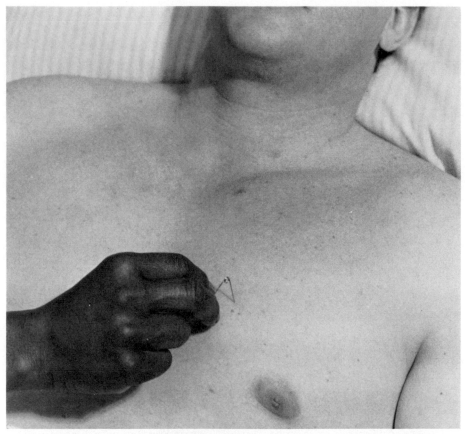

2 To test the spinothalmic tract, you can use both the pointed and blunt (below left) ends of a safety pin. Instruct the client to keep his eyes closed, and then stimulate anatomic locations at random, using both ends of the pin. Ask the client whether he feels a sharp or dull sensation. An abnormal response necessitates a more thorough assessment. Record the dermatome zone(s) in which the client has a diminished, heightened, or absent sensation. *Note: Because the spinothalmic tract transmits both pain and temperature, you can assess sensory function with warmth and coolness, for example by using test tubes filled with warm and cool water. The use of both testing modalities is rarely necessary, however.*

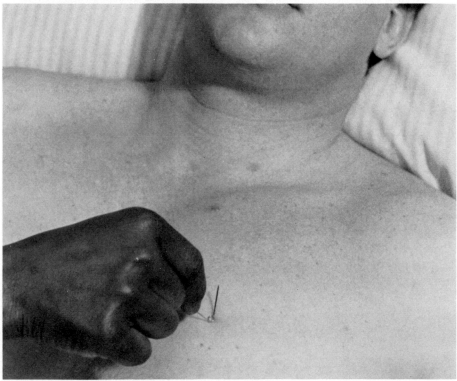

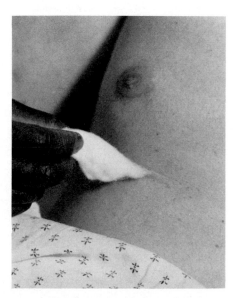

3 The dorsal column tract is assessed for light touch perception by brushing a cotton wisp against the client's skin. Again, test random areas and ask the client to alert you as soon as the sensation is felt. Record the dermatome zone(s) in which the client has diminished, heightened, or absent sensations.

Evaluating Deep Tendon Reflexes

Deep tendon reflexes (DTRs) are present in all normal adults. An absence of or heightened reflexes denote a pathology associated with an interruption of an impulse at the associated anatomic site in the spinal cord. Evaluate your client's DTRs according to the following scale:

0 Nonreflexive
1 Hyporeflexive—diminished response, can occur normally in the older client
2 Normal
3 Brisk—not always associated with a pathology
4 Hyperreflexive

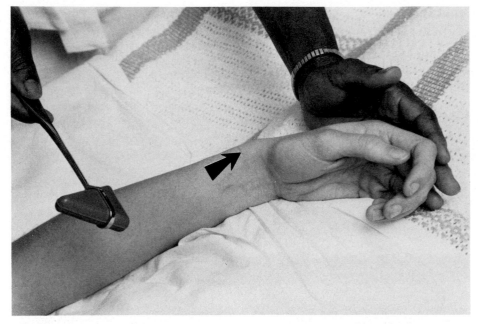

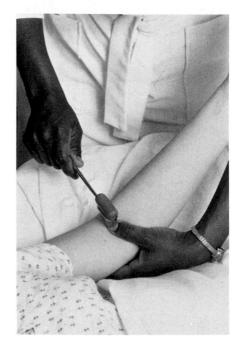

1 To test the biceps reflex (C5–C6 innervation), place your thumb over the client's biceps tendon at the antecubital fossa. Flex the client's elbow slightly, and then percuss your thumb with the pointed end of the reflex hammer. In a normal response, the client's elbow will flex and you should feel the tendon contract. Repeat the test on the tendon in the opposite extremity, noting the tone and symmetry of the reflex.

2 To test the brachioradialis (supinator) reflex (C5–C6 innervation), rest the client's forearm on a flat surface such as the bed or the client's lap, maintaining the hand in a moderate curve. Using the blunt end of the reflex hammer, percuss the brachioradialis tendon, which is located 2.5–5 cm (1–2 in.) above the wrist over the radius (see arrow). In a normal response, the client's elbow will flex and the forearm will rotate laterally. Test the reflex of the tendon in the opposite extremity, noting the tone and symmetry of the response.

3 To test the triceps reflex (C6–C7–C8 innervation), flex the client's elbow. Using the pointed end of the reflex hammer, percuss the triceps tendon just proximal to the olecranon between the epicondyles (see arrow). The elbow should extend as the triceps tendon contracts. Repeat the test on the tendon in the opposite extremity, noting the tone and symmetry of the reflex.

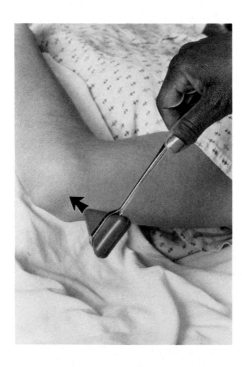

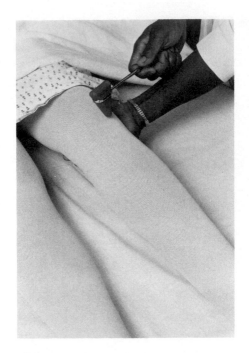

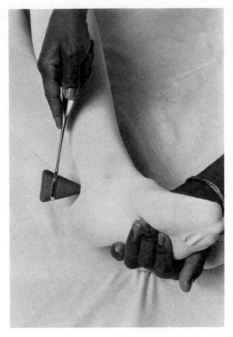

ASSESSING CRANIAL DRAINAGE FOR THE PRESENCE OF CEREBROSPINAL FLUID

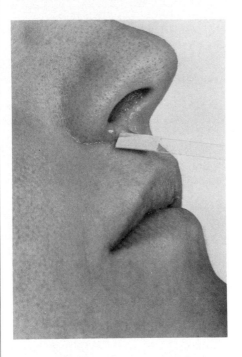

4 To test the patellar reflex (L2–L3–L4 innervation), have the client sit on the edge of the bed. If the client is unable to sit, flex and support the knee at the popliteal space (as shown) and percuss the patellar tendon just distal to the patella. Use the pointed end of the reflex hammer and tap the site lightly. The knee should extend and the quadriceps muscle should contract. Test the reflex on the tendon in the opposite extremity, noting the tone and symmetry of the reflex. *Note: In the elderly client, the response may normally be hyporeflexive.*

5 To test the ankle reflex (S1–S2 innervation), place the knee in slight flexion and then externally rotate and dorsiflex the ankle. Percuss the Achilles tendon with the pointed end of the reflex hammer. The client's ankle should plantarflex as the tendon contracts. Repeat the test on the tendon in the opposite extremity, noting the tone and symmetry of the reflex. Document the results of the assessment procedure.

If your client has sustained a craniocerebral injury or is recovering from a craniotomy, careful observation of any drainage from the eyes, ears, nose, or traumatic area is critical. Cerebrospinal fluid is colorless, generally nonpurulent, and its presence is indicative of a serious breach of cranial integrity. Because the risk of bacteria entering into the brain is very high if a tract exists, *any* suspicious drainage should be reported immediately.

Since cerebrospinal fluid contains glucose, you can test clear, nonsanguineous drainage with a glucose reagent stick and compare the results to the back of the reagent container. The test results will be positive for the presence of glucose if the drainage contains cerebrospinal fluid.

Caring for Clients with Neurologic Disorders

ASSISTING THE CLIENT WITH A TRANSCUTANEOUS ELECTRICAL NERVE STIMULATOR DEVICE

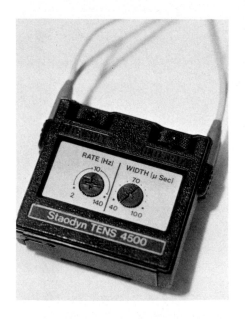

A transcutaneous electrical nerve stimulator (TENS) device is battery-operated, and it is used to deliver electrical impulses to the body to relieve pain. A client experiencing acute or chronic pain, for whom narcotics are contraindicated or ineffective, will especially benefit from this device. It is used most frequently for chronic back pain or headaches. It should not be used, however, for clients with cardiac pacemakers because the electrical impulses it generates can interrupt pacing. In addition, it should be avoided for clients who are pregnant, or who have arrhythmias or myocardial ischemia.

Assessing and Planning

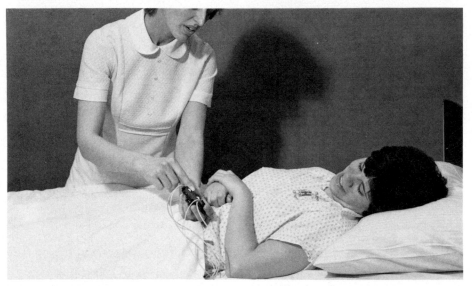

1 If your client has been using a TENS device, chances are she has already been trained in its use and application by a TENS specialist. Consult with the TENS specialist or read the manufacturer's instructions for operating the device before explaining it to your client.

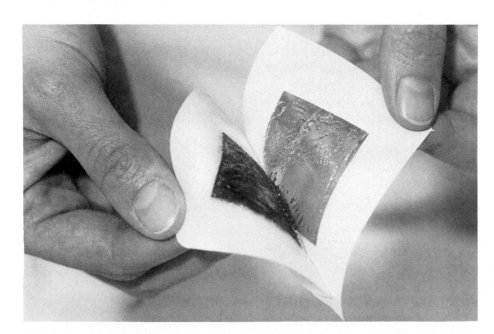

2 The electrodes are either reusable or disposable. They require the use of a conducting gel, or else they are water conductive and will need moistening with water. Many disposable electrodes, such as that in the photo, already contain the conducting gel and are self-adhering.

Implementing

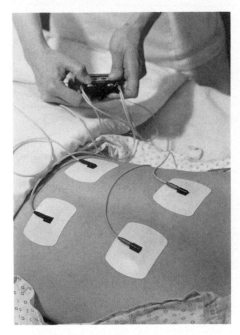

3 Attach the electrodes to the client's skin according to the pattern designed for your client. For example, for postoperative clients, place the electrodes on both sides of the incision. For clients with radiating pain, place the electrodes over the involved nerve roots along the spine. Attach the lead wires, making sure they are securely connected at both ends.

Evaluating

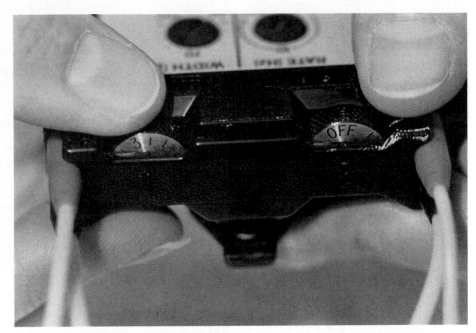

4 Many TENS devices have two dials that are labeled "intensity," "energy," or "amplitude," and each operates a set of two electrodes. In addition, most devices have a rate (frequency) dial that can be adjusted to deliver the desired number of electrical impulses per second, as well as a pulse-width dial that adjusts the impulse duration. If the client experiences a burning or itching sensation, lower the pulse-width dial. If the sensation is too intense, lower both the amplitude and pulse-width dials and adjust the rate accordingly. A mild to moderate sensation is the goal with this therapy. A sensation that is too intense can result in muscle spasms caused by over-stimulation of the nerve.

APPLYING INTERMITTENT PNEUMATIC COMPRESSION (ANTIEMBOLIC) CUFFS

Assessing and Planning

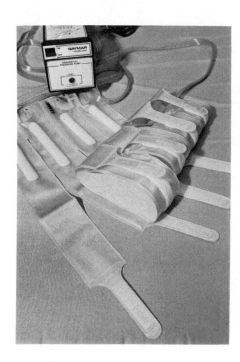

Clients who are immobile for an extended period of time are at risk of developing deep venous thrombosis due to stasis in the lower extremities. Intermittent calf compression via sequential pressure cuffs can be employed to empty the calf veins, thereby minimizing venous stasis. By allowing better drainage of the veins, the fibrinolytic (anticlotting) system is improved, as well. Because the cuffs work on the principle of compression, they are contraindicated in disorders associated with venous thrombosis or arterial insufficiency.

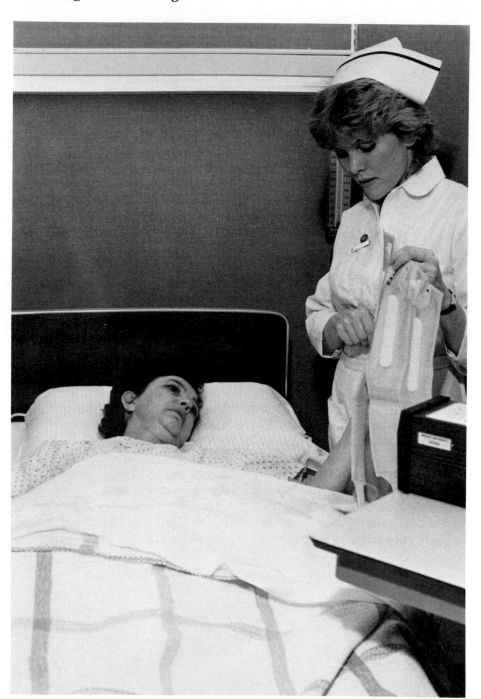

1 Assemble the equipment and explain the procedure to your client. Let her know that the cuffs are quite comfortable and that they will be worn during the period of time she is on bed rest.

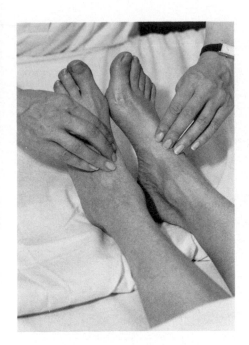

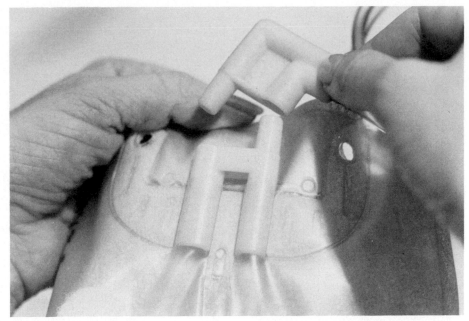

2 Palpate both pedal pulses (as shown) and popliteal pulses, and perform baseline neurovascular assessments in both feet (review the procedure in Chapter 9) before applying the cuffs. If the client shows evidence of marked arterial insufficiency or has a positive Homan's sign (see Chapter 7), notify the physician because the application of the cuffs might be contraindicated.

3 Attach the tubing to each cuff. The unit in these photos is marked "ankle" or "knee" at the appropriate connector cell to ensure that the tubing is connected to the proper ankle or knee plug.

Implementing

4 Place one of the cuffs over the client's lower leg, with the tubing positioned at the medial aspect. Position the padded side against the client's leg so that the Velcro is on the exterior of the cuff. Note that with the Thrombogard device, the end tabs are identified as either "ankle" (as shown) or "knee." With other brands the narrower straps are placed over the ankle, and the wider straps are positioned over the calf.

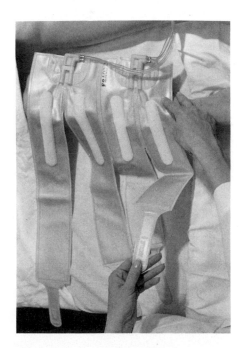

(Continued on p. 610)

Evaluating

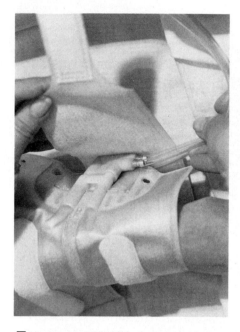

5 Wrap the cuff around the client's leg and the connector cell (as shown). Place two fingers over the cell before attaching the Velcro strip to ensure proper slack in the cuff.

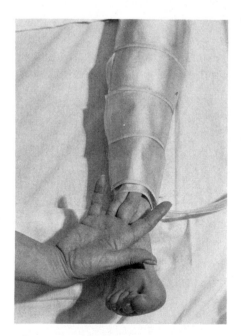

6 Once the straps have been attached to the cuff, again <u>ensure</u> <u>that two fingers fit between the</u> <u>client's skin and the cuff at both</u> <u>the ankle and knee before turn-</u> <u>ing on the unit.</u>

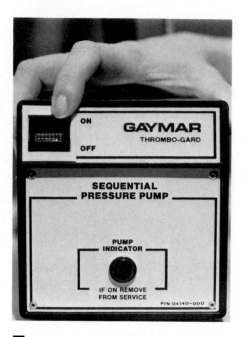

7 Plug the unit into a grounded outlet and press the switch to "on" to activate the device. Observe each cuff for at least two cycles to evaluate its functioning. Be sure that only one cuff is filled at a time. The ankle cell should fill first, followed by the inflation of the second, third, and knee cell. All the cells will remain inflated until the system vents, at which time all the cells should deflate. The cuff on the opposite leg should then begin its sequential filling in the same manner. If the sequence is reversed, remove the cuff and correct the problem. Document the procedure, being certain to note the client's baseline neurovascular assessment and the condition of the skin on both legs.

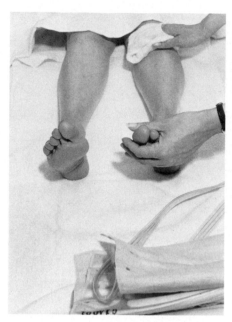

8 At prescribed intervals, unplug the unit and remove the cuffs after they have deflated. Inspect the skin and provide skin care. However, avoid <u>massaging</u> <u>the skin because vigorous rubbing</u> <u>can dislodge a thrombus.</u> Perform a neurovascular assessment to evaluate the color, temperature, sensation, pulses, and capillary refill of the distal extremities and compare the assessment to the baseline assessment.

PROVIDING CARE DURING A SEIZURE

Assessing and Planning

1 A client history of seizure disorders or the potential for a seizure should alert you to the need for protective measures. These include a padded tongue blade at the bedside table or taped to the headboard, and raised and padded siderails. Children with seizure disorders can wear soft seizure helmets (as shown) when they are ambulatory.

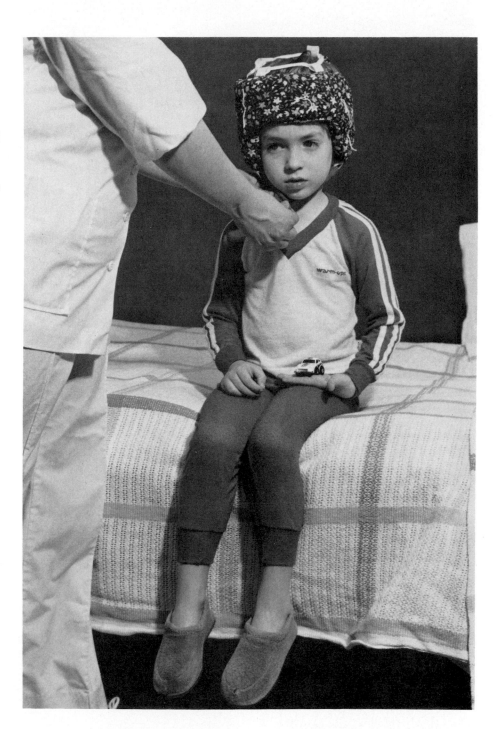

(Continued on p. 612)

Implementing

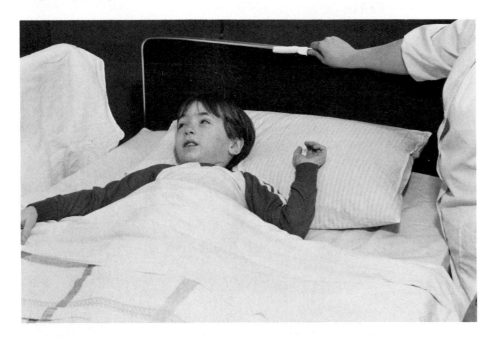

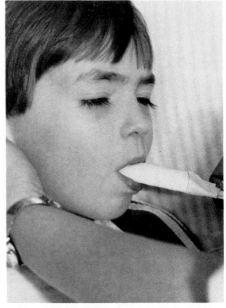

2 If your client has a seizure, remove the padded tongue blade from the headboard or bedside table, and cautiously insert it between his back teeth to prevent him from biting his tongue (right). If a padded tongue blade is unavailable, insert a firm padded object such as a belt as a substitute. Never insert a finger or a metal object, however. Position the head toward the side to facilitate drainage of secretions and to prevent aspiration into the lung.

3 A single seizure can last from 2–5 minutes. Always stay with the client, noting the onset, duration, and type of seizure. Do not attempt to restrain him, since this can increase the risk of injury. Observe the client's posture, pupillary changes, skin color, and the extremities involved. When the seizure has ceased, comfort and reorient the client, noting any cyanosis or difficult respiratory patterns. If the cyanosis persists, be sure to have oxygen available.

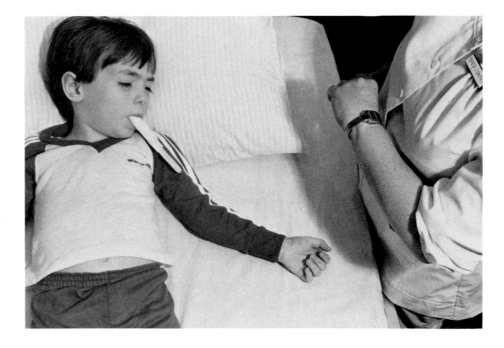

Evaluating

Document the seizure carefully, using descriptive terminology, the time of onset and duration, and any information about possible precipitating events.

USING A HYPERTHERMIA OR HYPOTHERMIA SYSTEM

Assessing and Planning

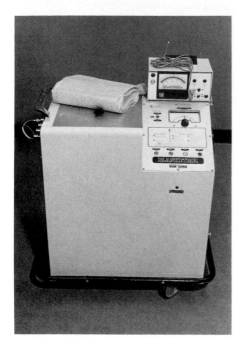

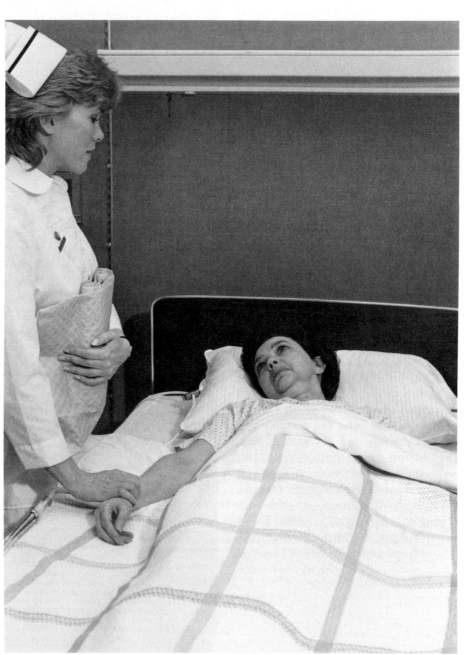

Many neurologic disorders involve the hypothalamus, the part of the brain that regulates body temperature. When vast fluctuations in body temperature occur, a hyperthermia or hypothermia system such as the Blanketrol® in these photos can be used to help keep your client's temperature within normal range, thereby minimizing the risk of irreversible brain damage.

1 Explain the procedure to the client and inform her that she will feel either warmth or coolness. Instruct her to alert you if the temperature becomes too extreme. Perform and record baseline assessments of the client's vital signs and neurologic status.

Note the integrity of the skin and document its condition prior to initiating the treatment. *Note: If the client's temperature will be greatly decreased, coat the skin with a thin layer of lanolin ointment to help prevent cold burns.*

(Continued on p. 614)

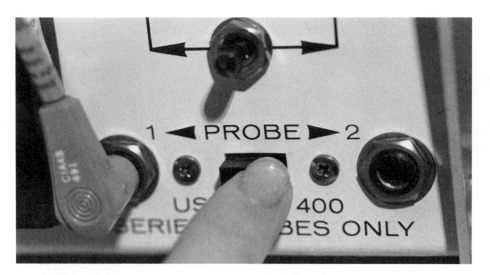

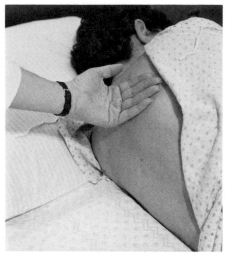

6 Insert the rectal probe plug (shown on the left) into one of the probe receptacles. Then turn the probe selector toward the corresponding receptacle (as shown).

9 Perform and document neurologic checks and vital signs and compare them to the client's baseline. Assess the client's skin integrity and temperature and be alert to alterations such as swelling or color changes that could indicate frostbite or burns. Check the servo controller reading to ensure that the client's temperature is reaching the desired level.

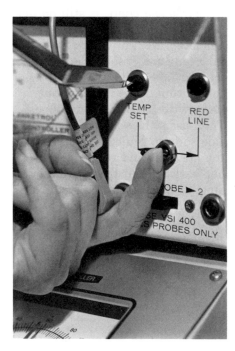

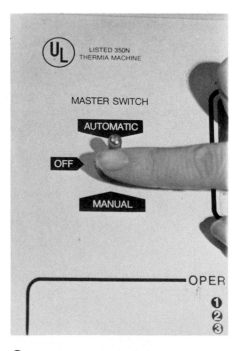

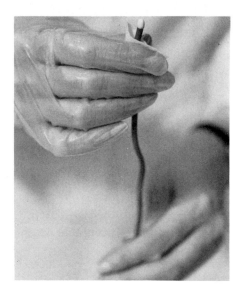

7 Set the prescribed temperature by pushing the temperature set switch to the left and turning the temperature set control screw with your scissors to the prescribed temperature (as shown). When the switch is released, the needle pointer will show the core temperature. This is the same switch you will push to check the calibrations by adjusting the needle to the red line.

8 Move the master control switch on the Blanketrol® to "automatic." Document the procedure, the client's baseline assessment, and the response and tolerance to the treatment.

10 Periodically remove the rectal probe and assess the client's body temperature with a rectal thermometer to ensure that the probe is accurately recording the client's actual body temperature. Clean and reinsert the probe.

Nursing Guidelines for the Care of Clients on Special Beds and Frames

Complications of immobility such as atelectasis, pneumonia, decubitus ulcers, and renal calculi are frequent occurrences in clients with neurologic disorders. Because many of these clients are unable to actively participate in their own turning, and yet may require frequent turning without the interruption of their alignment, special beds are often indicated to facilitate nursing care and to prevent or minimize the complications of prolonged bed rest. The Stryker Wedge Turning Frame, Circle Bed, and Roto Rest Kinetic Treatment Table are three types of beds or frames that may be used by your agency. Follow manufacturer's instructions carefully to ensure the proper care and/or safe turning for your clients.

Stryker Wedge Turning Frame and Circle Bed

The Stryker Wedge Turning Frame allows you to change the client's position from either prone or supine without disrupting alignment. It has both anterior and posterior frames that attach to a pivotal apparatus. The Circle Bed is electrically operated and it provides a vertical alteration of the client's position from either supine or prone via a supporting mattress and an anterior frame that attach to a circular outer frame. Follow operating instructions carefully when turning clients on these devices.

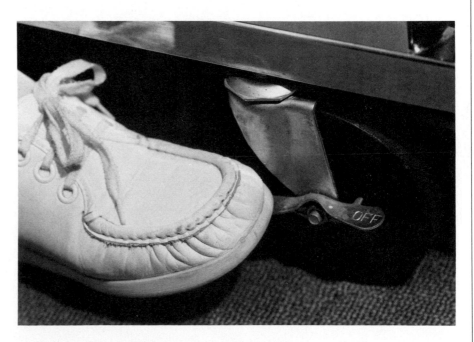

- Make sure the wheels are in a locked position prior to every turn. The wheels should always be maintained in a locked position unless the device is to be moved to another area.

(Continued on p. 618)

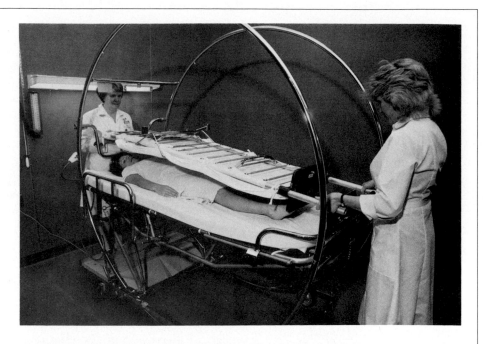

■ In most agencies, safety standards require that two people operate both devices.

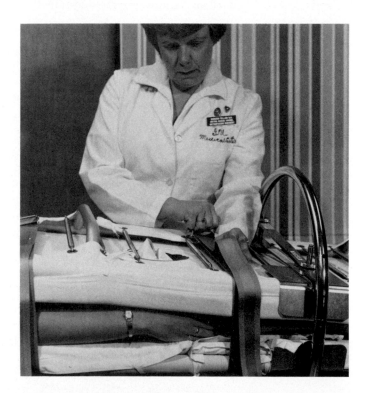

■ As an added safety measure, once the two frames are bolted or screwed together, wrap safety straps around both frames prior to every move. If the client lacks mobility in the upper extremities, position the straps at the shoulders, hands, and knees. If the client does have upper body mobility, keep the hands free so that she can embrace the frame for support if she desires.

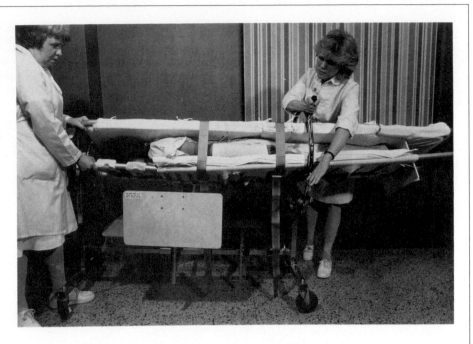

■ In the Stryker Wedge Turning Frame, the client will often feel more secure if you turn the frame toward yourself during every turn.

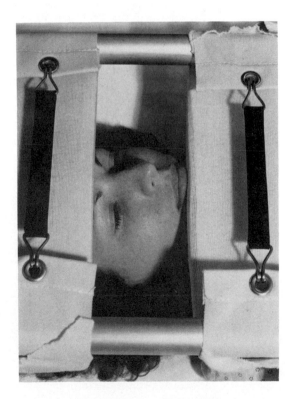

■ Ensure that the anterior frame is correctly positioned so that the forehead and chin bands do not obstruct the client's respirations in any way.

(Continued on p. 620)

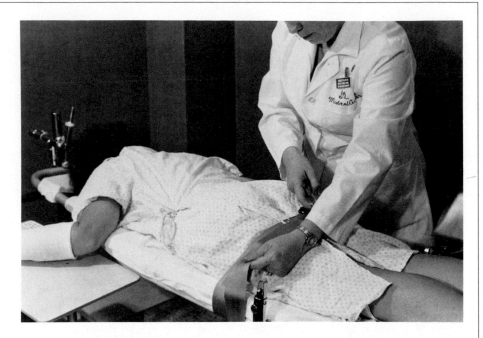

■ When the client is in the prone position on either device, wrap a safety belt around the thighs. To help prevent shoulder contractures, position the armrests so that they are below the level of the shoulders. (In the supine position they can be level with the shoulders.) Remove the footboard and allow the client's feet to hang over the frame. See Chapter 2 for positioning the prone client.

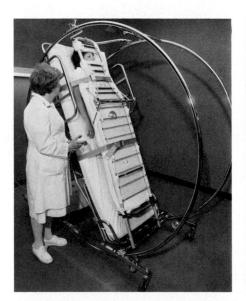
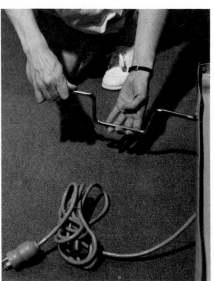

■ When turning the client on the Circle Bed, perform the move in one continuous movement. This will help to minimize nausea or dizziness.

■ If there is a motor malfunction or power failure, the Circle Bed can be turned manually by detaching the hand crank from under the head of the bed, inserting it into the proper slot, and turning it accordingly.

Roto Rest Kinetic Treatment Table

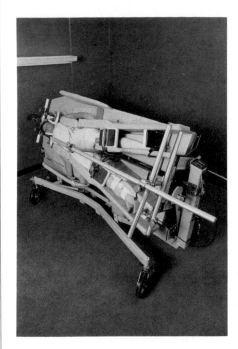

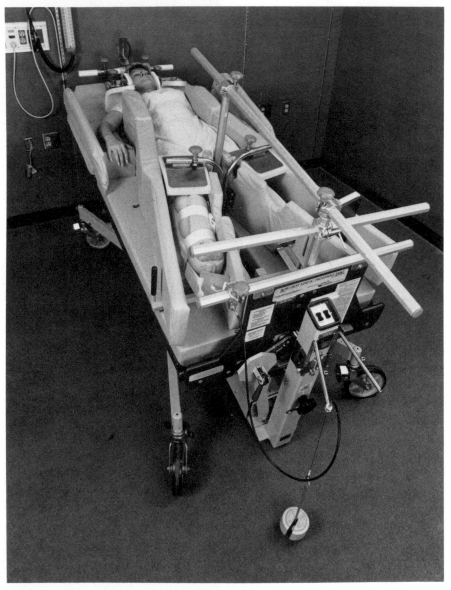

The Roto Rest is an automatic turning table that continuously rotates the client from side to side every 3.5 minutes, achieving a 62° lateral angle (see left). This continuous lateral rotation can enhance the distribution of pulmonary blood flow. The client is secured to the table via closely fitting pads that conform to the extremities and trunk. When the table achieves its most lateral position, the padded knee and shoulder braces give added security. Safety straps are also available for confused or combative clients. In addition to cervical traction, the table also allows the application of traction to all extremities.

(Continued on p. 622)

Caring for Clients With Disorders of the Sensory System

ASSESSING AUDITORY FUNCTION

There are several methods for assessing your client's hearing acuity. The simplest method is to stand approximately 60 cm (2 ft) from the client and out of his or her vision. Instruct the client to cover one ear as you whisper two-syllable words such as "baseball" or "armchair." With normal hearing, the client should be able to hear and repeat at least 50% of your words at this distance. If the client is unable to hear the whispered word, gradually increase the intensity of your voice until your words are heard and repeated. Perform the same test on the client's opposite ear, using different words.

Performing the Watch Test

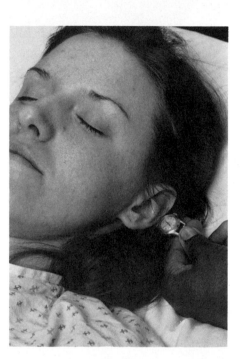

Another method for testing hearing acuity is the watch test, whereby the client covers one ear as you position a ticking watch approximately 2.5–5 cm (1–2 in.) from her uncovered ear. Instruct the client to alert you when she can no longer hear the watch, and slowly move the watch away from the ear. With normal hearing, the client should be able to hear the ticking 5 cm from her ear, provided she is in a quiet room. Repeat the test on the opposite ear and record the farthest distance at which the client was able to hear the ticking for both ears.

Performing the Weber and Rinne Tests

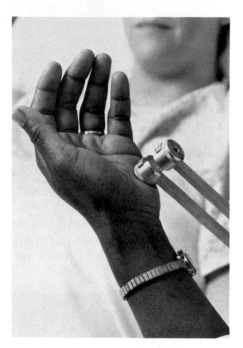

1 The Weber and Rinne tests are more sophisticated assessments of your client's auditory function. A combination of the two tests can help to categorize an auditory dysfunction as either conductive or sensorineural (perceptive). With conductive hearing loss, there is a physical obstruction of the sound such as a fusion of the stapes or a foreign body in the external canal. With a sensorineural hearing loss, the dysfunction can occur with the eighth cranial nerve, or in the cortex itself. To perform either the Weber or the Rinne test, first activate a tuning fork by holding it by its base and gently striking the prongs against the palmar surface of your hand. This will cause the prongs to vibrate.

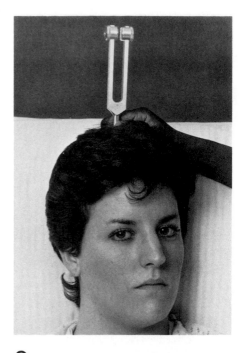

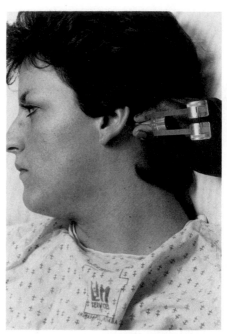

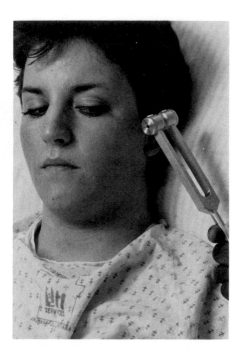

2 To perform the Weber test, activate the tuning fork, and position the base of the fork on the top of the client's head (as shown) or at the top of the forehead. Normally, the client will hear the sound equally in both ears. This is recorded as Weber negative. With conductive loss the sound will lateralize to the poorer ear. This occurs because the normal ear is penetrated by ordinary room noise, masking hearing in that ear. The poorer ear, on the other hand, is not penetrated by ordinary room noise and thus can hear the bone-conducted sound. Document the results as either "Weber negative" or "Lateralization Right" (or "Left").

3 To perform the Rinne test, instruct the client to cover one ear. After activating the tuning fork, position its base on the mastoid process of the uncovered ear. Instruct the client to alert you once she can no longer hear the sound. As soon as she alerts you, make a mental note of the amount of time during which she heard the sound.

4 Immediately move the prongs of the tuning fork in front of the uncovered ear, approximately 1.25–2.5 cm ($\frac{1}{2}$–1 in.). Because air conduction lasts at least twice as long as bone conduction, the client should be able to hear the sound twice as long in this position. The reverse is true if the client has conductive hearing loss. Repeat the test in the opposite ear. Document the results as positive if the client has normal hearing, or negative if the results are reversed.

IRRIGATING THE EYE

Assessing and Planning	**Implementing**	**Evaluating**

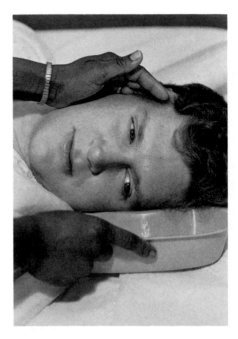

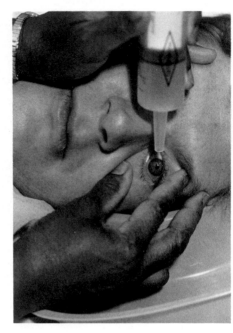

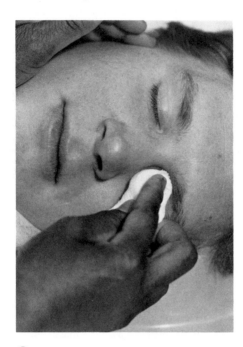

1 If an eye irrigation has been prescribed for your client, assemble the sterile irrigating solution warmed to room temperature, a sterile 50-mL syringe (or sterile infusion tubing if larger amounts of irrigant are to be used), sterile gauze pads, bed-saver pads, and an emesis basin. Fill the syringe with the irrigant. Explain the procedure to your client and position him so that he is on his side with his affected eye lowermost. Position the emesis basin underneath the affected eye and drape the client's gown and bed with the bed-saver pads. Then wash your hands.

2 Retract the upper and lower eyelids with your thumb and index finger, and administer the irrigant so that it flows from the inner to the outer canthus.

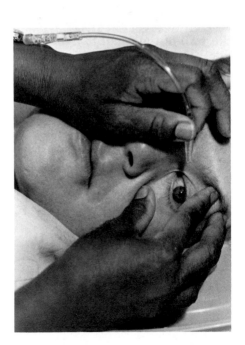

Note: Follow the same procedure if you are using infusion tubing to deliver the irrigant.

3 After completing the procedure, blot the client's eye gently with a sterile gauze pad, wiping from the inner to the outer canthus. Document the procedure, noting the type and amount of irrigant, and the client's tolerance to the irrigation.

USING OP-SITE ON DECUBITUS ULCERS

Op-Site is a transparent polyure-thane self-adhering dressing. Because it prevents the escape of fluid, it provides a moist environment that is thought to enhance granulation and epithelization for optimal wound healing.

Assessing and Planning

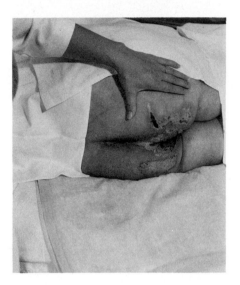

1 Wash your hands and position and drape the client so that you have good visualization of and access to the decubitus ulcer. Determine the size of dressing that will effectively cover the wound and yet provide at least a 5-cm (2-in.) border around the site, if possible. Op-Site dressings are available in a variety of sizes, ranging from 5 × 7.5 cm–28 × 30 cm.

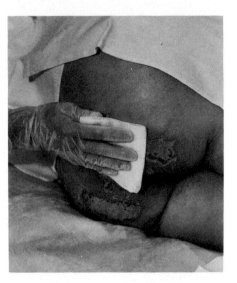

2 Thoroughly cleanse the wound and rinse it well with normal saline. To ensure complete adherence of the dressing, you must be sure to dry the site completely. If the wound is on the buttocks of a client with frequent episodes of diarrhea, it may be necessary to apply a thin layer of liquid skin barrier around the periphery of the area to improve dressing adherence. *Note: Gloves are recommended when client secretions, excretions, blood, or body fluids are touched (see p. 10).*

←

3 Peel the protective paper backing from the Op-Site sheet, just enough to adhere a small section of the dressing to the client's skin. Avoid peeling back more than 2.5 cm (1 in.).

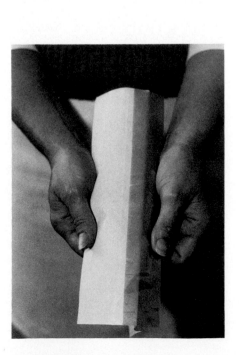

(Continued on p. 632)

Implementing

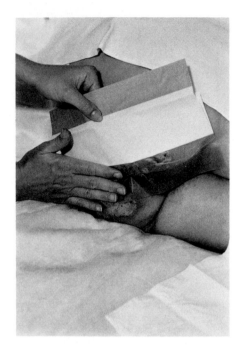

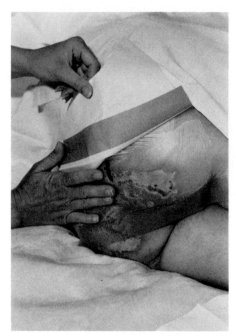

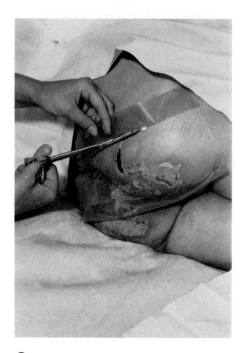

4 Position the sticky side of the dressing over the interior border of the wound site, allowing a 5-cm (2-in.) border to extend beyond the wound site, if possible. If the wound is on the buttocks, it may help to place the Op-Site sheet slightly on the diagonal, with a second sheet crossing it at the sacral area. Adhere the exposed section of the dressing to the client's skin.

5 Gradually peel away the protective paper as you smooth the dressing over the wound and surrounding area. Although you should avoid stretching the dressing, gentle tension will help prevent wrinkling. If a wrinkle does appear, however, pinch it together.

6 Once the dressing has been smoothed on the client's skin, use bandage scissors to cut off the green tabs. *Note: After use, it is always a good idea to clean the scissor blades with an alcohol wipe.*

Evaluating

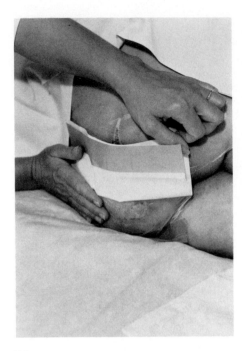

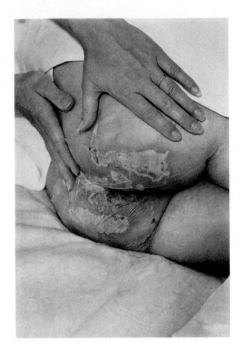

7 In the same manner, apply a second sheet if needed, and cut away the green tabs. If the dressing is on the buttocks, be sure to trim the dressing, as necessary, to accommodate the anus.

8 Ensure that the entire wound site is covered; then wash your hands and document the procedure. Be sure to note the size and character of the decubitus ulcer. It is not necessary to cover Op-Site with gauze or tape. Leaving the dressing uncovered allows observation of the wound without disruption of the dressing. Expect to see exudate forming under the dressing. This is normal and it is the mechanism for moist wound healing. Leave the dressing on until it begins to slough away. This usually takes 4–5 days. If you need to remove the dressing prior to this time, soak the dressing with a solution of soap and water and peel back the edges.

O'Shaughnessy, Carol

References

Ahmed, M. C. Jan. 1982. Op-Site for decubitus care. *AJN* 82: 61–64.

Friedman, F. B. Feb. 1982. An innovation in decubitus treatment sparks debate. *RN* 45:46–47, 118.

Hilt, N., and Cogburn, S. 1979. *Manual of orthopedics*. St. Louis: C. V. Mosby.

King, R. C. Dec. 1982. Checking the patient's neurological status. *RN* 45:57–62.

King, R. C. Feb. 1982. Taking a close look at the eye. *RN* 45:49–56.

Luckmann, J., and Sorensen, K. 1980. *Medical-surgical nursing: a psychophysiologic approach*. Philadelphia: W. B. Saunders.

Malkiewicz, J. March 1982. How to assess the ears and test hearing acuity. *RN* 45:56–63.

Meyer, T. M. Sept. 1982. TENS: relieving pain through electricity. *Nursing '82* 12:57–59.

Norman, S. April 1982. The pupil check. *AJN* 82: 588–591.

Nursing Photobook. 1981. *Assessing your patients*. Horsham, Pa: Intermed Communications.

Nursing Photobook. 1982. *Caring for surgical patients*. Springhouse, Pa: Intermed Communications.

Nursing Photobook. 1982. *Coping with neurologic disorders*. Springhouse, Pa: Intermed Communications.

Rantz, M., and Courtial, D. 1981. *Lifting, moving, and transferring patients*. St. Louis: C. V. Mosby.

Saxton, D., et al. 1983. *The Addison-Wesley manual of nursing practice*. Menlo, Park, Calif.: Addison-Wesley Publishing.

Schimmel, L., et al. 1977. A new mechanical method to influence pulmonary perfusion in critically ill patients. *Crit Care Med* 5:277–279.

Smith, S. F., and Duell, D. 1982. *Nursing skills and evaluation*. Los Altos, Calif.: National Nursing Review.

Spence, A. P. 1982. *Basic human anatomy*. Menlo Park, Calif.: Benjamin/Cummings Publishing.

Taylor, J. W., and Ballenger, S. 1980. *Neurological dysfunction and nursing intervention*. New York: McGraw-Hill Book Company.

Thompson, J. and Bowers, A. 1980. *Clinical manual of health assessment*. St. Louis: C. V. Mosby.

Tilton, C., and Maloof, M. April 1982. Diagnosing the problems in stroke. *AJN* 82:596–601.

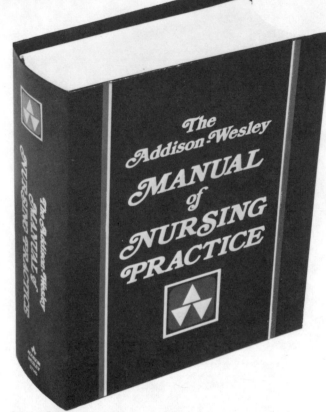

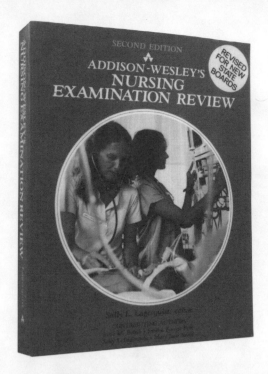

Addison-Wesley's
Nursing Examination Review

REVISED FOR NEW STATE BOARDS

PREPARE FOR THE BOARDS WITH THE BOOK THAT HAS ALL THESE FEATURES:

★ Coverage of Growth and Development Through the Life Span ● Life Cycle Theories ● Body Image ● Human Sexuality ● Health Teaching ● Psychiatric Nursing ● Maternity Nursing ● Pediatric Nursing ● Medical-Surgical Nursing ● Ethical and Legal Aspects of Nursing ● Cultural Diversity in Nursing Practice.

★ Over 1000 questions and answers with *rationales* that fully explain the reasoning behind every correct *and* incorrect answer. Most other books do not have this feature.

★ Annotated Bibliographies and Extensive Appendices

★ Special Orientation Section provides hints for scoring higher on the Boards plus *advice for foreign-educated nurses*

★ Integrated *Case Studies* test both cognitive abilities and nursing behaviors

Index